SpringerWienNewYork

Acta Neurochirurgica
Supplements

Editor: H.-J. Steiger

Early Brain Injury or Cerebral Vasospasm
Volume 1: Pathophysiology

Edited by
Hua Feng, Ying Mao, John H. Zhang

Acta Neurochirurgica
Supplement 110/1

SpringerWienNewYork

Hua Feng
Department of Neurosurgery, Southwest Hospital, Third Military Medical University,
Gaotanyan 30, Chongqing 400038, China, fenghua8888@yahoo.com.cn

Ying Mao
Department of Neurosurgery, Huashan Hospital, Fudan University, Shanghai,
China, yingmao@vnet.citiz.net

John H. Zhang
Departments of Physiology and Neurosurgery, Loma Linda University School of Medicine,
Risley Hall, Room 223, 92354 Loma Linda, California, USA, jhzhang@llu.edu

This work is subject to copyright.
All rights are reserved, whether the whole or part of the material is concerned, specifically those of translation, reprinting, re-use of illustrations, broadcasting, reproduction by photocopying machines or similar means, and storage in data banks.

Product Liability: The publisher can give no guarantee for all the information contained in this book. This does also refer to information about drug dosage and application thereof. In every individual case the respective user must check its accuracy by consulting other pharmaceutical literature. The use of registered names, trademarks, etc. in this publication does not imply, even in the absence of a specific statement, that such names are exempt from the relevant protective laws and regulations and therefore free for general use.

© 2011 Springer-Verlag/Wien
Printed in Germany
SpringerWienNewYork is part of Springer Science+Business Media
springer.at

Typesetting: SPI, Pondichery, India

Printed on acid-free and chlorine-free bleached paper
SPIN: 80015290

With 58 (partly coloured) Figures

ISSN 0065-1419
ISBN 978-3-7091-0352-4   e-ISBN 978-3-7091-0353-1
DOI: 10.1007/978-3-7091-0353-1
SpringerWienNewYork

Preface

On October 9–11, 2009, the Tenth International Conference on Cerebral Vasospasm was held for the first time in Chongqing, China. Literally translated to mean "double happiness", Chongqing was the perfect venue to host members of the community from all over the world to witness and participate in such a historic event. Just like the city's meaning would have you to believe, the conference was a joyous time for both the Chinese neurosurgery researchers who organized this well established conference and the vasospasm researchers from other countries who were delighted to have a meeting on a tour boat called the Misty Star. For many, being on a ship was a new experience, while for others, it was a time to soak in the beauty of China. The conference catered to more than 90 researchers from various countries around the world, presenting over 90 articles ranging from clinical trials to molecular biology experiments. This was all done while enjoying a cruise down the largest river in China, the Yangtze River, and experiencing the greatness of China's historic hydroelectric dams, the Three Gorges and the Three Little Gorges.

The meeting focused on subarachnoid hemorrhage research with topics divided into two main subcategories – early brain injury and delayed vasospasm. Since 1972 when the first conference on cerebral vasospasm took place, delayed vasospasm has been regarded as the single most important treatable cause of mortality and morbidity after subarachnoid hemorrhage. However, since the successfulness of steering patients out of vasospasm by an endothelin receptor antagonist failed to reduce mortality, more attention was placed on global cerebral injury, which was termed early brain injury. Since then, more than 20% of all published studies on subarachnoid hemorrhage in the last 3 years have been focused on early brain injury, with 45% targeting delayed vasospasm. As a result, the Tenth International Conference on Cerebral Vasospasm dedicated close to one third of all presentations to early brain injury.

The conference followed the Misty Star into the Chinese ghost city of Fengdu, which is located high atop a beautiful hill. Meeting attendees were able to take a gondola ride and dashed into the "Gates of Hell". Chinese people worship and respect the notion of death and for this reason, many believe that is why they built the "Gates of Hell" on a beautiful hill – like Heaven on Earth. This seems to be a coincident with the research on subarachnoid hemorrhage; it was believed over 50 years ago that delayed vasospasm was the major cause of death in victims. Nevertheless, the failure of Clazosentan to reduce mortality led researchers to shy away from the theory of delayed cerebral vasospasm, and transformed subarachnoid hemorrhage research into the birth of early brain injury.

Towards the end of the conference, the Misty Star led the meeting participants to a vast clearing of water, before the greatest dam on earth, the Three Gorges Dam appeared before them. Crossing the greatest dam during the evening provided a magnificent view for the participants and set the mood for the researchers.

In closing, it is with great pleasure that we would like to present the Volume One entitled "Pathophysiology" a collection of 43 chapters showcasing the magnificent works conducted by the conference participants. These chapters include studies on early brain injury, the pathophysiology of delayed cerebral vasospasm, the clinical manifestations of subarachnoid hemorrhage, and the latest strategies on treatments. Additionally, we are delighted to present two historic review articles conducted by our honored guest, Dr. Nicolas Dorsch and our distinguished keynote speaker, Dr. Ryszard Pluta. These chapters also include bench investigations conducted by researchers and scientists from all across Asia, North America, and European countries highlighting the achievements in subarachnoid hemorrhage since the Ninth International Conference on Cerebral Vasospasm in Istanbul, Turkey almost 3 years ago.

And finally, to our dear participating colleagues, we would like to thank YOU especially for your participation and support of the Tenth International Conference on Cerebral Vasospasm. We look forward to seeing you in Cincinnati, OH, USA at the 11th Conference in 2011.

Chongping, People's Republic of China	Hua Feng
Shanghai, People's Republic of China	Ying Mao
Loma Linda, CA, USA	John H. Zhang

Acknowledgement

International Organization Committee
Hua Feng (Chairman), Chognqing
Jian-Min Liu (Co-Chairman), Shanghia
Talat Kırış, Istanbul
Shigeru Nishizawa, Kitakyushu
Ryszard Pluta, Bethesda
Volker Seifert, Frankfurt
John Zhang (Secretary), Loma Linda
Gang Zhu, Chognqing

International Scientific Committee
Austin R.T. Colohan, Loma Linda
Jens Dreier, Berlin
Nick Dorsch, Sydney
Hua Feng, Chognqing
Satoshi Iwabuchi, Tokyo
Carla Jung, Heidelberg
Kenji Kanamaru, Suzuka
Hidetoshi Kasuya, Tokyo
Chunjin Kim. Chonbu
Kevin S. Lee, Charlottesville
Jianmin Liu, Shanghia
Ying Mao, Shanghai
Shigeru Nishizawa, Kitakyushu
Hiroki Ohkuma, Hirosaki
Ryszard M. Pluta, Bethesda
Wai Poon, Hong Kong
Gustavo Pradilla, Johns Hopkins
Jacob Hansen-Schwartz, Glostrup
Fatima Sehba, New York
Volker Seifert, Frankfurt
Wei Shi, Xian
Hans-Jakob Steiger, Düsseldorf
Xiaochuan Sun, Chongqing
Claudius Thome, Heidelberg
Hartmut Vatter, Frankfort
George Wellman, Vermont
Changman Zhou, Beijing
John Zhang, Loma Linda
Mario Zuccarello, Cincinnati

Contents

Part I: Advances in Subarachnoid Hemorrhage and Cerebral Vasospasm

Section I: Honored Guest & Honored Speaker Speeches

A Clinical Review of Cerebral Vasospasm and Delayed Ischaemia
Following Aneurysm Rupture 5
Dorsch, N.

New Regulatory, Signaling Pathways, and Sources of Nitric Oxide 7
Pluta, R.M.

Section II: Advances in Subarachnoid Hemorrhage Research

Advances in Experimental Subarachnoid Hemorrhage 15
Zhou, Y., Martin, R.D., and Zhang, J.H.

Advances in Treatment of Cerebral Vasospasm: an Update 23
Hansen-Schwartz, J.

Roles of Signal Transduction Mechanisms in Cerebral Vasospasm
Following Subarachnoid Hemorrhge: Overview 27
Nishziawa, S.

Part II: Mechanistic Studies

Section III: Early Brain Injury After Subarachnoid Hemorrhage

Hypoperfusion in the Acute Phase of Subarachnoid Hemorrhage 35
Schubert, G.A., Seiz, M., Hegewald, A.A., Manville, J., and Thomé, C.

Association of APOE Polymorphism with the Change of Brain Function
in the Early Stage of Aneurysmal Subarachnoid Hemorrhage 39
Lin, B., Dan, W., Jiang, L., Yin, X.-h., Wu, H.-t., and Sun, X.-c.

Apoptotic Mechanisms for Neuronal Cells in Early Brain Injury
After Subarachnoid Hemorrhage 43
Hasegawa, Y., Suzuki, H., Sozen, T., Altay O., and Zhang, J.H.

Early Micro Vascular Changes After Subarachnoid Hemorrhage 49
Sehba, F.A. and Friedrich, V.

Immunological Response in Early Brain Injury After SAH 57
Sozen, T., Tsuchiyama, R., Hasegawa, Y., Suzuki, H., Jadhav, V.,
Nishizawa, S., and Zhang, J.H.

Mechanisms of Early Brain Injury After SAH: Matrixmetalloproteinase 9 63
Guo, Z.-d., Sun, X.-c., and Zhang, J.H.

**Tyrosine Phosphatase Inhibition Attenuates Early Brain Injury
After Subarachnoid Hemorrhage in Rats** 67
Hasegawa, Y., Suzuki, H., Sherchan, P., Zhan, Y., Duris, K., and Zhang, J.H.

**Protection of Minocycline on Early Brain Injury After Subarachnoid
Hemorrhage in Rats** 71
Guo, Z.-d., Wu, H.-t., Sun, X.-c., Zhang, X.-d., and Zhang, J.H.

**Role of Osteopontin in Early Brain Injury After Subarachnoid
Hemorrhage in Rats** 75
Suzuki, H., Ayer, R., Sugawara, T., Chen, W., Sozen, T., Hasegawa, Y.,
Kanamaru, K., and Zhang, J.H.

**Matrix Metalloproteinase 9 Inhibition Reduces Early Brain Injury
in Cortex After Subarachnoid Hemorrhage** 81
Guo, Z.-d., Zhang, X.-d., Wu, H.-t., Lin, B., Sun, X.-c., and Zhang, J.H.

**Section IV: Nitric Oxide & Cortical Spreading Depolarization After
Subarachnoid Hemorrhage**

Nitric Oxide Synthase Inhibitors and Cerebral Vasospasm 87
Jung, C.S.

**The Role of Nitric Oxide Donors in Treating Cerebral Vasospasm
After Subarachnoid Hemorrhage** 93
Fathi, A.R., Bakhtian, K.D., and Pluta, R.M.

Nitric Oxide in Early Brain Injury After Subarachnoid Hemorrhage 99
Sehba, F.A., and Bederson, J.B.

**Nitric Oxide Related Pathophysiological Changes Following
Subarachnoid Haemorrhage** 105
Sabri, M., Ai, J., and Macdonald, R.L.

Endothelin-1$_{(1-31)}$ Induces Spreading Depolarization in Rats 111
Jorks, D., Major, S., Oliveira-Ferreira, A.I., Kleeberg, J., and Dreier, J.P.

**The Gamut of Blood Flow Responses Coupled to Spreading Depolarization
in Rat and Human Brain: from Hyperemia to Prolonged Ischemia** 119
Offenhauser, N., Windmüller, O., Strong, A.J., Fuhr, S., and Dreier, J.P.

**Cerebral Microdialysis in Acutely Brain-Injured Patients
with Spreading Depolarizations** 125
Krajewski, K.L., Orakcioglu, B., Haux, D., Hertle, D.N., Santos, E.,
Kiening, K.L., Unterberg, A.W., and Sakowitz, O.W.

Section V: Pathophysiology of Cerebral Vasospasm

Mitogen-Activated Protein Kinases in Cerebral Vasospasm After Subarachnoid Hemorrhage: A Review 133
Suzuki, H., Hasegawa, Y., Kanamaru, K., and Zhang, J.H.

Association of Apolipoprotein E Polymorphisms with Cerebral Vasospasm After Spontaneous Subarachnoid Hemorrhage 141
Wu, H.-t., Zhang, X.-d., Su, H., Jiang, Y., Zhou, S., and Sun, X.-c.

Impact of Subarachnoid Hemorrhage on Local and Global Calcium Signaling in Cerebral Artery Myocytes 145
Koide, M., Nystoriak, M.A., Brayden, J.E., and Wellman, G.C.

Enhanced Angiogenesis and Astrocyte Activation by Ecdysterone Treatment in a Focal Cerebral Ischemia Rat Model 151
Luo, C., Yi, B., Fan, W., Chen, K., Gui, L., Chen, Z., Li, L., Feng, H., and Chi, L.

Bilirubin Oxidation Products Seen Post Subarachnoid Hemorrhage Have Greater Effects on Aged Rat Brain Compared to Young 157
Clark, J.F., Harm, A., Saffire, A., Biehle, S.J., Lu, A., and Pyne-Geithman, G.J.

Preliminary Results of an ICP-Controlled Subarachnoid Hemorrhage Rabbit Model for the Study of Delayed Cerebral Vasospasm 163
Marbacher, S., Sherif, C., Neuschmelting, V., Schläppi, J.-A., Takala, J., Jakob, S., and Fandino, J.

PKGIα Inhibits the Proliferation of Cerebral Arterial Smooth Muscle Cell Induced by Oxyhemoglobin After Subarachnoid Hemorrhage 167
Luo, C., Yi, B., Chen, Z., Tang, W., Chen, Y., Hu, R., Liu, Z., Feng, H., and Zhang, J.H.

Characteristics of In Vivo Animal Models of Delayed Cerebral Vasospasm 173
Marbacher, S., Fandino, J., and Kitchen, N.

Endothelin Related Pathophysiology in Cerebral Vasospasm: What Happens to the Cerebral Vessels? 177
Vatter, H., Konczalla, J., and Seifert, V.

Expression and Role of COMT in a Rat Subarachnoid Hemorrhage Model 181
He, Z., Sun, X., Guo, Z., and Zhang, J.H.

Section VI: Clinical Manifestations of Subarachnoid Hemorrhage

Monitoring of the Inflammatory Response After Aneurysmal Subarachnoid Haemorrhage in the Clinical Setting: Review of Literature and Report of Preliminary Clinical Experience 191
Muroi, C., Mink, S., Seule, M., Bellut, D., Fandino, J., and Keller, E.

Perimesencephalic Subarachnoid Hemorrhage: Risk Factors, Clinical Presentations, and Outcome 197
Kong, Y., Zhang, J.H., and Qin, X.

The Relationship Between IL-6 in CSF and Occurrence of Vasospasm
After Subarachnoid Hemorrhage 203
Ni, W., Gu, Y.X., Song, D.L., Leng, B., Li, P.L., and Mao, Y.

Non-Aneurysm Subarachnoid Hemorrhage in Young Adults 209
Wang, T., Zhang, J.H., and Qin, X.

Cardiac Damage After Subarachnoid Hemorrhage 215
Wu, B., Wang, X., and Zhang, J.H.

Analysis on Death-Associated Factors of Patients with Subarachnoid
Hemorrhage During Hospitalization 219
Wang, T., Zhang, J.H., and Qin, X.

Clinical Study of Changes of Cerebral Microcirculation in Cerebral
Vasospasm After SAH 225
Chai, W.-n., Sun, X.-c., Lv, F.-j., Wan, B., and Jiang, L.

Effect of Weekend Admission on in-Hospital Mortality After
Subarachnoid Hemorrhage in Chongqing China 229
Zhang, G., Zhang, J.H., and Qin, X.

The Correlation Between COMT Gene Polymorphism and Early
Cerebral Vasospasm After Subarachnoid Hemorrhage 233
He, Z., Sun, X., Guo, Z., and Zhang, J.H.

Fever Increased In-Hospital Mortality After Subarachnoid Hemorrhage 239
Zhang, G., Zhang, J.H., and Qin, X.

Subarachnoid Hemorrhage in Old Patients in Chongqing China 245
Zhang, Y., Wang, T., Zhang, J.H., Zhang, J., and Qin, X.

Author Index 249

Subject Index 251

Table of Contents (Vols. 1 and 2) 257

Part I: Advances in Subarachnoid Hemorrhage and Cerebral Vasospasm

Section I: Honored Guest & Honored Speaker Speeches

A Clinical Review of Cerebral Vasospasm and Delayed Ischaemia Following Aneurysm Rupture

Nicholas Dorsch

Abstract The continuation of a review of delayed vasospasm after aneurysmal subarachnoid haemorrhage, originally published in 1994 and partially updated at the ninth vasospasm conference in Turkey, is presented. Further online and physical searches have been made of the relevant literature. The incidence of delayed ischaemic deficit (DID) or symptomatic vasospasm reported in 1994 was 32.5% in over 30,000 reported cases. In recent years, 1994–2009, it was 6,775/23,806, or 28.5%. Many of the recent reports did not specify whether a calcium antagonist was used routinely, and when this was stated (usually nimodipine or nicardipine), DID was noted in 22.0% of 10,739 reported patients. The outcome of delayed ischaemia in the earlier survey was a death rate of 31.6%, with favourable outcomes in 36.2%. In recent reports, though with fewer than 1,000 patients, the outcome is possibly better, with death in 25.6% and good outcome in 54.1%.

It thus appears likely that delayed vasospasm is still common but less so, and that the overall outcome has improved. This may be due to the more widespread use of calcium antagonists and more effective fluid management. A number of other mechanical and drug treatments are also mentioned.

Keywords Calcium antagonists · Incidence of delayed ischaemia · Outcome of vasospasm

Introduction

The incidence, effects and management of delayed cerebral ischaemia following aneurysmal subarachnoid haemorrhage from the time of first reports up to the early 1990s have been extensively reviewed, and published elsewhere [1–3]. Following further review presented at the ninth International Conference on Cerebral Vasospasm in 2006 in Istanbul [4], the information has now been brought more up to date, by means of a Medline search and physical review of the neurosurgical literature from 1993 on, including relevant conference proceedings.

Incidence of Vasospasm

Angiographic Spasm

In the earlier review angiographic vasospasm was noted in 43.3% or 13,490 of 31,168 patients reported, but when angiography was specified as performed during the second week after SAH, when vasospasm is most likely, the incidence was 67% in 2,738 cases [3].

Nowadays patients are more likely to be investigated by transcranial Doppler or CT angiography than by formal DSA. Also, any form of angiography is less likely to be used, the diagnosis of delayed ischaemia being more often made by exclusion. The overall incidence of "angiographic" spasm reported between 1993 and 2009 (31 publications) was 49.0% in 4,238 reported cases.

Delayed Ischaemic Deficits

The incidence of delayed ischaemic deficit (DID) or symptomatic vasospasm reported in recent years, in 171 publications, was 6,775 in 23,806 patients, or 28.5%. This is somewhat lower than the incidence of 32.4% reported for the natural history in the earlier study (10,445 DID in 32,188 cases).

N. Dorsch
Department of Neurosurgery, Westmead Hospital, University of Sydney, Sydney, NSW, Australia
e-mail: ndorsch@ozemail.com.au

Many of the recent reports did not specify whether or not prophylactic use of a calcium antagonist was a routine part of management. In 32 publications, calcium antagonist use (usually nimodipine or nicardipine) was specified, in 10,739 patients or 44.3% of the total; in these patients DID was reported in 2,362 (22.0%). In the other 13,267 the incidence of DID was 4,413 (33.3%), very similar to the 32.4% previously reported. The reduced incidence of delayed ischaemia with calcium antagonists in these large numbers of patients supports their usefulness as noted in many publications.

Delayed ischaemia was apparently less common when aneurysms were treated by interventional techniques rather than by open surgery – in 11 mostly unrandomised series totalling 6,013 patients, DID occurred in 31% after surgery and 23% after coiling. Again the proportion treated with a calcium antagonist is uncertain, although it was presumably similar in coiled and surgical patients.

Other forms of prophylaxis continue to attract interest. These include intravenous magnesium sulphate, with six reports showing 10% less delayed ischaemia with treatment; the statins, with over one-third less DID again in six studies; cisternal drainage or drug treatment including two studies of implanted pellets; intraventricular drug treatment; and a variety of other drugs and techniques.

Outcome

The outcome of delayed ischaemia in the earlier survey, in over 4,000 reported patients, was a death rate of 31.6%, while favourable outcomes were noted in 36.2%. The numbers reported in more recent studies are much smaller, but suggest a trend towards improved outcome – death rate in 168 patients was 25.6%, and favourable outcome was reported in 49.8% of 850 patients.

In the 1994 review, treatment with variations of HHH therapy was associated with a death rate of 18.1% and good outcome in 54.1% [1]. The recent improved outcome figures may be associated with general improvements in fluid management in patients with DID. The more common use of balloon and/or chemical angioplasty (in eight recent reports involving 161 patients with "intractable" ischaemia, 69 (43%) improved or recovered), and other techniques including hypothermia, may also be factors.

Conclusion

Although most of the figures presented here are from small or large uncontrolled studies, the large numbers involved do suggest conclusions from these results. The overall incidence of delayed ischaemia is almost certainly lower now than it was 15 or more years ago. It is likely that this, and possibly the suggested improvement in outcome of established DID, are due largely to improvements in the fluid management of SAH patients in general, avoiding the active dehydration therapy that used to be seen, and to the more widespread use of calcium antagonists.

While these figures are to some extent encouraging, there is obviously still a long way to go to improve SAH outcome in general, particularly from the point of view of delayed deterioration. As pointed out at the last two conferences on vasospasm and in review publications in between [5–7], many factors other than delayed vasospasm itself are involved, and these are attracting increasing attention.

Conflict of interest statement I declare that I have no conflict of interest.

References

1. Dorsch NWC. A review of cerebral vasospasm in aneurysmal subarachnoid haemorrhage. II. Management. J Clin Neurosci. 1994;1:78–92.
2. Dorsch NWC. A review of cerebral vasospasm in aneurysmal subarachnoid haemorrhage. III. Mechanisms of action of calcium antagonists. J Clin Neurosci. 1994;1:151–60.
3. Dorsch NWC, King MT. A review of cerebral vasospasm in aneurysmal subarachnoid haemorrhage. Part I: incidence and effects. J Clin Neurosci. 1994;1:19–26.
4. Murray M, Dorsch NWC. Advances in vasospasm research. In: Kiriş T, Zhang JH, editors. Cerebral vasospasm. New strategies in research and treatment. Acta Neurochir (Wien) Suppl 104. Vienna: Springer; 2008. p. 1–4.
5. Hansen-Schwartz J, Vajkoczy P, Macdonald RL, Pluta RM, Zhang JH. Cerebral vasospasm: looking beyond vasoconstriction. Trends Pharmacol Sci. 2007;28:252–6.
6. Macdonald RL, Pluta RM, Zhang JH. Cerebral vasospasm after subarachnoid hemorrhage: the emerging revolution. Nat Clin Pract Neurol. 2007;3:256–63.
7. Pluta RM, Hansen-Schwartz J, Dreier J, Vajkoczy P, Macdonald RL, Nishizawa S, et al. Cerebral vasospasm following subarachnoid hemorrhage: time for a new world of thought. Neurol Res. 2009; 31:151–8.

New Regulatory, Signaling Pathways, and Sources of Nitric Oxide

Ryszard M. Pluta

Abstract Discovered in 1980 by the late Robert F. Furchgott, endothelium-derived relaxing factor, nitric oxide (NO), has been in the forefront of vascular research for several decades. What was originally a narrow approach, has been significantly widened due to major advances in understanding the chemical and biological properties of NO as well as its signaling pathways and discovering new sources of this notorious free radical gas. In this review, recent discoveries regarding NO and their implications on therapy for delayed cerebral vasospasm are presented.

Keywords Hemoglobin · Neuroglobin · Nitric oxide · SAH · Vasospasm

Nitric oxide (NO), a gas with a half-life of milliseconds in blood is continuously synthesized from L-arginine by NO-synthases (NOS), a family of complex multifactorial enzymes that include neuronal and endothelial (both constitutive) and inducible NOS (Fig. 1). NO released from the endothelium can act locally or can exercise distant effects via activation of soluble guanylyl cyclase after binding to its heme moiety, resulting in increased cGMP, activation of GMP-dependent kinases and different biological effects such as vasodilation, increased blood flow, inhibition of platelet activation, and modulation of inflammatory reaction. Additionally, NO can produce biological effects via cGMP-independent pathways, acting as a neurotransmitter, quenching oxygen free radicals, modulating activity of genes and enzymes, evoking the lipid peroxidation cascade, and modulating apoptosis and angiogenesis [1].

In the blood vessels' lumen NO is oxidated to form nitrite and nitrate, reacts with oxyhemoglobin to form nitrate and methemoglobin, and it nitrosates the thiols and amines to nitrosothiols and nitrosamines, as well as it reacts with metals forming for instance the iron-nitrosyl compounds with heme proteins [1, 2]. It has been a longstanding notion that in the presence of erythrocytes, NO is ultra-rapidly consumed or "inactivated" to nitrate, an inert NO metabolite and removed via the kidneys [3]. Recent experiments revolutionized our understanding of this molecule's biological characteristics and effects.

New Regulatory, Signaling Pathways

NOSes are a family of complex dimeric enzymes that are multifactorial and contain several co-enzymes. This family consists of neuronal NOS (nNOS), endothelial NOS (eNOS) and inducible (iNOS). nNOS, type I or NOS1 is constitutive and coded by the gene on chromosome 12. iNOS, type II or NOS2 is inducible and its gene is on chromosome 17. eNOS, type III or NOS3 is also constitutive and coded by the gene on chromosome 7.

NOS Synthesis and Regulation

eNOS Single Nucleotide Polymorphism (SNP)

SNP is a change of the DNA sequence that leads to substitution, deletion or insertion of a single nucleotide. Results of the SNP can be silent or produce an inadequate action of the particular gene-product or complete inhibit activity of the coded protein. The eNOS gene promoter T-786C single nucleotide polymorphism (eNOS T-786C SNP) was shown to predict susceptibility to post-subarachnoid hemorrhage (SAH) vasospasm [4]. These authors reported that a single nucleotide polymorphism (T/C) was observed in all patients who developed clinical symptoms of vasospasm. Unfortunately, nitrite levels were not measured in this study. Thus,

R.M. Pluta
Surgical Neurology Branch, National Institute of Neurological Disorders and Stroke, National Institutes of Health, 10 Center Drive, Room 3D20, Bethesda, MD, 20892-1414, USA
e-mail: Ryszard.Pluta@jama-archives.org

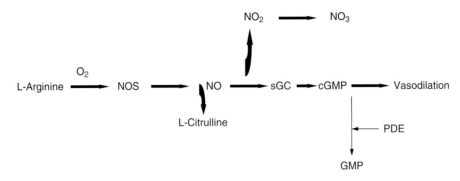

Fig. 1 NO production and metabolism. NO released from the endothelium acts locally or exercises a distant effect by activating soluble guanylyl cyclase after binding to its heme moiety, resulting in increased cGMP, activation of GMP-dependent kinases and different biological effects such as vasodilation, increased blood flow, inhibition of platelet activation, and modulation of inflammatory reaction. But, NO can also produce biological effects via cGMP-independent pathways, acting as a neurotransmitter, quenching oxygen free radicals, regulating gene and enzyme activity, evoking lipid peroxidation cascade, and modulating apoptosis and angiogenesis [1]. When NO is released into the vessel's lumen, several biochemical reactions occur, including NO oxidation to form nitrite and nitrate, reaction with oxyhemoglobin to form nitrate and methemoglobin, nitrosation of thiols and amines to form nitrosothiols and nitrosamines, and formation of iron-nitrosyl compounds with heme proteins [1, 2]. It has been a longstanding idea that, in the presence of erythrocytes, NO is ultra-rapidly consumed or "inactivated" to nitrate, an inert NO metabolite of NO and removed via the kidneys [3]. Recently, our understanding of this molecule's biological characteristics and effects has changed significantly

one can only hypothesize that this nucleotide substitution resulted in decreased production of NO and subsequent development of delayed cerebral vasospasm.

eNOS Phosphorylation

Phosphorylation by kinases and de-phosphorylation by phosphatases are two processes that activate or deactivate different enzymes. Activation of eNOS and increased production of NO have been attributed to its phosphorylation in response to physiological (shear stress, ischemia) or pharmacological (lipopolysaccharide, bradykinin, statins, sildenafil) stimuli that activate kinases Akt, AMPK, CaMK-2, PK A and PK G. However, eNOS is unique among other enzymes since the effect of phosphorylation depends on its locus. Phosphorylation of Ser 615, Ser633, or Ser1177 activates the enzyme but phosphorylation of Thr495 inhibits its activity. Nevertheless, dephosphorylation of the enzyme always decreases NO production [5]. Preventing and reversing delayed cerebral vasospasm by stimulating eNOS phosphorylation has been intensively investigated.

NO Synthesis

Asymmetric Dimethylarginine (ADMA)

L-arginine is a substrate not only for NOS but also for several other enzymes and metabolic pathways. In 1992, P. Valance and colleagues [6] discovered an endogenous NOS competitive inhibitor, double methylated L-arginine by protein arginine *N*-methyltransferase (PRMT I) ADMA; this recently received significant attention because it has been linked to development of vasospasm [7]. Despite the negative results of an experimental study to inhibit ADMA's effect [8], the recently confirmed prevention of vasospasm by statins has led to increased interest in this endogenous NOS inhibitor.

Arginase

Arginine is a semi-essential or conditionally essential amino acid that is used for NO production, protein synthesis, creatine, agmantine and the urea cycle [9]. When arginase is activated and produces ornithine and urea, such up-regulation may deplete eNOS of its substrate and indirectly decrease NO production that in turn may produce or aggravate the vasospasm after SAH. This hypothesis is currently being investigated.

Substrate and Coenzyme Deficiency

Each member of the NOS family is a complex (Fig. 2) enzyme that consists of several co-enzymes including flavin adenine dinucleotide (FAD), flavin mononucleotide (FMN), and co-factors, tetrahydrobiopterin (BH4), calmodulin (CAM), heme, and calcium. NOS produces NO by cleaving terminal nitrogen from arginine in the presence of nicotinamide adenine dinucleotide phosphate (NADPH) and oxygen. But, eNOS not only produces NO. When it is deprived of L-arginine, oxygen [10] or co-factor tetrahydrobiopterin, it produces hydrogen peroxide H_2O_2 [11], a potent vasoconstrictive and neurotoxic agent. Furthermore, in the presence

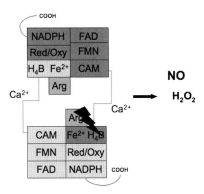

Fig. 2 Nitric oxide synthase (NOS) structure. Each member of the NOS family is a complex enzyme that consists of several co-enzymes including: flavin adenine dinucleotide (FAD), flavin mononucleotide (FMN), and co-factors, tetrahydrobiopterin (BH4), calmodulin (CAM), heme, and calcium. NOS produces NO by cleaving terminal nitrogen from arginine in the presence of nicotinamide adenine dinucleotide phosphate (NADPH) and oxygen. eNOS not only produces NO. When it is deprived of L-arginine, oxygen [10] or the co-factor tetrahydrobiopterin, it produces H_2O_2 [11], a potent vasoconstrictive and neurotoxic agent. Furthermore, in the presence of equal volumes of NO, H_2O_2 reacts with the NO to yield the extremely cytotoxic peroxynitrite (ONOO). This pathway as a source of vasospasm has been investigated only in relation to the unlikely depletion L-arginine [12]

of equal volumes of NO, H_2O_2 reacts with it, yielding the extremely cytotoxic peroxynitrite (ONOO). This pathway, as a source of vasospasm, has been investigated only in relation to the unlikely depletion of L-arginine [12]. However, it might be interesting because of the neuronal death that was reported both in the cortex and adventitia of cerebral vessels after SAH [13].

Erythropoietin (EPO)

Influence of EPO on NO production by eNOS remains unclear. There are at least three mechanisms that have been investigated. A. Desai and colleagues showed that in vitro EPO at low and high concentrations does not affect eNOS formation, but at a middle concentration (5 U/ml, it down-regulated expression of eNOS protein [14]. This confirmed the authors' hypothesis that administration of EPO accelerates atherosclerosis via decreased NO availability. Decreased availability of NO in the arterial wall was proposed as a mechanism for developing delayed cerebral vasospasm [13]. Thus, EPO could contribute to the increased severity of vasospasm after SAH. On the other hand, A–L Siren and her colleagues reported that EPO provides neuroprotection against ischemic insults inhibiting apoptosis [15], one of the purported pathomechanisms of vasospasm. Furthermore, in the in vitro study, 4 U/ml EPO (almost the same dose that was used in the Desai et al. experiment) induced

eNOS activity in several human cells lines [16] by EPO-related NOS phosphorylation [5]. There have been several experimental and clinical trials investigating the possible therapeutic effect of EPO on vasospasm after SAH.

Soluble Guanylyl Cyclase (sGC) and cGMP Regulation

J. Isenberg and colleagues [17] discovered that transpondin-1, a multi-domain glycoprotein, inhibits neovascularization and tumorigenesis. Reacting with multiple receptors including the integrin-associated protein (IAP), AKA CD47, transpondin-1 inhibits sGC. This binding makes it impossible for NO to exercise its vasodilatory effect via the cGMP pathway. Recently, this pathway was examined experimentally (Fathi et al. in preparation) but did not confirm a direct relationship with vasospasm in a primate model of SAH.

Up-regulation of phopshodiesterases, enzymes responsible for cGMP metabolism, has been known for several years as being a good experimental target to treat vasospasm [18]. This was of interest because cGMP levels are decreased in the artery in spasm [19, 20] but the presence and activity of eNOS remained unaffected despite the decrease of cGMP [21]. Different enzymes have been targeted (PDEV by Sildenafil, PDEIII by Cilostazol, and PDE IV by multiple agents) [22, 23] in experimental and clinical trials but the results remain questionable.

New Sources of Nitric Oxide Biological Activity

Since the discovery that NO is cleaved from L-arginine by NOS, studies assessing NO activity focused on protein synthesis and regulation of the enzyme. However, as reported by Malinski et al. [24] release of NO from the tissue could not be explained adequately by increased NO production by NOS. This effect occurred too quickly, almost immediately (within milliseconds) after ischemic injury to the brain. Thus, there was a lot of speculation about other sources of NO activity that included the presence of S-NO thiols, Fe–NO hemoglobin or S–NO hemoglobin, nitrite or even nitrate. Recently, such speculation has ended because it has been experimentally [25, 26] and clinically proven [27] (Pluta et al. in preparation) that deoxygenated hemoglobin in an acidic environment reduces nitrite to NO.

Nitrite an On-Demand NO Donor

When NO is released into the vessel's lumen, several biochemical reactions occur, including NO oxidation to form nitrite, reaction with oxyhemoglobin to form nitrate, nitrosation of thiols and amines to form nitrosothiols and nitrosamines, and formation of iron-nitrosyl compounds with heme proteins [1, 2]. It has been a longstanding notion that in the presence of erythrocytes, NO is ultra-rapidly consumed or "inactivated" to nitrate, the inert NO metabolite of NO [3]. However, this hemoglobin "sink effect" [28] has been questioned. A recent report showed that during inhalation of NO there was a subtle increase in forearm blood flow despite regional inhibition of NO synthase. This blood flow increase was associated with a concomitant rise in both heme-bound NO and nitrite [29] evoking artery-to-vein gradients and suggesting that nitrite produces vasodilation [2, 26, 30, 31]. Thus, nitrite represents a major bioavailable pool of NO and deoxygenated hemoglobin acts as nitrite reductase in vivo contributing to hypoxic vasodilation. Reversing and preventing cerebral vasospasm by NO/NO donors strongly suggest that decreased availability of NO is at least contributing to delayed vasospasm after SAH [32, 33]. Thus, we hypothesized that nitrite should act as the "on-demand" NO donor in the presence of deoxyhemoglobin [34] and lower pH [35, 36] in the subarachnoid space after SAH. We tested this hypothesis and demonstrated that intravenous, continuous long-lasting infusion of sodium nitrite prevented development of vasospasm [26]. This encouraging result was followed by a Phase I toxicity and safety study of prolonged intravenous sodium nitrite infusion in healthy volunteers (Pluta et al. in preparation) and a Phase II efficacy study in patients following an aneurismal SAH.

Nitrate as a Source of NO

Nitrate has been known as a metabolically inert end-product of NO oxidation that is removed by the kidneys. However, this opinion has dramatically changed when a panel of researchers "advocate(d) consumption of a diet high in nitrate(s) to protect individuals at risk of adverse vascular events" [37]. This revolutionary change was spearheaded by the studies of Jon Lundeberg and Eddie Weitzberg [38]. As with the earlier discovery that nitrite can become an NO donor, this time it was nitrate that became a source of nitrite and NO. The authors proposed a "recycling" process (Fig. 3) in which both nitrate and nitrite from food are reduced by the nitrate reductase present in bacteria residing in the mouth. After the saliva is swallowed, the nitrite is reduced to NO by chemical disproportionation in the acidic milieu of the stomach. The residual nitrate/nitrite is absorbed in the intestines and part of it is excreted as nitrate by the kidneys. The remaining in plasma exogenous nitrate combined with the nitrite and nitrate produced from the endogenous NO is "recycled" by being absorbed into the salivary glands and then excreted back into the saliva [38]. This very efficient cycle protects nitrite and facilitates its delivery to the plasma to be stored for "on-demand" NO delivery.

However, the mechanism of nitrite reduction to NO is not limited to the red blood cells and the presence of deoxygenated hemoglobin. Recently, it was shown that xanthine oxydo-reductase in plasma also can also act as a nitrite reductase [39]. In addition, neuroglobin [40], the newly discovered member of the globin family, specific for neurons,

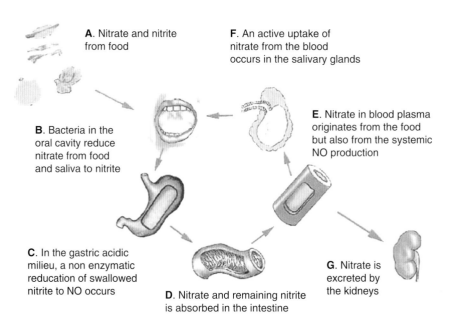

Fig. 3 Nitrite/nitrate "recycling" from [38]

may also reduce nitrite [41]. The latter provides additional support for neuroglobin's protective mechanisms against ischemia proposed several years ago; it also explains the reported high levels of NO-heme in the brain [42].

Conclusion

New pathways and sources of NO activity as well as a deeper understanding of the biological effects of NO have enabled us to develop a new group of therapeutic agents that, by regulating the presence of NO can provide therapeutic effects against vasospasm but may also be useful against the injuries from ischemia/reperfusion, high blood pressure, pulmonary hypertension, cancer development and metastasis, as well as organ transplants.

Acknowledgment This research was supported by the Intramural Research Program of the National Institute of Neurological Disorders and Stroke at the NIH.

Conflict of interest statement The author is one of holders of the international patent on sodium nitrite use in cerebrovascular diseases.

References

1. Ignarro L. Nitric oxide as a unique signaling molecule in the vascular system: a historical overview. J Physiol Pharmacol. 2002;53:503–14.
2. Gladwin M, Crawford J, Patel R. The biochemistry of nitric oxide, nitrite, and hemoglobin: role in blood flow regulation. Free Rad Biol Med. 2004;36:707–16.
3. Liu X, Miller MJS, Joshi MS, Sadowska-Krowicka H, Clark DD, Lancaster Jr JR. Diffusion-limited reaction of free nitric oxide with erythrocytes. J Biol Chem. 1998;273:18709–13.
4. Khurana VG, Sohni YR, Mangrum WI, McClelland RL, O'Kane DJ, Meyer FB, et al. Endothelial nitric oxide synthase gene polymorphism predict susceptibility to aneurismal subarachnoid hemorrhage and cerebral vasospasm. J Cereb Blood Flow Metabol. 2004;24:291–7.
5. Kukreja RC, Xi L. eNOS phosphorylation: a pivotal molecular switch in vasodilation and cardioprotection? J Mol Cell Cardiol. 2007;42(2):280–2.
6. Vallance P, Leone A, Calver A, Collier J, Moncada S. Endogenous dimethylarginine as an inhibitor of nitric oxide synthesis. J Cardiovasc Pharmacol. 1992;20(Suppl 12):S60–2.
7. Jung CS, Oldfield EH, Harvey-White J, Espey MG, Zimmermann M, Seifert V, et al. Association of an endogenous inhibitor of nitric oxide synthase with cerebral vasospasm in patients with aneurysmal subarachnoid hemorrhage. J Neurosurg. 2007;107(5):945–50.
8. Pluta RM, Jung CS, Judith Harvey-White J, Whitehead A, Espey MG, et al. In vitro and in vivo effects of probucol on hydrolysis of asymmetric dimethyl l-arginine and vasospasm in primates. J Neurosurg. 2005;103:731–8.
9. Morris SM Jr. Recent advances in arginine metabolism: roles and regulation of the arginases. Br J Pharmacol. 2009;157(6):922–30.
10. Stuehr S, Pou S, Rosen G. Oxygen reduction by nitric oxide synthases. J Biol Chem. 2001;276:14533–6.
11. Cai H. Hydrogen peroxide regulation of endothelial function: origins, mechanisms, and consequences. Cardiovasc Res. 2005;68(1):26–36.
12. Pluta RM, Afshar JK, Thompson BG, Boock RJ, Harvey-White J, Oldfield EH. Increased cerebral blood flow but no reversal or prevention of vasospasm in response to L-arginine infusion after subarachnoid hemorrhage. J Neurosurg. 2000;92:121–6.
13. Pluta R. Delayed cerebral vasospasm and nitric oxide: review, new hypothesis, and proposed treatment. Pharmacol Ther. 2005;105:23–56.
14. Desai A, Zhao Y, Heather A, Lankford HA, Warren JS. Nitric oxide suppresses EPO-induced monocyte chemoattractant protein-1 in endothelial cells: implications for atherogenesis in chronic renal disease. Lab Invest. 2006;86(4):369–79.
15. Sirén AL, Fratelli M, Brines M, Goemans C, Casagrande S, Lewczuk P, et al. Erythropoietin prevents neuronal apoptosis after cerebral ischemia and metabolic stress. Proc Natl Acad Sci USA. 2001;98(7):4044–9.
16. Banerjee D, Rodriguez M, Nag M, Adamson JW. Exposure of endothelial cells to recombinant human erythropoietin induces nitric oxide synthase activity. Kidney Int. 2000;57(5):1895–904.
17. Isenberg JS, Shiva S, Gladwin M. Thrombospondin-1-CD47 blockade and exogenous nitrite enhance ischemic tissue survival, blood flow and angiogenesis via coupled NO-cGMP pathway activation. Nitric Oxide. 2009;21(1):52–62.
18. Sobey C. Cerebrovascular dysfunction after subarachnoid hemorrhage: novel mechanisms and directions for therapy. Clin Exp Pharm Physiol. 2001;28:926–9.
19. Kim P, Schini VB, Sundt Jr TM, Vanhoutte PM. Reduced production of cGMP underlies the loss of endothelium-dependent relaxations in the canine basilar artery after subarachnoid hemorrhage. Circ Res. 1992;70:248–56.
20. Edwards D, Byrne J, Griffith T. The effect of chronic subarachnoid hemorrhage on basal endothelium-derived relaxing factor activity in intrathecal cerebral arteries. J Neurosurg. 1992;76:830–7.
21. Kasuya H, Weir BK, Nakane M, Pollock JS, Johns L, Marton LS, et al. Nitric oxide synthase and guanylate cyclase levels in canine basilar artery after subarachnoid hemorrhage. J Neurosurg. 1995;82:250–5.
22. Yamaguchi-Okada M, Nishizawa S, Mizutani A, Namba H. Multifaceted effects of selective inhibitor of phosphodiesterase III, cilostazol, for cerebral vasospasm after subarachnoid hemorrhage in a dog model. Cerebrovasc Dis. 2009;28(2):135–42.
23. Willette RN, Shiloh AO, Sauermelch CF, Sulpizio A, Michell MP, Cieslinski LB, et al. Identification, characterization, and functional role of phosphodiesterase type IV in cerebral vessels: effects of selective phosphodiesterase inhibitors. J Cereb Blood Flow Metab. 1997;17(2):210–9.
24. Malinski T, Bailey F, Zhang ZG, Chopp M. Nitric oxide measured by a porphyrinic microsensor in rat brain after transient middle cerebral artery occlusion. J Cereb Blood Flow Metab. 1993;13:355–8.
25. Doyle M, Hoekstra J. Oxidation of nitrogen oxides by bound dioxygen in hemoproteins. J Inorg Biochem. 1981;14:351–8.
26. Pluta RM, Dejam A, Grimes G, Gladwin MT, Oldfield EH. Nitrite infusions prevent cerebral artery vasospasm in a primate model of subarachnoid aneurismal hemorrhage. JAMA 2005;293:1477–84.
27. Gladwin MT, Kim-Shapiro DB. The functional nitrite reductase activity of the heme-globins. Blood 2008;112(7):2636–47.
28. Ignarro L. Biosynthesis and metabolism of endothelium-derived nitric oxide. Annu Rev Pharmacol Toxicol. 1990;30:535–60.
29. Gladwin MT, Shelhamer JH, Schechter AN, Pease-Fye ME, Waclawiw MA, Panza JA, et al. Role of circulating nitrite and S-nitrosohemoglobin in the regulation of regional blood flow in humans. Proc Natl Acad Sci USA. 2000;97:11482–7.

30. Cosby K, Partovi KS, Crawford JH, Patel RP, Reiter CD, Martyr S, et al. Nitrite reduction to nitric oxide by deoxyhemoglobin vasodilates the human circulation. Nat Med. 2003; 9:1498–505.
31. Dejam A, Hunter CJ, Schechter AN, Gladwin MT. Emerging role of nitrite in human biology. Blood Cell Mol Dis. 2004;32:423–9.
32. Afshar JK, Pluta RM, Boock RJ, Thompson BG, Oldfield EH. Effect of intracarotid nitric oxide on primate cerebral vasospasm after subarachnoid hemorrhage. J Neurosurg. 1995;83:118–22.
33. Pluta R, Oldfield E, Boock R. Reversal and prevention of cerebral vasospasm by intracarotid infusions of nitric oxide donors in a primate model of subarachnoid hemorrhage. J Neurosurg. 1997;87:746–51.
34. Pluta RM, Afshar JK, Boock RJ, Oldfield EH. Temporal changes in perivascular concentrations of oxyhemoglobin, deoxyhemoglobin and, methemoglobin in subarachnoid hemorrhage. J Neurosurg. 1998;88:557–61.
35. Hashi K, Meyer JS, Shinmaru S, Welch KM, Teraura T. Cerebral hemodynamic and metabolic changes after subarachnoid hemorrhage. J Neurol Sci. 1972;17:1–14.
36. Khaldi A, Zauner A, Reinert M, Woodward JJ, Bullock MR. Measurements of nitric oxide and brain tissue oxygen tension in patients after severe subarachnoid hemorrhage. Neurosurgery 2001;49:33–40.
37. Webb AJ, Patel N, Loukogeorgakis S, Okorie M, Aboud Z, Misra S, et al. Acute blood pressure lowering, vasoprotective, and antiplatelet properties of dietary nitrate via bioconversion to nitrite. Hypertension 2008;51(3):784–90.
38. Lundberg JO, Weitzberg E. NO generation from inorganic nitrate and nitrite: role in physiology, nutrition and therapeutics. Arch Pharm Res. 2009;32(8):1119–26.
39. Jansson EA, Huang L, Malkey R, Govoni M, Nihlén C, Olsson A, et al. A mammalian functional nitrate reductase that regulates nitrite and nitric oxide homeostasis. Nat Chem Biol. 2008;4(7):411–7.
40. Burmester T, Hankeln T. Neuroglobin: a respiratory protein of the nervous system. News Physiol Sci. 2004;19:110–3.
41. Petersen MG, Dewilde S, Fago A. Reactions of ferrous neuroglobin and cytoglobin with nitrite under anaerobic conditions. J Inorg Biochem. 2008;102(9):1777–82.
42. Bryan NS, Rassaf T, Maloney RE, Rodriguez CM, Fumito Saijo, Juan R. Rodriguez, et al. Cellular targets and mechanism of nitros(yl)ation: an insight into their nature and kinetics in vivo. PNAS. 2004;101:4308–13.

a # Section II: Advances in Subarachnoid Hemorrhage Research

Advances in Experimental Subarachnoid Hemorrhage

Yilin Zhou, Robert D. Martin, and John H. Zhang

Abstract Subarachnoid hemorrhage (SAH) remains to be a devastating disease with high mortality and morbidity. Two major areas are becoming the focus of the research interest of SAH: these are cerebral vasospasm (CVS) and early brain injury (EBI). This mini review will provide a broad summary of the major advances in experimental SAH during the last 3 years. Treatments interfering with nitric oxide (NO)- or endothelin-pathways continue to show antispasmotic effects in experimental SAH. HIF 1 may play both a detrimental and beneficial role in the setting of SAH, depending on its activation stage. Inflammation and oxidative stress contribute to the pathophysiology of both CVS and EBI. Apoptosis, a major component of EBI after SAH, also underlie the etiology of CVS. Since we recognize now that CVS and EBI are the two major contributors to the significant mortality and morbidity associated with SAH, ongoing research will continue to elucidate the underlying pathophysiological pathways and treatment strategies targeting both CVS and EBI may be more successful and improve outcome of patients with SAH.

Keywords Cerebral vasospasm (CVS) · Early brain injury (EBI) · Subarachnoid hemorrhage (SAH)

Y. Zhou and R.D. Martin
Department of Anesthesiology, Loma Linda University School of Medicine, Loma Linda, CA 92354, USA

J.H. Zhang (✉)
Department of Anesthesiology, Loma Linda University School of Medicine, Loma Linda, CA 92354, USA
Department of Neurosurgery, Loma Linda University School of Medicine, Loma Linda, CA 92354, USA
Department of Physiology, Loma Linda University School of Medicine, Loma Linda, CA 92354, USA
e-mail: johnzhang3910@yahoo.com

Introduction

Aneurismal subarachnoid hemorrhage (SAH) remains to be a serious disease that carries a high mortality and morbidity and affects mainly those aged between 40 and 60 years [69]. The incidence is approximately 10/100,000 people years [39]. Nearly 12% of patients die before receiving medical attention, additional 40% of patients die within 1 month after admission to hospital [23]. Of the survivors, up to 30% exhibit significant morbidity and will be dependent on others for activities of daily living [69]. Up to 50% of the survivors develop cognitive dysfunction in the long time and never return to their previous employment [33]. Despite advances in diagnosis and surgical treatment of SAH, effective therapeutic interventions are still limited and clinical outcomes remain disappointing. To date, substantial evidence indicates that there are two main issues contribute to the significant mortality and morbidity associated with SAH: these are cerebral vasospasm (CVS) and early brain injury (EBI).

Cerebral vasospasm occurs usually on day 3 after SAH, peaks at days 6–8, and lasts for 2–3 weeks [70]. CVS has been considered as the major cause of high mortality and poor outcome [17], thus researches have been primarily focused on vasospasm and its sequelae during the last several decades. However, the success with regard to improve outcome is limited [57]. In addition, although around 70% of patients may present arterial narrowing (angiographic CVS) after SAH, only about 30% will exhibit neurological deficits [17]. Thus, whether CVS is the only major cause of significant mortality and morbidity associated with SAH is questionable. More recently, early brain injury following SAH has also been linked to mortality and morbidity in SAH patients [7, 21]. EBI refers to the immediate injury to the brain, within the first 72 h following SAH. The underlying pathophysiological mechanisms include the immediate global ischemic brain injury caused by an acute increase in intracranial cerebral pressure (ICP) and decrease in cerebral blood flow (CBF), initiation of cell death signaling, blood–brain barrier breakdown, brain edema and inflammation [5, 8, 10, 35, 51, 68]. In this mini-review, we aim to provide an overview of the major advances in experimental SAH, published during the last 3 years, with an emphasis on the major pathophysiological pathways involved in the development of CVS and EBI, as well as treatment strategies targeting CVS and EBI.

Underlying Pathophysiological Pathways and Treatment Strategies Targeting CVS and EBI in SAH

CVS and Nitric Oxide Synthase (NOS)–Nitric Oxide (NO) Pathway

The dysfunction of endothelial nitric oxide-dependent pathway has been implicated as a major pathophysiological mechanism for the development of CVS [16, 53]. NO, produced by the endothelial nitric oxide synthase (eNOS) in cerebrovascular endothelium, diffuses to adjacent smooth muscle cells and stimulates soluble guanyl cyclase (sGC), leading to generation of cGMP. cGMP activates intracellular calcium channels, transporting free Ca^{2+} into intracellular stores and relaxing smooth muscle cells [16]. Vatter et al. aimed to characterize the endothelium-NO-cGMP-dependent pathway of cerebral arteries altered by delayed CVS, since the efficacy of the treatment targeting CVS by interfering with the NO-pathway at different levels seems to be inconsistent [66]. Their results suggest that the endothelium-NO-cGMP dependent relaxation is morphologically and functionally conserved in the major cerebral arteries during CVS in a rat double-hemorrhage model, by immunohistochemical analysis of eNOS and sGC expression and measuring the vasorelaxing effect of sodium nitroprusside (SNP), acetylcholine and 8-bromo-cGMP on rat BA ring segments. Thereby, they drew the conclusion that treatment of CVS aiming at the endothelium-NO-cGMP-dependent pathway seems to be practicable [66]. In a rat single-hemorrhage model, Osuka et al. showed that eNOS was significantly activated in the basilar arteries at an early stage after the onset of SAH, accompanied by the upregulation of AMP-activated protein kinase (AMPK α) in a rat single-hemorrhage model [52]. So the AMPKα-eNOS signaling pathway might be important in modulating cerebral blood flow in mild vasospasm [52]. As therapeutic intervention, 17β-estradiol benzoate (E2) was reported to attenuate CVS and preserve the eNOS expression by activating estrogen receptor subtype α (ERα) in a rat double-hemorrhage model [38, 62]. Furthermore, the same laboratory demonstrated that E2 mediated vasoprotection through inhibiting SAH-induced increase in expression levels of inducible nitric oxide synthase (iNOS) via NF-κB signaling pathway [61].

CVS and Endothelin Pathway

It has been well established that endothelin plays a key role in the development of CVS after SAH. Endothelin-1, a potent vasoconstrictor, was isolated from cultured porcine endothelial cells by Yanagisawa and colleagues in 1988 [73] and it acts by two specific receptors, ET(A) and ET(B) [55]. Elevated levels of endothelin have been found in the cerebrospinal fluid of patient after SAH [71]. Activation of ET(A) receptor on the vascular smooth muscle cells results in vasoconstriction, whereas ET(B1) receptor subtype, expressed on the vascular endothelial cells, mediates the vasorelaxing effects of endothelin. ET(B2) receptor subtype is localized on smooth muscle cells and causes vasoconstriction [76]. Yet, the expression and function of the ET(B) receptor subtypes after SAH is not well known. Vatter et al. demonstrated an unchanged immunohistochemical expression of the ET(B) receptor, which was observed exclusively in the endothelium, during the development of delayed CVS in a rat double-hemorrhage model [67]. Furthermore, they showed that sarafotoxin 6c (S6c), an ET(B) receptor agonist, did not cause vasoconstriction under resting tension in basilar artery segments. However, after preconstriction, activation of ET(B) receptor by S6c results in a vasodilation in sham-operated rat, which decreased time-dependently after SAH [67]. Thereby, a functionally relevant ET(B2) receptor-mediated vasoconstriction of the cerebrovasculature during CVS seems to be absent [67]. In contrast, Ansar et al. reported that SAH induces the upregulation of ET(B) receptor (mRNA and protein levels) in the cerebrovascular smooth muscle cells over the first 48 h in a rat single-hemorrhage model [1]. The discrepancy between the findings may relate to differences in the SAH models (double- vs. single-hemorrhage) and time point of ET(B) receptor measurement (on day 3 and 5 vs. the first 48 h). In this regard, further investigations are warranted. Schubert et al. determined the role of endothelin in the acute phase (the first minutes to hours) after SAH in a rat single-hemorrhage model. Prophylactic treatment with clazosentan, the endothelin receptor antagonist, was shown not to affect peracute cerebral perfusion pressure (CPP)-dependent hypoperfusion, but will block the continuous cerebral blood flow (CBF) reduction [58].

CVS and Hypoxia Inducible Factor-1 (HIF-1)

HIF-1 is an important transcription factor and involved in various biological processes including energy metabolism, angiogenesis, erythropoiesis, cell survival and apoptosis [14, 54]. HIF-1 is a key molecule in the pathophysiological response to hypoxia and oxidative stress and regulates more than 40 genes including vascular endothelial growth factor (VEGF), erythropoietin, BNIP3, and glucose transporter-1 [59]. Previous experimental data suggest that HIF-1 may play a dual role by activating both prosurvival and prodeath pathways in the central nervous system in the settings of ischemic stroke and cerebral hemorrhage [3, 22, 28]. Likewise, HIF-1 protein expression was shown to be upregulated on Day 7 after SAH in a rat double-hemorrhage model [25]. Administration of deferoxamine (DFO), a HIF-1 activator, on Day 4 increased the HIF-1 protein expression and activity on Day 7 and attenuated the basilar artery vasospasm in the same SAH model [25]. However, Yan et al. reported that HIF-1protein expression and activity was significantly increased at 24 h after SAH in a rat monofilament puncture model. 2-Methxyestradiol (2ME2), a HIF-1 inhibitor, administered at 1 h after SAH attenuated the CVS and the neurological deficits [72]. We speculate that HIF-1 could also play a prosurvival and prodeath role in the context of SAH. Activation of HIF-1 at an early stage after SAH may be detrimental whereas HIF-1 stimulation at a later stage could be neuroprotective. However, the HIF-1 downstream cascades mediating these beneficial and detrimental effects after SAH remain to be further elucidated.

CVS and Inflammation

Substantial evidence implicates a critical role of pro-inflammatory cascades in the development and maintenance of CVS after SAH [18]. Administration of simvastatin after onset of SAH was shown to attenuate CVS and decrease perivascular granulocyte migration at 72 h after SAH in a rabbit single-hemorrhage model, suggesting the efficacy of simvastatin targeting CVS may dependent on its anti-inflammatory effects [46]. Zhou et al. demonstrated that SAH induces an increase in the NF-kB DNA-binding activity and the mRNA levels of TNFα, IL-1β, intercellular adhesion molecule-1 and vascular cell adhesion molecule-1 on Day 5 after SAH in a rabbit double-hemorrhage model [70]. Administration of pyrrolidine dithiocarbamate (PDTC), a NF-κB inhibitor, reversed the aforementioned SAH-induced effects and attenuated the CVS after SAH, indicating NF-κB mediated pro-inflammatory response in SAH may contribute to the development of CVS [75]. N-benzyl-oxycarbonyl-Val–Ala–Asp-fluoromethylketone (Z-VAD-FMK), a caspase inhibitor, was shown to reduce the CVS on Day 2 after SAH in a rabbit single-hemorrhage model, which is associated with a decrease in the IL-1β release into the cerebrospinal fluid and the levels of caspase-1 and IL-1β in macrophages infiltrating into the subarachnoid space [27]. Monocyte chemoattractant protein-1(MCP-1), a potent chemokine attracting macrophage, has been implicated in the detrimental inflammatory processes associated with stroke and other disorders in the central nervous system [11, 34]. Lu et al. found that the mRNA and protein levels of MCP-1 increased in a parallel time course to the development of CVS (peaked on day 5) in a rat double-hemorrhage model, suggesting that specific MCP-1 antagonists may be beneficial to prevent CVS caused by SAH [41]. Experimental data from Bowman et al. indicates that inflammatory cytokines, in particular IL-6, are involved in the development of CVS in the rat femoral artery model [6].

CVS/EBI and Oxidative Stress

Oxidative stress is the other key factor that has been suggested to contribute to the pathogenesis of cerebral vasospasm as well as early brain injury after SAH. Superoxide anion levels in the cerebrospinal fluid have been shown to be increased parallel to the development of CVS [47]. Treatment strategies inhibiting free radical generating enzymes or scavenging free radical have been reported to attenuate CVS in animal models of SAH [4, 26, 45]. Recently, Karaoglan et al. demonstrated that resveratrol, a stilbene polyphenol and tyrosine kinase inhibitor, reduced SAH-induced CVS in a rat single-hemorrhage model. This protective effect is associated with decreased lipid peroxidation levels in brain and serum, and increased superoxide dismutase expression compared to the untreated group [30]. Hypersensitivity of the basilar artery to hydroxyl radicals has been implicated to underlie the pathogenesis of CVS after SAH [48]. Furthermore, free radicals can damage neurons and other major cell types in the brain by enhancing lipid peroxidation, protein oxidation and degradation, and DNA damage, which results in endothelial injury and blood–brain barrier (BBB) breakdown by initiating apoptotic cascades or necrosis processes [2, 37, 42]. Inhibition of oxidative stress has been shown to prevent apoptosis and BBB permeability. Recently, Ersahin et al. showed that administration of antioxidant melatonin prevented BBB breakdown, reduced brain edema and neurological deficits in a rat single-hemorrhage model [20]. Using transgenic rats, Endo et al. demonstrated that reduction in oxidative stress by superoxide dismutase (SOD) over expression results in decreased apoptosis in an endovascular perforation SAH model [19]. And this antiapoptotic effect was contributed to the activation of Akt/glycogen synthase kinase-3beta (GSK-3β) signaling pathway [19]. Another antioxidant, Mexiletine was shown to attenuate apoptosis of endothelial cells and prevent CVS in a rabbit single-hemorrhage model [60], suggesting a cross-talk between CVS and EBI and that the attenuation of CVS may be contributed at least partially to the preservation of endothelium integrity due to the reduction in oxidative stress.

CVS/EBI and Apoptosis

Apoptosis is one of the major pathophysiological components of early brain injury, and may also play a significant role in the etiology of cerebral vasospasm in the setting of SAH. Zhou et al. demonstrated previously that treatment with caspase inhibitors reduced endothelial apoptosis and CVS in a dog model of experimental SAH [74]. Recently, recombinant human erythropoietin (rhEPO) has been shown to attenuate the CVS in a rabbit double-hemorrhage model by inhibiting the endothelial apoptosis and these beneficial effects may be mediated by the activation of JAK2/STAT3 signaling pathway [13]. Likewise, JAK2 has been shown to be activated in the arterial wall after SAH and inhibition of JAK2 by AG490 aggravated the endothelium apoptosis and CVS by downregulation of bcl-2 and bcl-xL [12]. Furthermore, reduction in apoptosis by administration of PFT-α, a p53 inhibitor, results in preventing severe CVS and blood–brain barrier (BBB) breakdown in a rat monofilament puncture model of SAH by down- regulating caspase 8, cytochrome C, apoptosis inducing factor (AIF) and caspase 3 in the basilar arteries [9]. The aforementioned study results and previously experimental data implicate that prevention of apoptosis might attenuate CVS after SAH [8, 12, 13, 56]. One of the possible mechanisms could be reduced function of endothelial cells in SAH to prevent smooth muscle cell proliferation and vasoconstriction by generating inhibiting factors such as endothelial NO synthase or absence of endothelial vasodilative ET(B) receptor-mediated vasorelaxation due to the endothelial cell injury. Further studies are warranted to explore the cross talk between EBI and CVS after SAH.

Statin and CVS/EBI

Data of previous experimental and clinical studies has suggested that treatment with 3-hydroxy-3-methylglutaryl coenzyme A (HMGCoA) reductase inhibitors, also referred to as statins, promotes endothelial function, and reduces CVS in the setting of SAH [36, 43, 44, 49]. Recently, Sugawara et al. demonstrated that administration of simvastatin attenuated CVS and improved neurological outcomes in a rat SAH endovascular perforation model. And this simvastatin-mediated neuroprotection depends on the activation of PI3K/Akt/eNOS pathway [63]. Furthermore, prophylactic treatment with atorvastatin has been shown to reduce apoptotic cell death, prevent blood–brain barrier disrupt, attenuate CVS and improve neurological outcome in a rat perforating SAH model. Down regulation of caspase 3 and caspase 8 may contribute to the atorvastatin-induced neuroprotection in the context of SAH [15].

Thrombin and CVS/EBI

Thrombin, a serine protease coagulation protein, has been previously implicated in the pathogenesis of CVS after SAH and blood–brain barrier permeability in animal models of ischemic stroke and intracerebral hemorrhage [32, 50]. Thrombin activity in patient cerebrospinal fluid has been shown to coincide with the development of CVS and the degree of SAH [31]. Inhibition of thrombin activity by antithrombin III attenuated CVS, which associated with decreased immunoactivity of MAPK in smooth muscle cells of basilar artery [65]. Recently, Kai et al. demonstrated that inhibition of proteinase–activated receptor 1 (PAR1), which mediates thrombin's vascular effects [24], by E5555 blocked the upregulation of PAR1 expression and the hypercontractile response of the basilar artery to thrombin in a rabbit double-SAH model [29]. Moreover, administration of argatroban, a direct thrombin inhibitor, has been shown to prevent early brain injury after SAH in a rat intravascular perforation model, including reduction in cell death, brain edema and expression of inflammatory marker, and preservation of BBB integrity [64]. These new data further provide evidence that inhibition of thrombin may exhibit powerful neuroprotection in the setting of SAH by targeting both CVS and EBI, the two major events of SAH, which contribute to the significant mortality and morbidity of SAH.

Conclusion

In summary, research efforts with regard to SAH during the last 3 years have been continued focusing on exploring the pathogenesis of CVS and more recently, that of EBI. Endothelium-NO-cGMP dependent vasodilation appears to be conserved in the major cerebral arteries during CVS and treatment strategies interfering this pathway seem to be practicable. Endothelin appears to play a significant role not only in the development of delayed CVS, but also in the acute vasoconstriction after SAH. Prophylactic endothelin antagonism has been shown to prevent the acute hypoperfusion after SAH. The role of endothelin B receptor subtype after SAH remains to be clarified. HIF-1 seems to play a dual role in the setting of SAH. Inhibition of HIF-1 at early stage and activation of HIF-1 at later stage have been shown to prevent vasospasm after SAH. Further researches to evaluate the involved HIF-1 downstream cascades are warranted. The inflammatory response as well as oxidative stress associated to SAH may play biphasical roles in the pathophysiology after SAH, as it has been suggested for ischemic stroke [40]. Pro-inflammatory reactions and free radicals at acute stage of SAH may contribute to cell death and CVS, whereas they might be required for neurovascular remodeling and neurogenesis in later stage. In this regard, further studies are needed to elucidate the time course and evaluate the optimal time windows for treatment targeting the inflammatory reactions and oxidative stress after SAH. Early brain injury and cerebral vasospasm are the two major components contributing to brain injury after SAH. Cell death after SAH plays an important role not only in the long-term morbidity of SAH, but also possibly in the etiology of CVS. CVS in turn results in hypoperfusion of the related brain areas and may also trigger cell death processes. Molecular pathways underlying EBI after SAH remains further to be elucidated. Given the complexity of the pathogenesis in SAH, therapeutic modalities interfering with different pathophysiological pathways of SAH, and interventions targeting both CVS and EBI appear to be more desirable.

Conflict of interest statement We declare that we have no conflict of interest.

References

1. Ansar S, Vikman P, Nielsen M, Edvinsson L. Cerebrovascular ETB, 5-HT1B, and AT1 receptor upregulation correlates with reduction in regional CBF after subarachnoid hemorrhage. Am J Physiol Heart Circ Physiol. 2007;293(6):H3750–8.
2. Ayer RE, Zhang JH. Oxidative stress in subarachnoid haemorrhage: significance in acute brain injury and vasospasm. Acta Neurochir Suppl. 2008;104:33–41.
3. Baranova O, Miranda LF, Pichiule P, Dragatsis I, Johnson RS, Chavez JC. Neuron-specific inactivation of the hypoxia inducible factor 1 alpha increases brain injury in a mouse model of transient focal cerebral ischemia. J Neurosci. 2007;27:6320–32.
4. Barbosa MD, Arthur AS, Louis RH, MacDonald T, Polin RS, Gazak C, et al. The novel 5-lipoxygenase inhibitor ABT-761 attenuates cerebral vasospasm in a rabbit model of subarachnoid hemorrhage. Neurosurgery 2001;49:1205–12.
5. Bederson JB, Germano IM, Guarino L. Cortical blood flow and cerebral perfusion pressure in a new noncraniotomy model of subarachnoid hemorrhage in the rat. Stroke 1995; 26:1086–91.
6. Bowman G, Bonneau RH, Chinchilli VM, Tracey KJ, Cockroft KM. A novel inhibitor of inflammatory production (CNI-1493) reduces rodent post-hemorrhagic vasospasm. Neurocrit Care. 2006;5(3): 22209.
7. Broderick JP, Brott TJ, Duldner JE, Tomsick T, Leach A. Initial and recurrent bleeding are the major causes of death following subarachnoid hemorrhage. Stroke 1994;25:1342–7.
8. Cahill J, Zhang JH. Subarachnoid hemorrhage: is it time for a new direction? Stroke 2009;40(suppl 1):S86–7.
9. Cahill J, Calvert JW, Solaroglu I, Zhang JH. Vasospasm and p53-induced apoptosis in an experimental model of subarachnoid hemorrhage. Stroke 2006;37(7):1868–74.
10. Cahill WJ, Calvert JH, Zhang JH. Mechanisms of early brain injury after subarachnoid hemorrhage. J Cereb Blood Flow Metab. 2006;26:1341–53.
11. Che X, Ye W, Panga L, Wu DC, Yang GY. Monocyte chemoattractant protein-1 expressed in neurons and astrocytes during focal ischemia in mice. Brain Res. 2001;902(2):171–7.
12. Chen G, Wu J, Sun C, Qi M, Hang C, Gong Y, et al. Potential role of JAK2 in cerebral vasospasm after experimental subarachnoid hemorrhage. Brain Res. 2008;1214:136–44.
13. Chen G, Zhang S, Shi J, Ai J, Hang C. Effects of recombinant human erythropoietin (rhEPO) on the JAK2/STAT3 pathway and endothelial apoptosis in the rabbit basilar artery after subarachnoid hemorrhage. Cytokine 2009;45(3):162–8.
14. Chen W, Ostrowski RP, Obenaus A, Zhang JH. Prodeath or pro-survival: two facets of hypoxia inducible factor-1 in perinatal brain injury. Exp Neurol. 2009;216(1):7–15.
15. Cheng G, Wei L, Zhi-Dan S, Shi-Guang Z, Xiang-Zhen L. Atorvastatin ameliorates cerebral vasospasm and early brain injury after subarachnoid hemorrhage and inhibits caspase-dependent apoptosis pathway. BMC Neurosci. 2009;10:7.
16. Dietrich HH, Dacey RG Jr. Molecular keys to the problems of cerebral vasospasm. Neurosurgery 2000;46(3):517–30.
17. Dorsch NW. Cerebral arterial spasm-a clinical review. Br J Neurosurg. 1995;9:403–12.
18. Dumont AS, Dumont RJ, Chow MM, Lin CL, Calisaneller T, Ley KF, et al. Cerebral vasospasm after subarachnoid hemorrhage: putative role of inflammation. Neurosurgery 2003;53(1):123–33.
19. Endo H, Nito C, Kamada H, Yu F, Chan PH. Reduction in oxidative stress by superoxide dismutase overexpression attenuates acute brain injury after subarachnoid hemorrhage via activation of Akt/glycogen synthase kinase-3beta survival signaling. J Cereb Blood Flow Metab. 2007;27(5):975–82.
20. Ersahin M, Toklu HZ, Cetinel S, Yuksel M, Yegen BC, Sener G. Melatonin reduces experimental subarachnoid hemorrhage-induced oxidative brain damage and neurological symptoms. J Pineal Res. 2009;46(3):324–32.
21. Frykholm P, Andersson JL, Langstrom B, Persson L, Enbald P. Haemodynamic and metabolic disturbances in the acute stage of subarachnoid haemorrhage demonstrated by PET. Acta Neural Scand. 2004;109:25–32.
22. Helton R, Cui J, Scheele JR, Ellison JA, Ames C, Gibson C, et al. Brain-specific knock-out of hypoxia-inducible factor-1 alpha reduces rather than increases hypoxic-ischemic damage. J Neurosci. 2005;25:4099–107.
23. Hijdra A, Braakman R, van Gijn J, Vermeulen M, van Crevel H. Aneurysmal subarachnoid hemorrhage. Complications and outcome in a hospital population. Stroke 1987;18(6):1061–7.
24. Hirano K, Kanaide H. Role of proteinase-activated receptors in the vascular system. J Atheroscler Thromb. 2003;10:211–25.
25. Hishikawa T, Ono S, Ogawa T, Tokunage K, Sugiu K, Date I. Effects of deferoxamine-activated hypoxia-inducible factor-1 on the brainstem after subarachnoid hemorrhage in rats. Neurosurgery 2008;62(1):232–40.
26. Horky LL, Pluta RM, Boock RJ, Oldfield EH. Role of ferrous iron chelator 2,2'-dipyridyl in preventing delayed vasospasm in a primate model of subarachnoid hemorrhage. J Neurosurg. 1998; 88:298–303.
27. Iseda K, Ono S, Onoda K, Satoh M, Manabe H, Nishiguchi M, et al. Antivasospastic and antiinflammatory effects of caspase inhibitor in experimental subarachnoid hemorrhage. J Neurosurg. 2007;107 (1):128–35.

28. Jiang Y, Wu J, Keep RF, Hua Y, Hoff JT, Xi G. Hypoxia-inducible factor-1α accumulation in the brain after experimental intracerebral hemorrhage. J Cereb Blood Flow Metab. 2002;22: L689–96.
29. Kai Y, Hirano K, Maeda Y, Nishimura J, Sasaki T, Kanaide H. Prevention of the hypercontractile to thrombin by proteinase-activated receptor 1 antagonist in subarachnoid hemorrhage. Stroke 2007;38:3259–65.
30. Karaoglan A, Akdemir O, Barut S, Kokturk S, Uzun H, Tasyurekli M, et al. The effect of resveratrol on vasospasm after experimental subarachnoid hemorrhage in rats. Surg Neurol. 2008;70(4):337–43.
31. Kasuya H, Shimizu T, Takakura K. Thrombin activity in CSF after SAH is correlated with the degree of SAH the persistence of subarachnoid clot and the development vasospasm. Acta Neurochir (Wien). 1998;140(6):579–84.
32. Kitaoka T, Hua Y, Xi G, Hoff JT, Keep RF. Delayed argatroban treatment reduces edema in a rat model of intracerebral hemorrhage. Stroke 2002;33(12):3012–8.
33. Kreiter KT, Copeland D, Bernardini GL, Bates JE, Peery S, Claassen J, et al. Predictors of cognitive dysfunction after subarachnoid hemorrhage. Stroke 2002;33:200–8.
34. Kumagai N, Chiba Y, Hosono M, Fujii M, Kawamura N, Keino H, et al. Involvement of pro-inflammatory cytokines and microglia in an age-associated neurodegeneration model, the SAMP10 mouse. Brain Res. 2007;1185:75–85.
35. Kusaka G, Ishikawa M, Nanda A, Granger DN, Zhang JH. Signaling pathways for early brain injury after subarachnoid hemorrhage. J Cereb Blood Flow Metab. 2004;24:916–25.
36. Laufs U, Liao JK. Post-transcriptional regulation of endothelial nitric oxide synthase mRNA stability by Rho GTPase. J Bio Chem. 1998;273(37):24266–71.
37. Lewen A, Matz P, Chan PH. Free radical pathways in CNS injury. J Neurotrauma. 2000;17:871–90.
38. Lin CL, Shih HC, Dumont AS, Kassell NF, Lieu AS, Su YF, et al. The effect of 17beta-estradiol in attenuating experimental subarachnoid hemorrhage-induced cerebral vasospasm. J Neurosurg. 2006; 104(2):298–304.
39. Linn FH, Rinkel GJ, Algra A, Van Gijn J. Incidence of subarachnoid hemorrhage: role of region, year, and rate of computed tomography: a meta-analysis. Stroke 1996;27(4):625–9.
40. Lo EH. A new penumbra: transitioning from injury into repair after stroke. Nat Med. 2008;14(5):497–500.
41. Lu H, Shi JX, Chen HL, Hang CH, Wang HD, Yin HX. Expression of monocyte chemoattractant protein-1 inthe cerebral artery after experimental subarachnoid hemmorrhage. Brain Res. 2009;1262: 73–80.
42. Matz PG, Copin JC, Chan PH. Cell death after exposure to subarachnoid hemolysate correlates inversely with expression of CuZn-superoxide dismutase. Stroke 2000;31:2450–59.
43. McGirt MJ, Blessing R, Alexander MJ, Nimjee SM, Woodworth GF, Friedman AH, et al. Risk of cerebral vasospasm after subarachnoid hemorrhage reduced by statin therapy: a multivariate analysis of an institutional experience. J Neurosurg. 2006;105:671–74.
44. McGirt MJ, Lynch JR, Parra A, Sheng H, Pearlstein RD, Laskowitz DT, et al. Simvastatin increases endothelial nitric oxide synthase and ameliorates cerebral vasospasm resulting from subarachnoid hemorrhage. Stroke 2002;33:2950–56.
45. McGirt MJ, Parra A, Sheng H, Higuchi Y, Oury TD, Laskowitz DT, et al. Attenuation of cerebral vasospasm after subarachnoid hemorrhage in mice overexpressing extracellular superoxide dismutase. Stroke 2002;33:2317–23.
46. McGirt MJ, Pradilla G, Legnani FG, Thai QA, Recinos PF, Tamargo RJ, et al. Systemic administration of simavastatin after the onset of experimental subarachnoid hemorrhage attenuates cerebral vasospasm. Neurosurgery 2006;58(5):945–51.
47. Mori T, Nagata K, Town T, Tan J, Matsui T, Asano T. Intracisternal increase of superoxide anion production in a canine subarachnoid hemorrhage model. Stroke 2001;32:636–42.
48. Nishihashi T, Trandafir CC, Wang A, Ji X, Shimizu Y, Kurahashi K. Hypersensitivity to hydroxyl radicals in rat basilar artery after subarachnoid hemorrhage. J Pharmacol Sci. 2006;100(3):234–6.
49. O'Driscoll G, Green D, Taylor RR. Simvastatin, an HMG-coenzyme A reductase inhibitor, improves endothelial function within 1 month. Circulation 1997;95:1126–31.
50. Ohyama H, Hosomi N, Takahashi T, Mizushige K, Kohno M. Thrombin inhibition attenuates neurodegeneration and cerebral edema formation following transient forebrain ischemia. Brain Res. 2001;902(2):264–71.
51. Ostrowski RP, Colohan AR, Zhang JH. Mechanisms of hyperbaric oxygen-induced neuroprotection in a rat model of subarachnoid hemorrhage. J Cereb Blood Flow Metab. 2005;25:554–71.
52. Osuka K, Watanabe Y, Usuda N, Atsuzawa K, Yoshida J, Takayasu M. Modification of endothelial nitric oxide synthase through AMPK after experimental subarachnoid hemorrhage. J Neurotrauma. 2009;26(7):1157–65.
53. Pluta RM. Delayed cerebral vasospasm and nitric oxide: review, new hypothesis, and proposed treatment. Pharmacol Ther. 2005;105(1):23–56.
54. Pugh CW, Ratcliffe PJ. Regulation of angiogenesis by hypoxia: role of the HIF system. Nat Med. 2003;9:677–84.
55. Rubanyi GM, Polokoff MA. Endothelins: molecular biology, biochemistry, pharmacology, physiology, and pathophysiology. Pharmacol Rev. 1994;46:325–415.
56. Santhanam AV, Smith LA, Akiyama M, Rosales AG, Bailey KR, Katusic ZS. Role of endothelial NO synthase phosphorylation in cerebrovascular protective effect of recombinant erythropoietin during subarachnoid hemorrhage-induced cerebral vasospasm. Stroke 2005;36(12):2731–7.
57. Schievink WI. Intracranial aneurysms. N Engl J Med. 1997;336: 28–40.
58. Schubert GA, Schilling L, Thome C. Clazosentan, an endothelin receptor antagonist, prevents early hypoperfusion during the acute phase of massive experimental subarachnoid hemorrhage: a laser doppler flowmetry study in rats. J Neurosurg. 2008;109(6):1134–40.
59. Semenza GL. Signal transduction to hypoxia inducible factor 1. Biochem Pharmacol. 2002;64:993–8.
60. Sen O, Caner H, Aydin MV, Ozem O, Atalay B, Altinors N, et al. The effect of mexiletine on the level of lipid peroxidation and apoptosis of endothelium following experimental subarachnoid hemorrhage. Neurol Res. 2006;28:859–63.
61. Shih HC, Lin CL, Lee TY, Lee WS, Hsu C. 17beta-estradiol inhibits subarachnoid hemorrhage-induced inducible nitric oxide synthase gene expression by interfering with the nuclear factor kappa B transsaction. Stroke 2006;37(12):3025–31.
62. Shih HC, Lin CL, Wu SC, Kwan AL, Hong YR, Howng SL. Upregulation of estrogen receptor alpha and mediation of 17beta-estradiol vasoprotective effects via estrogen receptor alpha in basilar arteries in rats after experimental subarachnoid hemorrhage. J Neurosurg. 2008;109(1):92–9.
63. Sugawara T, Ayer R, Jadhav V, Chen W, Tsubokawa T, Zhang JH. Simvastatin attenuation of cerebral vasospasm after subarachnoid hemorrhage in rats via increased phosphorylation of Akt and endothelial nitric oxide synthase. J Neurosci Res. 2008;86(16):3635–43.
64. Sugawara T, Jadhav V, Ayer R, Chen W, Suzuki H, Zhang JH. Thrombin inhibition by argatroban ameliorate early brain injury and improves neurological outcomes after experimental subarachnoid hemorrhage in rats. Stroke 2009;40:1530–32.
65. Tsurutani H, Ohkuma H, Suzuki S. Effects of thrombin inhibitor on thrombin-related signal transduction and cerebral vasospasm in the rabbit subarachnoid hemorrhage model. Stroke 2003;34(6): 1497–500.

66. Vatter H, Weidauer S, Dias S, Preibisch C, Ngone S, Raabe A, et al. Persistence of the nitric oxide-dependent vasodilator pathway of cerebral vessels after experimental subarachnoid hemorrhage. Neurosurgery 2007;60(1):179–87.
67. Vatter H, Konczalla J, Weidauer S, Preibisch C, Raabe A, Zimmermann M, et al. Characterization of the endothelin-B receptor expression and vasomotor function during experimental cerebral vasospasm. Neurosurgery 2007;60(6):1100–8.
68. Voldby B, Enevoldsen EM. Intracranial pressure changes following aneurysm rupture. Part 1: clinical and angiographic correlations. J Neurosurg. 1982;56:186–96.
69. Wardlaw JM, White PM. The detection and management of unruptured intracranial aneurysms. Brain 2000;123:205–21.
70. Wilkins RH. Cerebral vasospasm. Crit Rev Neurobiol. 1990;6:51–77.
71. Yamaji T, Johshita H, Ishibashi M. Endothelin family in human plasma and cerebrospinal fluid. J Clin Endocrinol Metab. 1990;71:1611–15.
72. Yan J, Chen C, Lei J, Yang L, Wang K, Liu J, et al. 2-methoxyestradiol reduces cerebral vasospasm after 48 hours of experimental subarachnoid hemorrhage in rats. Exp Neurol. 2006;202(2):348–56.
73. Yanagisawa M, Kurihara H, Kimura S, Tomobe Y, Kobayashi M, Mitsui Y, et al. Novel potent vasoconstrictor peptide produced by vascular endothelial cells. Nature 1988;332(6163):411–5.
74. Zhou C, Yamaguchi M, Kusaka G, Schonholz C, Nanda A, Zhang JH. Caspase inhibitors prevent endothelial apoptosis and cerebral vasospasm in dog model of experimental subarachnoid hemorrhage. J Cereb Blood Flow Metab. 2004;24:419–31.
75. Zhou ML, Shi JX, Hang CH, Cheng HL, Qi XP, Mao L, et al. Potential contribution of nuclear factor-kappaB to cerebral vasospasm after experimental subarachnoid hemorrhage in rabbits. J Cereb Blood Flow Metab. 2007;27(9):1583–92.
76. Zimmermann M, Seifer V. Endothelin and subarachnoid hemorrhage: an overview. Neurosurgery 1998;43(4):863–75.

Advances in Treatment of Cerebral Vasospasm: an Update

Jacob Hansen-Schwartz

Abstract An update of published clinical advances in the treatment of cerebral vasospasm after subarachnoid haemorrhage was provided. Searching MEDLINE using the search terms "cerebral vasospasm" and "clinical trials" 46 papers were identified that had been published since the International Conference on Cerebral Vasospasm in Istanbul, Turkey in 2006. Of these 26 were either safety studies or case reports leaving 20 papers for consideration. The major topics covered were calcium antagonists, magnesium sulphate, statins, and fasudil hydrochloride. The studies published did not reach an impact justified recommended routine use, but certainly as options. Results of the CONSCIOUS trials on endothelin receptor antagonists are awaited.

Keywords Calcium · Endothelin · Fasudil · Magnesium · Statins · Vasospasm

Introduction

As is well known, clinicians and researchers alike are struggling to find an effective treatment of cerebral vasospasm subsequent to subarachnoid haemorrhage. In his paper from the ninth International Conference on Cerebral Vasospasm, held in Istanbul in 2006, Nick Dorsch summarised the overall status on vasospasm research [1]. The purpose of the present paper was to summarise the published advances in the years since 2006.

The major topics covered in the 2006 paper were calcium antagonists, endothelin receptor antagonists, magnesium sulphate and statins. In brief, topics such as CSF drainage, intraoperative implantation of papaverine pellets, head shaking and drainage techniques, and nitric oxide donors were also covered.

The field of advance was uncovered doing a MEDLINE search employing the search phrases "cerebral vasospasm" and "treatment outcome". In total, at the time of doing the search (September 2009) 42 studies published since the 2006 conference were identified. Of these, nine addressed the effect of calcium antagonists on cerebral vasospasm [2–10], five the effect of statin treatment [11–15], five the effect of magnesium sulphate [16–20], and four the effect of fasudil hydrochloride [21–24]. The remaining 17 papers addressed the effect of mechanical treatment [25], head shaking and CSF lavage [26], various methods of CSF drainage [27, 28], clasozentan [29], cilostazol [30], prostacyclin [31], erythropoietin [32], sodium nitroprusside [33], edavarone [34], milrinone [35], and eicosapentaenoic acid (a polyunsaturated fatty acid) [36]. Finally, two papers emerged as a result of reviewing the patient database gather from the tirilazad studies, one a meta-analysis of tirilazad and one identifying factors predicting outcome after subarachnoid haemorrhage [37, 38].

Comparing with the major topics covered in the paper from Murray and Dorsch the major topics remain the same except for the ongoing clazosentan study (the CONSCIOUS trials). The study published during the period of observation was a dose finding study in preparation for the CONSCIOUS II and III phase III trials. These results are pending.

Calcium Antagonists

In 2007 Barth et al. published a randomised phase IIa trial on the use of intraoperatively placed nicardipine pellets to prevent and treat cerebral vasospasm [10]. 32 patients with SAH Hunt and Hess grade 3 or 4 entered the study; 16 patients had the pellets along the conduit arteries exposed as part of the surgical clipping procedure. The control group

J. Hansen-Schwartz
Department of Neurosurgery, Glostrup University Hospital, DK-2600, Glostrup, Denmark
e-mail: jacob.schwartz@dadlnet.dk

had surgery performed without the placement of pellets. Otherwise the patients were treated according to the existing protocol for SAH patients. The results showed angiographic vasospasm in 7% of the treatment group vs. 73% in the control group. There was a lower incidence of CT verified ischemia; 14 vs. 47%, respectively. The short-term outcome rated on the Barthel index was "good" in 85 vs. 39%, respectively, and mortality was 6 vs. 38%, respectively. All differences were statistically significant. Two years later the same group published a follow-up study [2]. 18 of the original 32 patients were investigated (11 from the study group and 7 from the control group) at 1 year after aneurysm rupture. In terms of functional cognitive outcome the study group was, as reported in the initial study, superior to the control group (rated using the Karnofsky score and the MMSE test). Interestingly, however, in terms of the emotional outcome (anxiety, oblivion, and mild symptoms of depression) no statistically significant difference between the two groups was recorded. The authors concluded that quality of life seems related to the severity of the SAH itself. Although well designed and although the data are indeed very promising, the sample size is small necessitating validation in a phase III study. The use of pellets was also reported in a surgical series from Krischek et al. [7]. In a consecutive series of 100 surgically treated Fisher grade 3 SAH patients, they reported that 83 patients were independent at 3-month follow-up.

Five papers reported the use of intra-arterial and intra-thecal use of calcium antagonists (nimodipine and nicardipine) [4–6, 9, 39]. The studies were either case reports or safety and feasibility studies without a control group.

Kronvall et al. published a randomized study evaluating the possible difference in between intravenous and oral administration of nimodipine. 103 patients were included – no difference in outcome was observed [40].

Statins

During the time of observation two randomised controlled studies have been published [11, 14]. The first came from Tseng et al. covering 80 consecutive with SAH randomised to treatment with pravastatin 40 mg orally daily or to placebo treatment. Medication was initiated on average 2 days after debut and was continued until day 14. They found a significantly reduced need for triple-H therapy and a significantly reduced mortality as a well as incidence of sepsis. At 6 months follow-up the treated group experienced a 73% reduction in unfavourable outcome (measured using Short Form 36, differences noted in the psychosocial and physical dimensions). In another study on the same patient group the authors concluded that statin treatment improved cerebral autoregulation after SAH [15].

In contrast, Vergouwen et al. covering 32 consecutive patients with SAH randomised to treatment with simvastatin 80 mg orally daily or to placebo treatment, did not find any effect in terms of incidence of cerebral vasospasm during in-patient stay and neither in terms of long-term outcome.

Conflicting studies is second nature in academia, and in such cases meta-analysis may be attempted. Sillberg et al. did this in their 2008 meta-analysis including three randomized controlled studies published in 2005 and 2006 [13]. The studies included had conflicting conclusions, yet using meta-analysis method the authors found that on balance, routine use of statins was recommended. The mentioned study did not, however, include the latter of the aforementioned study indicating no effect of statin treatment on the outcome of SAH.

Based on the initial results the West Australian Neurosurgical Service of Sir Charles Gairdner and Royal Perth Hospitals, Australia decided to implement routine use of statins in the treatment of SAH patients [12]. Reviewing patient outcome as a field study 1 year after this change (72 patients) and comparing the data with historical controls treated 1 year before the change (58 patients) the authors did not find any difference in vasospasm parameters during in-stay and neither in long term outcome.

Magnesium Sulphate

The possible effect of magnesium sulphate is thought of as a competitive calcium antagonist. There is, however, precedence that it be treated as separate compared to calcium antagonists as such.

Wong et al. published a double blind study enrolling 60 SAH patients [20]. The treatment group had 80 mmol Mg^{2+} administered daily over a period of 14 days. Symptomatic vasospasm was observed in 23% of the patients in the treatment group vs. 46% in the placebo group. The duration of symptomatic vasospasm was also shorter in the treatment group. However, the differences did not reach statistical significance, and neither was any difference observed regarding neurological outcome after 6 months rated with the Barthel index and Glasgow outcome scale.

In 2006 Schmid–Elsaesser published a double blind study randomising 104 patients with SAH to either $MgSO_4$ (20 mmol/day) or nimodipine treatment [15] for at least 7 days after securing the aneurysm. In terms of both short and long term outcome no significant differences were observed.

Stippler et al. administered 100 mmol/day $MgSO_4$ over 12 days to 38 SAH patients, and compared the treatment effect with matched historical controls [18]. End points were on short term symptomatic vasospasm and mortality, and on long term outcome as rated with the Barthel index and Glasgow outcome score. A trend toward lower incidence of vasospasm and improved long term outcome was observed though not on a statistically significant level.

The latest study is from Muroi et al. who performed a single blind study on 64 SAH patients receiving either placebo or MgSO$_4$ [17]. Dose regimens were individualised to double the plasma Mg^{2+} concentration. On average 64 mmol were administered daily, and the treatment was continued for 12 days. Results were similar to the afore mentioned studies with the notable difference that in 16 patients treatment had to be abandoned before day 12 due to adverse effects (primarily hypotension and hypocalcemia). Interestingly, this does not appear to have been a significant problem in the other studies mentioned despite even higher doses of calcium were administered.

Intrathecal administration of MgSO$_4$ has also been reported. Mori et al. published a safety study where Mg^{2+} was administered to ten patients as part of a CSF lavage treatment (ventricular infusion and lumber drainage) [16]. Treatment was well tolerated and the incidence of symptomatic vasospasm was reduced compared to clinical experience.

Fasudil Hydrochloride

Fasudil hydrochloride has entered standard clinical use in Easter Asia in much the same fashion as nimodipine is used. Zhao et al. did a randomised comparative study between the two treatments enrolling 72 patients [24]. No significant difference was observed between the two groups, and thus fasudil hydrochloride seems to be equipotent to nimodipine.

Two post-marketing studies were published that confirmed the conclusions at the time of the phase III studies.

Conclusion

In terms of evidence based treatment of cerebral vasospasm matters are status quo compared to 2006. The mainstays of vasospasm treatment thus remain unchanged and they are in short keeping the patient well hydrated and correcting sodium levels as needed. According to local consensus either nimodipine or fasudil is administered for the prevention of cerebral vasospasm. There is an option for treating with calcium antagonist pellets, statins and magnesium sulphate.

Conflict of interest statement I declare that I have no conflict of interest.

References

1. Murray M, Dorsch NWC. Advances in vasospasm research. Acta Neurochir Suppl. 2008;104:1–4.
2. Barth M, Thome C, Schmiedek P, Weiss C, Kasuya H, Vajkoczy P. Characterization of functional outcome and quality of life following subarachnoid hemorrhage in patients treated with and without nicardipine prolonged-release implants. J Neurosurg. 2009;110:955–60.
3. Conti A, Angileri FF, Longo M, Pitrone A, Granata F, La Rosa G. Intra-arterial nimodipine to treat symptomatic cerebral vasospasm following traumatic subarachnoid haemorrhage. Technical case report. Acta Neurochir (Wien). 2008;150:1197–202.
4. Hanggi D, Beseoglu K, Turowski B, Steiger HJ. Feasibility and safety of intrathecal nimodipine on posthaemorrhagic cerebral vasospasm refractory to medical and endovascular therapy. Clin Neurol Neurosurg. 2008;110:784–90.
5. Mayer TE, Dichgans M, Straube A, Birnbaum T, Muller-Schunk S, Hamann GF, et al. Continuous intra-arterial nimodipine for the treatment of cerebral vasospasm. Cardiovasc Intervent Radiol. 2008;31:1200–4.
6. Goodson K, Lapointe M, Monroe T, Chalela JA. Intraventricular nicardipine for refractory cerebral vasospasm after subarachnoid hemorrhage. Neurocrit Care. 2008;8:247–52.
7. Krischek B, Kasuya H, Onda H, Hori T. Nicardipine prolonged-release implants for preventing cerebral vasospasm after subarachnoid hemorrhage: effect and outcome in the first 100 patients. Neurol Med Chir (Tokyo). 2007;47:389–94.
8. Dorhout Mees SM, Rinkel GJ, Feigin VL, Algra A, van den Bergh WM, Vermeulen M, et al. Calcium antagonists for aneurysmal subarachnoid haemorrhage. Cochrane Database Syst Rev. 2007; CD000277.
9. Tejada JG, Taylor RA, Ugurel MS, Hayakawa M, Lee SK, Chaloupka JC. Safety and feasibility of intra-arterial nicardipine for the treatment of subarachnoid hemorrhage-associated vasospasm: initial clinical experience with high-dose infusions. AJNR Am J Neuroradiol. 2007;28:844–8.
10. Barth M, Capelle HH, Weidauer S, Weiss C, Munch E, Thome C, et al. Effect of nicardipine prolonged-release implants on cerebral vasospasm and clinical outcome after severe aneurysmal subarachnoid hemorrhage: a prospective, randomized, double-blind phase IIa study. Stroke 2007;38:330–6.
11. Vergouwen MD, Meijers JC, Geskus RB, Coert BA, Horn J, Stroes ES, et al. Biologic effects of simvastatin in patients with aneurysmal subarachnoid hemorrhage: a double-blind, placebo-controlled randomized trial. J Cereb Blood Flow Metab. 2009; 29:1444–53.
12. Kern M, Lam MM, Knuckey NW, Lind CR. Statins may not protect against vasospasm in subarachnoid haemorrhage. J Clin Neurosci. 2009;16:527–30.
13. Sillberg VA, Wells GA, Perry JJ. Do statins improve outcomes and reduce the incidence of vasospasm after aneurysmal subarachnoid hemorrhage: a meta-analysis. Stroke 2008;39:2622–6.
14. Tseng MY, Hutchinson PJ, Czosnyka M, Richards H, Pickard JD, Kirkpatrick PJ. Effects of acute pravastatin treatment on intensity of rescue therapy, length of inpatient stay, and 6-month outcome in patients after aneurysmal subarachnoid hemorrhage. Stroke 2007;38:1545–50.
15. Tseng MY, Czosnyka M, Richards H, Pickard JD, Kirkpatrick PJ. Effects of acute treatment with statins on cerebral autoregulation in patients after aneurysmal subarachnoid hemorrhage. Neurosurg Focus. 2006;21:E10.
16. Mori K, Yamamoto T, Nakao Y, Osada H, Hara Y, Oyama K, et al. Initial clinical experience of vasodilatory effect of intra-cisternal infusion of magnesium sulfate for the treatment of cerebral

vasospasm after aneurysmal subarachnoid hemorrhage. Neurol Med Chir (Tokyo). 2009;49:139–44.
17. Muroi C, Terzic A, Fortunati M, Yonekawa Y, Keller E. Magnesium sulfate in the management of patients with aneurysmal subarachnoid hemorrhage: a randomized, placebo-controlled, dose-adapted trial. Surg Neurol. 2008;69:33–9.
18. Stippler M, Crago E, Levy EI, Kerr ME, Yonas H, Horowitz MB, et al. Magnesium infusion for vasospasm prophylaxis after subarachnoid hemorrhage. J Neurosurg. 2006;105:723–9.
19. Schmid-Elsaesser R, Kunz M, Zausinger S, Prueckner S, Briegel J, Steiger HJ. Intravenous magnesium versus nimodipine in the treatment of patients with aneurysmal subarachnoid hemorrhage: a randomized study. Neurosurgery 2006;58:1054–65.
20. Wong GK, Chan MT, Boet R, Poon WS, Gin T. Intravenous magnesium sulfate after aneurysmal subarachnoid hemorrhage: a prospective randomized pilot study. J Neurosurg Anesthesiol. 2006;18:142–8.
21. Suzuki Y, Shibuya M, Satoh S, Sugiyama H, Seto M, Takakura K. Safety and efficacy of fasudil monotherapy and fasudil-ozagrel combination therapy in patients with subarachnoid hemorrhage: sub-analysis of the post-marketing surveillance study. Neurol Med Chir (Tokyo). 2008;48:241–7.
22. Suzuki Y, Shibuya M, Satoh S, Sugimoto Y, Takakura K. A postmarketing surveillance study of fasudil treatment after aneurysmal subarachnoid hemorrhage. Surg Neurol. 2007;68:126–31.
23. Iwabuchi S, Yokouchi T, Hayashi M, Uehara H, Ueda M, Samejima H. Intra-arterial administration of fasudil hydrochloride for vasospasm following subarachnoid hemorrhage – analysis of time-density curve with digital subtraction angiography. Neurol Med Chir (Tokyo). 2006;46:535–9.
24. Zhao J, Zhou D, Guo J, Ren Z, Zhou L, Wang S, et al. Effect of fasudil hydrochloride, a protein kinase inhibitor, on cerebral vasospasm and delayed cerebral ischemic symptoms after aneurysmal subarachnoid hemorrhage. Neurol Med Chir (Tokyo). 2006;46:421–8.
25. Haque R, Kellner CP, Komotar RJ, Connolly ES, Lavine SD, Solomon RA, et al. Mechanical treatment of vasospasm. Neurol Res. 2009;31:638–43.
26. Hanggi D, Liersch J, Turowski B, Yong M, Steiger HJ. The effect of lumboventricular lavage and simultaneous low-frequency head-motion therapy after severe subarachnoid hemorrhage: results of a single center prospective Phase II trial. J Neurosurg. 2008;108:1192–9.
27. Mura J, Rojas-Zalazar D, Ruiz A, Vintimilla LC, Marengo JJ. Improved outcome in high-grade aneurysmal subarachnoid hemorrhage by enhancement of endogenous clearance of cisternal blood clots: a prospective study that demonstrates the role of lamina terminalis fenestration combined with modern microsurgical cisternal blood evacuation. Minim Invasive Neurosurg. 2007;50:355–62.
28. Otawara Y, Ogasawara K, Kubo Y, Sasoh M, Ogawa A. Effect of continuous cisternal cerebrospinal fluid drainage for patients with thin subarachnoid hemorrhage. Vasc Health Risk Manag. 2007;3:401–4.
29. Macdonald RL, Kassell NF, Mayer S, Ruefenacht D, Schmiedek P, Weidauer S, et al. Clazosentan to overcome neurological ischemia and infarction occurring after subarachnoid hemorrhage (CONSCIOUS-1): randomized, double-blind, placebo-controlled phase 2 dose-finding trial. Stroke 2008;39:3015–21.
30. Yoshimoto T, Shirasaka T, Fujimoto S, Yoshidumi T, Yamauchi T, Tokuda K, et al. Cilostazol may prevent cerebral vasospasm following subarachnoid hemorrhage. Neurol Med Chir (Tokyo). 2009;49:235–40.
31. Koskinen LO, Olivecrona M, Rodling-Wahlstrom M, Naredi S. Prostacyclin treatment normalises the MCA flow velocity in nimodipine-resistant cerebral vasospasm after aneurysmal subarachnoid haemorrhage: a pilot study. Acta Neurochir (Wien). 2009;151:595–9.
32. Tseng MY, Hutchinson PJ, Richards HK, Czosnyka M, Pickard JD, Erber WN, et al. Acute systemic erythropoietin therapy to reduce delayed ischemic deficits following aneurysmal subarachnoid hemorrhage: a Phase II randomized, double-blind, placebo-controlled trial. Clinical article. J Neurosurg. 2009;111:171–80.
33. Agrawal A, Patir R, Kato Y, Chopra S, Sano H, Kanno T. Role of intraventricular sodium nitroprusside in vasospasm secondary to aneurysmal subarachnoid haemorrhage: a 5-year prospective study with review of the literature. Minim Invasive Neurosurg. 2009;52:5–8.
34. Munakata A, Ohkuma H, Nakano T, Shimamura N, Asano K, Naraoka M. Effect of a free radical scavenger, edaravone, in the treatment of patients with aneurysmal subarachnoid hemorrhage. Neurosurgery 2009;64:423–8.
35. Fraticelli AT, Cholley BP, Losser MR, Saint Maurice JP, Payen D. Milrinone for the treatment of cerebral vasospasm after aneurysmal subarachnoid hemorrhage. Stroke 2008;39:893–8.
36. Yoneda H, Shirao S, Kurokawa T, Fujisawa H, Kato S, Suzuki M. Does eicosapentaenoic acid (EPA) inhibit cerebral vasospasm in patients after aneurysmal subarachnoid hemorrhage? Acta Neurol Scand. 2008;118:54–9.
37. Fergusen S, Macdonald RL. Predictors of cerebral infarction in patients with aneurysmal subarachnoid hemorrhage. Neurosurgery 2007;60:658–67.
38. Jang YG, Ilodigwe D, Macdonald RL. Metaanalysis of tirilazad mesylate in patients with aneurysmal subarachnoid hemorrhage. Neurocrit Care. 2009;10:141–7.
39. Hanggi D, Turowski B, Beseoglu K, Yong M, Steiger HJ. Intra-arterial nimodipine for severe cerebral vasospasm after aneurysmal subarachnoid hemorrhage: influence on clinical course and cerebral perfusion. AJNR Am J Neuroradiol. 2008;29:1053–60.
40. Kronvall E, Undren P, Romner B, Saveland H, Cronqvist M, Nilsson OG. Nimodipine in aneurysmal subarachnoid hemorrhage: a randomized study of intravenous or peroral administration. J Neurosurg. 2009;110:58–63.

Roles of Signal Transduction Mechanisms in Cerebral Vasospasm Following Subarachnoid Hemorrhage: Overview

Shigeru Nishziawa

Abstract The concept of "cortical spreading depression" following subarachnoid hemorrhage (SAH) drastically tends to change the direction of vasospasm research. It has been rather confuse whether classical idea, delayed long-lasting major cerebral arterial contraction is real cerebral vasospasm or it occurs just after SAH and classical arterial contraction is an epiphenomenon. However, it is true that such sustained arterial contraction occurs following SAH, and the mechanisms still remain unclear. Intracellular signal transduction plays a pivotal role in long-lasting arterial contraction. Although scientific research advances, each role of signal transduction system has been getting clarified; overview or interrelations among such systems have to be more investigated. Based on the previous results, some aspect or part of streams of interrelation of signal transduction systems can be getting clearer. Such way to clarify the overview is extremely important to understand the real mechanisms of long-lasting arterial contraction following SAH ("classical cerebral vasospasm").

Keywords Cerebral vasospasm · Signal transduction · Subarachnoid hemorrhage

Introduction

As scientific researches in cerebral vasospasm following subarachnoid hemorrhage (SAH) advance, the fundamental definition of cerebral vasospasm itself is now rather in confusion. Most researches have been done to clarify why and how cerebral major arteries continue contraction for long time following SAH. However, the concept of "cortical spreading depression" or "cortical depolarization wave" make the heading of research about cerebral vasospasm drastically changed [1, 2]. "Three or 4 days delayed onset" following SAH and long-lasting major cerebral arterial constriction have been basic principles of cerebral vasospasm. Nowadays, it is the time to re-consider what is cerebral vasospasm and delayed ischemic neurological deficits (DIND) caused by cerebral vasospasm [2].

On the other hand, it is also true that long-term potent constriction of major cerebral arteries following SAH definitely occurs and the mechanisms of such phenomenon have not been clarified. Classical "cerebral vasospasm" may contribute on DIND. In that sense, it is still significantly important to understand the mechanisms of long-lasting arterial contraction.

Signal transduction mechanisms play pivotal roles in such contraction. Each role of kinases or phosphorylated proteins has been clarified, but it is not clear how they integrate or regulate each other in the development and maintenance of cerebral vasospasm. Interrelation of the roles of kinases or phosphorylated proteins should be overviewed for understanding the mechanisms of long-lasting arterial constriction [3]. The purpose of this article is to introduce and review just some parts of such interrelations.

Overview

Protein Kinase C (PKC)

It is no doubt that PKC plays a significant role in the cerebral vasospasm [4–6]. Among PKC isoforms, four PKC isoforms are identified in canine cerebral arteries (basilar artery) such as PKCα, δ, ζ, and η. In those four isoforms,

S. Nishziawa
Department of Neurosurgery, University of Occupational and Environmental Health, Iseigaoka, Yahata-Nishi, Kitakyushu, Fukuoka, 807-8555, Japan
e-mail: snishizawa@nifty.com

PKCδ is involved in the development of cerebral vasospasm, and PKCα in its maintenance [7, 8].

In canine "two-hemorrhage" model, cerebral vasospasm in basilar artery continues until day 14. However, the translocation of both PKCδ and PKCα down-regulate on day 14, and return to the control levels. It means another factors have to consider for sustaining the cerebral vasospasm. Furthermore, it is unclear which protein is substrate of each PKC isoform.

Myosin Light Chain Phosphorylation

The MLC phosphorylation has been believed as an essential and fundamental factor in the vascular contraction. However, it has been reported that myosin light chain (MLC) phosphorylation level is not parallel with the extent of cerebral vasospasm at all [9]. In the treatment study using PKC-inhibitors, cheleryhtrine, it completely inhibits the whole course of cerebral vasospasm in canine "two-hemorrhage" model, although high MLC phosphorylation level continues [9]. In another word, MLC phosphorylation and maintenance of cerebral vasospasm are not correlated at all. The role of MLC phosphorylation has still been a controversial issue [9, 10].

From these results, the role of actin-side for sustaining cerebral vasospasm is considered to be important. Especially, the role of caldesmone has been focused on as a mechanism of long-lasting cerebral arterial contraction following SAH [11].

Rho-Kinase and Rho A

It is also true that Rho is very important for the mechanisms of cerebral vasospasm. In clinical field, Rho-kinase inhibitor, fasudil hydrochloride is widely used for the treatment of cerebral vasospasm. Intra-arterial administration of fasudil shows significant vasodilatory effect, but the effect is just temporary, not long-lasting.

In the consideration between Rho A and PKC, the treatment study using Rho-kinase inhibitor, Y-27632 inhibits arterial contraction on day 4 of canine "two-hemorrhage" model, but not on day 7. It suggests that Rho A also contributes on the development of cerebral vasospasm, but not on the maintenance. Y-27632 inhibits the intracellular distribution of PKCδ on day 4. However, Y-27632 has no effect of such intracellular distribution of PKCα. PKCδ-inhibitor, rottlerin does not inhibit the translocation of Rho A. These results indicate that Rho-kianse/Rho A system locates in the upstream of PKCδ, and regulates the activity of PKCδ [11]. On the other hand, PKCα and Rho-k6nase/Rho A are completely independent [9]. The development of cerebral vasospasm in canine "two-hemorrhage" model introduces by PKCδ under regulation of Rho-kinase/Rho A.

Protein Tyrosine Kinase (PTK)

As described, PKC activity and arterial contraction in canine "two-hemorrhage" model are not parallel after day 7. As down-regulation of PKC activities occurs even in the continuation of the cerebral vasospasm after day 7, PTK starts to be activated from day 7, and its activation continues until day 14. Protein tyrosine kinase (PTK) might modulate various intracellular signal transduction systems, such as sustaining long-term arterial contraction, and vascular smooth muscle thickening.

It is probably suggested that the main role to keep arterial contraction following SAH might shift from PKC to PTK [12]. There is evidence that activity of PTK is regulated by PKCδ activity. During the first 7 days, activated PKCδ regulates the activation of PTK, resulting in PTK activation [12].

Phenotypic Change of the Vascular Smooth Muscle Cells

There are two types of vascular smooth muscle cells, contractile and synthetic types. The contractile type of vascular smooth muscle cells are normal one. On the other hand, synthetic type of vascular smooth muscle cells is identified in the embryo, and such type of vascular smooth muscle cells are induced once the cells are injured. According to our experimental results, vascular smooth muscle cells of canine basilar arteries in "two-hemorrhage model", phenotypic change from contractile type to synthetic type is clearly seen on day 7, and such changes are most prominent on day 14 and 21. Thereafter, the phenotypic change returns to the normal contractile type on day 28 [13]. These time courses are very similar with those of PTK activation. It is also seen that the stiffness of the vascular smooth muscle is very significant when the synthetic type of vascular smooth muscle cells are prominent [13]. As the phenotypic change returns to the normal, the stiffness of the artery also returns to the normal.

These results indicate that the vascular smooth muscle phenotypic changes occurs in the long-lasting cerebral vasospasm, and such phenotypic changes probably is induced by the activation of PTK as PTK activation closely relates to the cell-growth, or phenotypic change. Those phenotypic changes contribute to the long-lasting cerebral arterial contraction such as cerebral vasospasm. This is a cause of non-myogenic mechanism of cerebral vasospasm [13].

Mitogen-Activated Protein (MAP)/MAP Kinase (MAPK)

MAPK/MAP are considered as a final pathway of intracellular signal transduction, and they play a role of regulation of cell growth and cellular mitosis. There have been reported that inhibition of MAPK/MAP significantly suppresses the cerebral vasospasm following subarachnoid hemorrhage [14, 15]. However, as mentioned, MAPK/MAP regulates cell growth and mitosis. The reason why the inhibition of MAPK/MAP induces reduction of cerebral vasospasm is not clear.

Among isoforms of MAPK, ERK1/2 pays an important role in regulation of cellular proliferation of vascular smooth muscle cells, and inhibition of ERK1/2 induces significant inhibition of cellular proliferation of vascular smooth muscle cells in vasospastic arteries in rabbit model [16]. These data support that a single stream of intracellular signal transduction such as Rho-PKCδ-PTK-MAPK/MAP following SAH induces vascular phenotypic change and thickness of medial muscle layer in vasospastic arteries.

Conclusion

The roles of signal transduction mechanisms in the cerebral vasospasm following SAH described above are just a part of them. Figures 1 and 2 show some aspects or streams of such interrelation. To investigate and clarify the interrelated/integrated roles of each signal transduction system, and how they positively or negatively regulate each other are extremely important to understand the mechanisms of long-lasting major arterial contraction such as "cerebral vasospasm" following SAH.

Conflict of interest statement I declare that I have no conflict of interest.

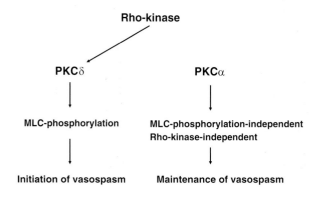

Fig. 1 Interrelation between Rho-kinase and PKC isoforms

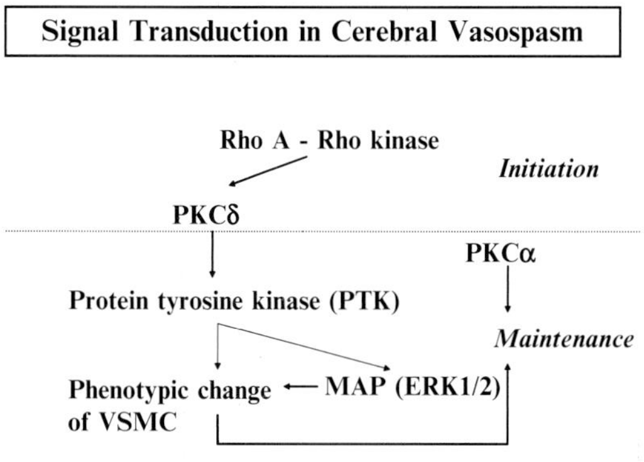

References

1. Dreier JP, Major S, Manning A, Woitzik J, Drenckhahn C, Steinbrink J, et al. COSBID study group: cortical spreading ischaemia is a novel process involved in ischaemic damage in patients with aneurismal subarachnoid haemorrhage. Brian 2009;132:1866–81.
2. Pluta RM, Hansen-Schwartz J, Dreier J, Vajkoczy P, Macdonald RL, Nishizawa S, et al. Cerebral vasospasm following subarachnoid hemorrhage: time for a new world of thought. Neurol Res. 2009;31:151–8.
3. Nishizawa S, Koide M, Yamaguchi-Okada M. The roles of cross-talk mechanisms in the signal transduction systems in the pathophysiology of the cerebral vasospasm after subarachnoid haemorrhage – what we know and what we do not know. Acta Neurochir Suppl (Wien). 2008;104:59–63.
4. Nishizawa S, Nezu N, Uemura K. Direct evidence for a key role of protein kinase C in the development of vasospasm after subarachnoid hemorrhage. J Neurosurg. 1992;76:635–9.
5. Nishizawa S, Peterson JW, Shimoyama I, Uemura K. Relation between protein kinase C and calmodulin systems in cerebrovascular contraction: investigation of the pathogenesis of vasospasm after subarachnoid hemorrhage. Neurosurgery 1992;31:711–6.
6. Nishizawa S, Yamamoto S, Yokoyama T, Ryu H, Uemura K. Chronological changes of arterial diameter, cGMP, and protein kinase C in the development of vasospasm. Stroke 1995;26: 1916–21.
7. Nishizawa S, Obara K, Nakayama K, Koide M, Yokoyama T, Yokota N, et al. Protein kinase C δ and α are involved in the development of vasospasm after subarachnoid hemorrhage. Eur J Pharmacol. 2000;398:113–9.

Fig. 2 Signal Transduction in Cerebral Vasospasm

8. Nishizawa S, Obara K, Nakayama K, Koide M, Yokoyama T, Ohta S. Which protein kinase C isoforms are involved in the development of vasospasm after subarachnoid hemorrhage ? Acta Neurochir (Wien). 2001;77(suppl):21–4.
9. Nishizawa S, Obara K, Koide M, Nakayama K, Ohta S, Yokoyama T. Attenuation of canine cerebral vasospasm after subarachnoid hemorrhage by protein kinase C inhibitors despite augmented phosphorylation of myosin light chain. J Vasc Res. 2003;40:168–79.
10. Butler WE, Psterson JW, Zervas NT, Morgan KG. Intracellualr calcium, myosin light chain phosphorylation, and contractile force in experimental cerebral vasospasm. Neurosurgery 1996;38:781–8.
11. Obara K, Nishizawa S, Koide M, Nozawa K, Mitate A, Ishikawa T, et al. Interactive role of protein kinase Cδ with Rho-kinase in the development of cerebral vasospasm in a canine-hemorrhage model. J Vasc Res. 2005;42:67–76.
12. Koide M, Nishizawa S, Ohta S, Yokoyama T, Namba H. Chronological changes of the contractile mechanism in prolonged vasospasm after subarachnoid hemorrhage: from protein kinase C to protein tyrosine kinase. Neurosurgery 2002;51:1468–76.
13. Yamaguchi-Okada M, Nishizawa S, Koide M, Nonaka Y. Biomechanical and phenotypic changes in the vasospastic canine basilar artery after subarachnoid hemorrhage. J Appl Physiol. 2005;99:2045–52.
14. Aoki K, Zubkov AY, Tibbs RE, Zhang JH. Role of MAPK in chronic cerebral vasospasm. Life Sci. 2002;70:1901–8.
15. Yatsushige H, Yamaguchi M, Zhou C, Calvert JW, Zhang JH. Roles of c-Jun N-terminal kinase in cerebral vasospasm after experimental subarachnoid hemorrhage. Stroke 2005;36:1538–43.
16. Chen D, Chen JJ, Yin Q, Guan JH, Liu YH. Role of ERK1/2 and vascular cell proliferation in cerebral vasospasm after experimental subarachnoid hemorrhage. Acta Neurochir (Wien). 2009;151:1127–34.

Part II: Mechanistic Studies

Section III: Early Brain Injury After Subarachnoid Hemorrhage

Hypoperfusion in the Acute Phase of Subarachnoid Hemorrhage

Gerrit Alexander Schubert, Marcel Seiz, Aldemar Andrés Hegewald, Jérôme Manville, and Claudius Thomé

Abstract *Purpose*: Acute disruption of cerebral perfusion and metabolism is a well-established hallmark of the immediate phase after subarachnoid hemorrhage (SAH). It is thought to contribute significantly to acute brain injury, but despite its prognostic importance, the exact mechanism and time course is largely unknown and remains to be characterized.

Methods: We investigated changes in cerebral perfusion after SAH in both an experimental and clinical setting. Using an animal model of massive, experimental SAH ($n = 91$), we employed Laser-Doppler flowmetry (LDF), parenchymal microdialysis (MD; $n = 61$), Diffusion-weighted imaging (DWI) and MR spectroscopy (MRS; $n = 30$) to characterize the first hours after SAH in greater detail. The effect of prophylactic treatment with hypothermia (HT; 32°C) and an endothelin-A (ET-A) receptor antagonist (Clazosentan) was also studied. In a group of patients presenting with acute SAH ($n = 17$) we were able to determine cerebral blood flow (CBF) via Xenon-enhanced computed tomography (XeCT) within 12 h after the ictus. Results: The acute phase after SAH is characterized both experimentally and clinically by profound and prolonged hypoperfusion independent from current intracranial pressure (ICP), indicating acute vasospasm. Experimentally, when treated with hypothermia or a ET-A receptor antagonist prophylactically, acute hypoperfusion improved rapidly. DWI showed a generalized, significant decline of the apparent diffusion coefficient (ADC) after SAH, indicating cytotoxic edema which was not present under hypothermia. SAH causes a highly significant reduction in glucose, as well as accumulation of lactate, glutmate and aspartate (MD and MRS). HT significantly ameliorated these metabolic disturbances.

Conclusion: Acute vasospasm, cytotoxic edema and a general metabolic stress response occur immediately after experimental SAH. Prophylactic treatment with hypothermia or ET-A antagonists can correct these disturbances in the experimental setting. Clinically, prolonged and ICP-independent hypoperfusion was also confirmed. As the initial phase is of particular importance regarding the neurological outcome and is amenable to beneficial intervention, the acute stage after SAH demands further investigation and warrants the exploration of measures to improve the immediate management of SAH patients.

Keywords Acute phase · Hypoperfusion · Subarachnoid hemorrhage · Vasospasm

Introduction

Cumulative morbidity and mortality after subarachnoid hemorrhage remain high despite considerable research efforts of neuroclinicians worldwide. The kind of intervention (clipping vs. coiling) and the prevention of secondary ischemia due to delayed vasospasm are within the main focus of current investigations. However, despite the well-established fact that the acute phase after SAH itself – defined by the initial neurological presentation – is highly predictive to the overall outcome of a patient [1], only limited effort has been put into its pathophysiological characterization.

This review is intended to summarize our recent research efforts regarding the changes in physiology, namely perfusion and metabolism immediately after SAH, both within the experimental and clinical setting. The aim was to better understand those first minutes to hours after SAH which are known to have a significant impact for both primary and secondary brain injury.

G.A. Schubert (✉), M. Seiz, A.A. Hegewald, J. Manville, and C. Thomé
Department of Neurosurgery, Universitätsmedizin Mannheim, University of Heidelberg, Theodor-Kutzer-Ufer 1-3, 68167 Mannheim, Germany

Methods

In an experimental model of massive SAH (induced by injection of 0.5 ml of autologous blood into the cisterna magna of adult, male Sprague-Dawley rats; n = 91), we recorded cortical LDF as well as ICP and mean arterial blood pressure in one group of animals (group A; n = 61), which is described elsewhere in greater detail [2]. Measurements lasted from 30 min prior to 180 min after induction of SAH. Analysis was complemented by the acquisition of a parenchymal microdialysates to determine changes in metabolism (glucose, lactate, glutamate and aspartate). In a second group of animals (group B; n = 30), we performed DWI and MRS (2.35T experimental Bruker Biospec Scanner) while inducing SAH, within the same time frame [3]. In a subset of each group, we also investigated the effect of prophylactic treatment with moderate hypothermia (group A-HT; group B-HT; 32°C) and with an anti-vasoconstrictive agent, an endothelin-A receptor antagonist (clazosentan; group A-ET) [4].

In 17 patients with acute SAH (HH 1–3: n = 9; HH 4–5: n = 8) and in four healthy controls we performed Xenon-enhanced CT (XeCT) scans to measure absolute CBF values. Cortical regions of interest (ROI) of anterior, middle and posterior cerebral artery territories, but also infratentorially and within the basal ganglia were averaged and compared.

Mann–Whitney and t-test were used as applicable to estimate differences between groups (SigmaStat®, Systat Software GmbH, Erkrath, Germany). Statistical significance was set at $p < 0.05$, $p < 0.01$ and $p < 0.001$ respectively.

Results

CBF decreases significantly immediately after experimental SAH (group A, Fig. 1), and hypoperfusion with disrupted autoregulation prevails for over 3 h in normothermia (group A-NT), but recovers rapidly to baseline values with both prophylactic HT and an ET-A antagonist (group A-HT, A-ET). Changes in CBF are independent from current ICP. DWI showed comparable pattern of a generalized, significant decline in ADC after SAH, which was not present under hypothermia. MRS and MD were able to demonstrate a significant accumulation of lactate for normothermia only; at the same time, a highly significant reduction in glucose as well as increase in glutmate and aspartate was observed (MD). HT significantly ameliorated these metabolic disturbances. Experimental findings of changes in perfusion and metabolism are summarized in Table 1.

While ICP was not significantly elevated, absolute CBF values were significantly lower in patients with acute SAH (mean time since hemorrhage 7.6 ± 3.7 h), when compared to healthy controls (64 ml/100 g*min) (Figs. 2 and 3). Cortical CBF decreases profoundly within the first 12 h after the insult (HH 1–3: 42 ml/100 g*min; HH 4–5: 25 ml/100 g*min), and statistical significance increases with severity of initial neurological deficit ($p < 0.05$, and $p < 0.001$ respectively). Changes within the basal ganglia and infratentorial structures are less severely disrupted (data not shown).

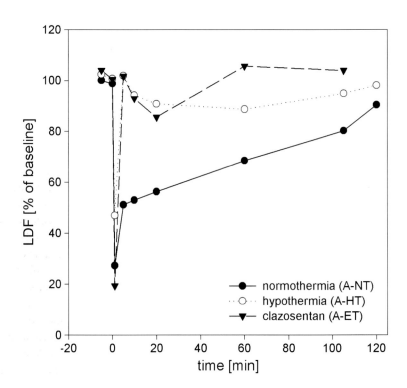

Fig. 1 This figure illustrates severe hypoperfusion in all experimental groups immediately after SAH. After normalization of ICP (not shown), CBF improves promptly in the hypothermia- and clazosentan-group (A-HT and A-ET), while hypoperfusion persists in normothermia (A-NT)

Table 1 Summary of perfusion and metabolism

		Group A				Group B	
		NT	HT	ET		NT	HT
CBF	At 5 min	↓↓↓	≈	≈	ADC	↓	≈
	At 60 min	↓	≈	≈		↓	≈
Autoregulation		↓	≈	≈		NA	NA
Microdialysis	Glucose	↓↓↓	≈	NA	MRS	NA	NA
	Lactate	↑↑	≈	NA		↑↑	≈
	Glutamate	↑↑	≈	NA			
	Aspartate	↑↑↑	≈	NA			

This table summarizes all experimental findings regarding changes in perfusion, autoregulation and metabolism. ↑ = increase, ↓ = decrease, ≈ = unchanged, *NA* nonapplicable

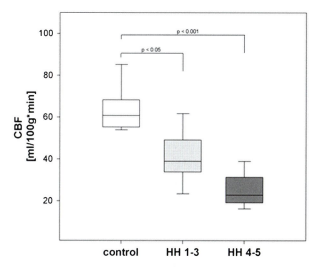

Fig. 2 CBF is significantly decreased in all patients after SAH; significance increases with the severity of the neurological deficit (HH 1–3 vs. HH 4–5)

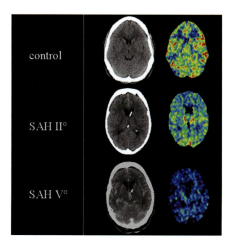

Fig. 3 This figure shows color-coded, exemplatory XeCT scans of a control patient, a patient HH II° and V°. Darker colors such as *blue* and *green* show lower levels of perfusion than warmer colors such as *yellow* and *red*

Discussion

Clinical grade at admission has been established as one of the major predictors regarding overall outcome after SAH [5, 6]. For the very first minutes, CPP-dependent hypoperfusion has been demonstrated repeatedly [7, 8]; pathophysiological changes thereafter, however, are less clearly defined. Our group has now been able to demonstrate – both experimentally and clinically – a phase of prolonged and profound hypoperfusion, which is ICP-independent and most likely is the result of peripheral constriction of the microvasculature. Reduction of CBF is paralled by a significant decrease in ADC, indicating cytotoxic edema. Another indication for a metabolic stress and misery perfusion is both a severe reduction in glucose, as well as a simultaneous increase in lactate, glutamate and aspartate. This metabolic disruption is amenable to early intervention, as shown in our studies with prophylactic administration of hypothermia, which improves the crucial supply/demand ratio. Prolonged hypoperfusion can be effectively forestalled by prophylactic administration of both hypothermia and an ET-A receptor antagonist, the latter being extensively studied as an effective agent in the treatment of delayed vasospasm [9]. As perfusion recovers promptly, autoregulation is maintained and intracranial pressure is not elevated, a causative role for acute vasoconstriction must be considered, a hypothesis that is enforced by the finding of cortically pronounced, peripheral hypoperfusion on Xenon-CT scanning, while more proximal territories, such as the basal ganglia are spared (data not shown). The degree of hypoperfusion, and therefore the degree of vasoconstriction clinically appears to correlate with the neurological deficit on admission (Fig. 3). As the initial neurological presentation is considered predictive as to the overall outcome [10], recovery of perfusion and metabolic disruption appear to be essential and promising targets for future therapy and intervention.

Conclusion

Acute and ICP-independent hypoperfusion occurs immediately after SAH both in the experimental and the clinical setting. Cytotoxic edema and a general metabolic stress response are further hallmarks of the acute phase, which is amenable to prophylactic treatment with hypothermia or ET-A antagonists within the experimental setting. The acute stage after SAH warrants further investigation, as it is of particular importance regarding the overall outcome.

Conflict of interest statement We declare that we have no conflict of interest.

References

1. Jakobsen M, Enevoldsen E, Bjerre P. Cerebral blood flow and metabolism following subarachnoid haemorrhage: cerebral oxygen uptake and global blood flow during the acute period in patients with SAH. Acta Neurol Scand. 1990;82:174–82.
2. Schubert GA, Poli S, Mendelowitsch A, Schilling L, Thome C. Hypothermia reduces early hypoperfusion and metabolic alterations during the acute phase of massive subarachnoid hemorrhage: a laser-Doppler-flowmetry and microdialysis study in rats. J Neurotrauma. 2008;25:539–48.
3. Schubert GA, Poli S, Schilling L, Heiland S, Thome C. Hypothermia reduces cytotoxic edema and metabolic alterations during the acute phase of massive SAH: a diffusion-weighted imaging and spectroscopy study in rats. J Neurotrauma. 2008;25:841–52.
4. Schubert GA, Schilling L, Thome C. Clazosentan, an endothelin receptor antagonist, prevents early hypoperfusion during the acute phase of massive experimental subarachnoid hemorrhage: a laser Doppler flowmetry study in rats. J Neurosurg. 2008;109:1134–40.
5. Roos YB, de Haan RJ, Beenen LF, Groen RJ, Albrecht KW, Vermeulen M. Complications and outcome in patients with aneurysmal subarachnoid haemorrhage: a prospective hospital based cohort study in the Netherlands. J Neurol Neurosurg Psychiatry. 2000;68:337–41.
6. Rosenstein J, Suzuki M, Symon L, Redmond S. Clinical use of a portable bedside cerebral blood flow machine in the management of aneurysmal subarachnoid hemorrhage. Neurosurgery 1984;15:519–25.
7. Bederson JB, Germano IM, Guarino L. Cortical blood flow and cerebral perfusion pressure in a new noncraniotomy model of subarachnoid hemorrhage in the rat. Stroke 1995;26:1086–91; discussion 1091–1082.
8. Thomé C, Schubert GA, Piepgras A, Elste V, Schilling L, Schmiedek P. Hypothermia reduces acute vasospasm following SAH in rats. Acta Neurochir Suppl. 2001;77:255–8.
9. Vajkoczy P, Meyer B, Weidauer S, Raabe A, Thomé C, Ringel F et al,. Clazosentan (ASV-034343), a selective endothelin A receptor antagonist, in the prevention of cerebral vasospasm follwoing severe aneurysmal subarachnoid hemorrrhage: results of a randomized, double-blind, placebo-controlled, multicenter Phase IIa study. J Neurosurg. 2005;103:9–17.
10. Proust F, Hannequin D, Langlois O, Freger P, Creissard P. Causes of morbidity and mortality after ruptured aneurysm surgery in a series of 230 patients. The importance of control angiography. Stroke 1995;26:1553–7.

Association of APOE Polymorphism with the Change of Brain Function in the Early Stage of Aneurysmal Subarachnoid Hemorrhage

Bin Lin, Wei Dan, Li Jiang, Xiao-hong Yin, Hai-tao Wu, and Xiao-chuan Sun

Abstract Recent studies have indicated that early brain injury may be responsible for the detrimental effects seen in patients after subarachnoid hemorrhage (SAH). In this study, we investigated the relationship between apolipoprotein E gene (APOE) polymorphism and the change of brain function in the early stage of aneurysmal SAH. A total of 79 patients admitted within 5 days after aneurysmal SAH were recruited in the study. Patient characteristics, such as age, gender, Fisher and Hunt–Hess grade were collected when admitted. Electroencephalogram (EEG) was recorded on admission and at 3–5 days after onset to assess the change of brain function of the patients in acute stage of SAH. The result of the second EEG recording was defined as EEG deterioration if the decrease in alpha wave frequency, increase in slow wave or decline in amplitude were observed when compared with the first EEG recording. The APOE polymorphism was determined in all patients by polymerase chain reaction-restriction fragment length polymorphism (PCR-RFLP). Ten of 17 patients with APOEε4 (58.8%) showed the deteriorated EEGs, which was significantly different from those without APOEε4 (18 of 62 patients, 29.0%, $p = 0.023$). However, neither the presence of ε2 nor of ε3 was significantly different from those absent of it ($p > 0.05$). Univariate logistic regression analyses showed that both high Fisher grade ($p = 0.028$, $OR = 2.917$, 95% $CI = 1.124–7.572$) and APOEε4 ($p = 0.027$, $OR = 3.492$, 95% $CI = 1.150–10.604$) were risk factors to EEG aggravation after aneurysmal SAH. The association of APOEε4 for deteriorated EEG was more significant after adjustment for age, gender, Hunt–Hess grade on admission, and Fisher grade ($p = 0.007$, $OR = 5.741$, 95% $CI = 1.625–20.280$). Our findings suggest that APOEε4 allele is a risk factor to brain function aggravation in the early stage of aneurysmal SAH, and it may contribute to early brain injury after SAH.

Keywords Apolipoprotein E · Early brain injury · Electroencephalogram · Subarachnoid hemorrhage

Introduction

Subarachnoid hemorrhage (SAH) due to ruptured intracranial aneurysms is a life-threatening disease with an annual incidence of 2–22.5/100,000 [1]. SAH accounts for only 1–7% of all strokes, but affects younger patients than other stroke subtypes, resulting in a greater loss of productive life. Approximately 12.4% of patients die of the initial hemorrhage before receiving medical attention, and a total of 40% of the hospitalized patients die within 1 month after onset [2]. More than one third of the survivors need lifelong care. Rebleeding and cerebral vasospasm have traditionally been recognized as the most cause of morbidity and mortality from SAH. Recent studies indicate that the early brain injury (EBI) after SAH which occur during the 24–72 h following aneurysm rupture, make significant contributions to patient outcomes, and may be responsible for the detrimental effects seen in patients after SAH [3].

The pathogenesis of aneurysmal SAH remains uncertain, and genetic factors may play a major role in the formation and rupture of aneurysms. Apolipoprotein E (apoE = protein, APOE = gene), encoded by a polymorphic gene, is produced by astrocytes and has a neuroprotective effect in the central nervous system. Recently, the APOE gene polymorphism has been reported to be associated with outcome after aneurysmal SAH, and the ε4 allele may increase the risk of early death [4, 5].

Over the past three decades, case fatality rates after SAH have decreased, owing to modern technological advancement and intentional treatment. But the decrease will probably be

B. Lin, W. Dan, L. Jiang, X.-h. Yin, H.-t. Wu, and X.-c. Sun (✉)
Department of Neurosurgery, the First Affiliated Hospital of Chongqing Medical University, Chongqing 400016, People's Republic of China
e-mail: sunxch1445@gmail.com

limited by the substantial proportion of patients who die before reaching hospital or reach hospital in poor neurological condition [6]. The aim of our study was to investigate whether the APOEε4 allele has detrimental effects on brain function in the early stage of SAH.

Materials and Methods

Patients

A total of 79 patients with aneurismal SAH admitted to the Department of Neurosurgery (the First Affiliated Hospital of Chongqing Medical University) from March 2008 to May 2009 were prospectively recruited. Study inclusion criteria were (1) admitted within 5 days after onset; (2) SAH was confirmed by computed tomographic scan or lumbar puncture; (3) intracranial aneurysm was verified by digital subtraction angiography (DSA) or CT angiography (CTA). The exclusion criteria were (1) patients with a history of neurological disorder; (2) SAH resulted from arteriovenous malformation, moyamoya disease, or trauma. All patients received standard nursing and medical care including blood glucose and blood pressure monitoring (systolic blood pressure was controlled under 140 mmHg), antifibrinolytic therapy, anticonvulsant prophylaxis, analgesia and prevention of cerebral vasospasm by intravenous nimodipine. Patient characteristics, such as age, gender, hypertension history, Fisher and Hunt–Hess grade were collected when admitted.

This study was approved by the Ethics Committee of the Department of Medical Research and informed consent was obtained from either the patients or their proxies.

APOE Genotyping

Genotyping was performed on DNA extracted from peripheral venous blood samples collected from patients on admission. APOE genotypes were determined by polymerase chain reaction-restriction fragment length polymorphism (PCR-RFLP) using methods and primers described previously [7].

EEG Detection and Interpretation

Electroencephalogram (EEG) was recorded on admission and at 3–5 days after onset to assess the change of brain function of the patients in acute stage of SAH. EEG data were acquired from 16 channels: Fp1, Fp2, F7, F3, F4, F8, T3, C3, C4, T4, T5, P3, P4, T6, O1 and O2, according to the international 10–20 system. All the EEG recordings last 10–15 min with the patient's eyes closed in a relaxed state. The result of the second EEG recording was defined as EEG deterioration if the decrease in alpha wave frequency, increase in slow wave or decline in amplitude were observed when compared with the first EEG recording, otherwise it was defined as EEG stabilization. Interpretations of EEG were performed blinded to the APOE genotype.

Statistical Analysis

Data were analyzed with SPSS for Windows, release 17.0. We compared the distribution of patient characteristics between the groups (EEG deterioration and EEG stabilization) using the Pearson χ^2 test and the Fisher Exact test when necessary. Univariate logistic regression was performed to determine the effect of sex, age, hypertension history, Hunt–Hess grade, Fisher grade and APOE genotype on the change of EEG after SAH. Then we analyzed the association of APOE polymorphism with the change of EEG by a multiple logistic regression (Forward: Wald). Variables entered the multivariate regression at $p < 0.05$ and were removed at $p > 0.10$.

Results

In this study, a total of 17 patients were APOEε4 allele carriers, and allele frequencies were as follows: 8.9% for ε2, 79.7% for ε3, and 11.4% for ε4. Genotypic distribution was consistent with Hardy–Weinberg equilibrium ($p > 0.05$) (Table 1).

Of 79 patients, 28 subjects presented with deteriorated EEG in acute stage of SAH. There were no statistically significant differences between the EEG deterioration and EEG stabilization groups in terms of sex, age, hypertension history, or Hunt–Hess grade. Patients in Fisher grade 3–4 were more common in the EEG deterioration group than in the EEG stabilization group ($p = 0.026$) (Table 2). Ten of 17 patients with APOEε4 (58.8%) showed the deteriorated EEGs, which was significantly different from those without APOEε4 (18 of 62 patients, 29.0%, $p = 0.023$). However, neither the presence of ε2 nor of ε3 was significantly differ-

Table 1 Distribution of APOE genotype

Genotype					Allele frequency		
ε2ε3	ε2ε4	ε3ε3	ε3ε4	ε4ε4	ε2	ε3	ε4
12	2	50	14	1	8.9%	79.7%	11.4%

Table 2 Comparison of characteristics between the EEG deterioration and EEG stabilization groups

Items	EEG deterioration	EEG stabilization	p-value
Sex			
Male	12	24	0.720
Female	16	27	
Age (years)			
<60	18	36	0.565
≥60	10	15	
Hypertension history			
Negative	15	32	0.427
Positive	13	19	
Hunt–Hess grade			
Grade 1–2	9	28	0.063
Grade 3–5	19	23	
Fisher grade			
Grade 1–2	12	35	0.026
Grade 3–4	16	16	

Table 3 Correlation of APOEε2, ε3, ε4 status with the change of EEG

EEG	ε2 allele ε2+…ε2−	ε3 allele ε3+…ε3−	ε4 allele ε4+…ε4−
Deterioration	3…25	26…2	10…18
Stabilization	11…40	50…1	7…44
p-value	0.368	0.591	0.023

ent from those absent of it ($p > 0.05$) (Table 3). Univariate logistic regression analyses showed that both high Fisher grade ($p = 0.028$, $OR = 2.917$, 95% $CI = 1.124–7.572$) and APOEε4 ($p = 0.027$, $OR = 3.492$, 95% $CI = 1.150–10.604$) were risk factors to EEG aggravation after aneurysmal SAH. The association of APOEε4 for deteriorated EEG was more significant after adjustment for age, gender, Hunt–Hess grade on admission, and Fisher grade ($p = 0.007$, $OR = 5.741$, 95% $CI = 1.625–20.280$).

Conclusion

Recent reports have tended to use the Glasgow Outcome Scale (GOS) to grade the clinical outcome in patients with aneurysmal SAH, but at the present time there is no standardized method of measuring the cognitive or neurobehavioral deficits [8]. EEG is particularly sensitive to cerebral ischemia, and has a clear association with the consciousness. In the acute stage of SAH, it may be more suitable than other means to assess the change of brain function of the patients.

In our study, EEG was recorded on admission and at 3–5 days after onset to evaluate brain function. We found that patients in poor Fisher grade were more common in the EEG deterioration group than in the EEG stabilization group, and univariate logistic regression analyses also showed it was a risk factor to brain function aggravation after aneurysmal SAH. This result may be explained by one prior study which shows the products of hemolysis in the subarachnoid space after SAH can lead to widespread necrosis of the cortex [9].

Genome-wide linkage analyses for familial intracranial aneurysm have revealed linkages to several chromosomal regions. Among them, 19q13 which APOE located on is potentially interesting because they have been replicated in several studies [10]. ApoE is a polymorphic protein with three common isoforms, encoded by three alleles of a single gene locus on chromosome 19q13.2. The neuroprotective effect of the apoE4 isoform is less than that of the others, and this has made the APOEε4 allele a risk factor candidate in the event of CNS insults. In the SAH population, the risk of an unfavorable outcome is 1.4 times higher among carriers of the ε4 allele than patients without the ε4 allele [11]. In Chinese population, the ε4 allele also is thought as a possible risk factor to poor outcome in aneurysmal SAH, and patients with ε4 allele are more susceptive to early clinical critical condition [12]. Some hospital-based studies have reported there is no association of APOE ε4 allele with the incidence of aneurysmal SAH. A conceivable explanation for this negative finding is the influence of the ε4 allele on early mortality after SAH could have introduced a selection bias in their studies [5]. One study on animals has shown mice expressing the apoE4 isoform have greater functional deficit, mortality, cerebral edema, and vasospasm as compared with their apoE3 counterparts during the 3 days after experimental SAH [13]. A study by Leung et al. [14] find the frequency of possession of the APOEε4 allele in patients who have died in 24 h after SAH is up to 37.5%. These studies support this hypothesis that the patients who possess the APOEε4 allele are more susceptible to early death. EBI, which describes the immediate injury to the brain after SAH, is the result of physiological derangements such as increased intracranial pressure and decreased cerebral blood flow that result in global cerebral ischemia, and lead to the acute development of edema, apoptosis, and infarction [3]. The consequence of these events is often death or significant neurological disability. In our study, the time of EEG detection was set within 5 days after SAH, due to the limitation of the patients admitted to our department, and we found that the ε4 allele is a risk factor to brain function aggravation in the early stage of aneurysmal SAH, and it may contribute to early brain injury after SAH.

GOS at 3 or 6 months post-hemorrhage is used as outcome measurement in recently studies on the association of the APOE with outcome after SAH. Though the exact mechanism of APOEε4 still remains unknown, these studies indicate the inhibitory effects of the ε4 allele are exerted later in the recovery process and impact long-term recovery [15]. Different from previous studies, we found the ε4 allele has exerted effects in the acute stage after aneurysmal SAH. As mechanistic pathways of APOEε4 to poor prognosis are identified, further studies should focus on developing therapeutics and interventions to weaken the inhibitory effects of the ε4 allele in the early stage of aneurysmal SAH.

Conflict of interest statement We declare that we have no conflict of interest.

References

1. Ingall T, Asplund K, Mahonen M, Bonita R. A multinational comparison of subarachnoid hemorrhage epidemiology in the WHO MONICA stroke study. Stroke 2000;31:1054–61.
2. Huang J, van Gelder JM. The probability of sudden death from rupture of intracranial aneurysms: a meta-analysis. Neurosurgery 2002;51:1101–7.
3. Aver RE, Zhanf JH. The clinical significance of acute brain injury in subarachnoid hemorrhage and opportunity for intervention. Acta Neurochir Suppl. 2008;105:179–84.
4. Sudlow C, Martinez Gonzalez NA, Kim J, Clark C. Does apolipoprotein E genotype influence the risk of ischemic stroke, intracerebral hemorrhage, or subarachnoid hemorrhage? Systematic review and meta-analyses of 31 studies among 5961 cases and 17,965 controls. Stroke 2006;37:364–70.
5. Dunn LT, Stewart E, Murray GD, Nicoll JA, Teasdale GM. The influence of apolipoprotein E genotype on outcome after spontaneous subarachnoid hemorrhage: a preliminary study. Neurosurgery 2001;48(5):1006–11.
6. Nieuwkamp DJ, Setz LE, Algra A, Linn FH, de Rooij NK, Rinkel GJ. Changes in case fatality of aneurysmal subarachnoid haemorrhage over time, according to age, sex, and region: a meta-analysis. Lancet Neurol. 2009;8:635–42.
7. Jiang Y, Sun X, Xia Y, Tang W, Cao Y, Gu Y. Effect of APOE polymorphisms on early responses to traumatic brain injury. Neurosci Lett. 2006;408:155–8.
8. Bederson JB, Connolly ES Jr, Batjer HH, Dacey RG, Dion JE, Diringer MN et al. Guidelines for the management of aneurysmal subarachnoid hemorrhage: a statement for healthcare professionals from a special writing group of the Stroke Council, American Heart Association. Stroke 2009;40:994–1025.
9. Dreier JP, Ebert N, Priller J, Megow D, Lindauer U, Klee R et al. Products of hemolysis in the subarachnoid space inducing spreading ischemia in the cortex and focal necrosis in rats: a model for delayed ischemic neurological deficits after subarachnoid hemorrhage? J Neurosurg. 2000;93:658–66.
10. Mineharu Y, Inoue K, Inoue S, Yamada S, Nozaki K, Takenaka K et al. Association analysis of common variants of ELN, NOS2A, APOE and ACE2 to intracranial aneurysm. Stroke 2006;37:1189–94.
11. Martinez-Gonzalez N A, Sudlow C L. Effects of apolipoprotein E genotype on outcome after ischaemic stroke, intracerebral haemorrhage and subarachnoid haemorrhage. J Neurol Neurosurg Psychiatry. 2006;77:1329–35.
12. Tang J, Zhao J, Zhao Y, Wang S, Chen B, Zeng W. Apolipoprotein E epsilon4 and the risk of unfavorable outcome after aneurysmal subarachnoid hemorrhage. Surg Neurol. 2003;60:391–7.
13. Gao J, Wang H, Sheng H, Lynch JR, Warner DS, Durham L et al. A novel apoE-derived therapeutic reduces vasospasm and improves outcome in a murine model of subarachnoid hemorrhage. Neurocrit Care. 2006;4:25–31.
14. Leung CH, Poon WS, Yu LM, Wong GK, Ng HK. Apolipoprotein e genotype and outcome in aneurysmal subarachnoid hemorrhage. Stroke 2002;33:548–52.
15. Gallek MJ, Conley YP, Sherwood PR, Horowitz MB, Kassam A, Alexander SA. APOE genotype and functional outcome following aneurysmal subarachnoid hemorrhage. Biol Res Nurs. 2009;10:205–12.

Apoptotic Mechanisms for Neuronal Cells in Early Brain Injury After Subarachnoid Hemorrhage

Yu Hasegawa, Hidenori Suzuki, Takumi Sozen, Orhan Altay, and John H Zhang

Abstract *Objects*: The major causes of death and disability in subarachnoid hemorrhage (SAH) may be early brain injury (EBI) and cerebral vasospasm. Although cerebral vasospasm has been studied and treated by a lot of drugs, the outcome is not improved even if vasospasm is reversed. Based on these data, EBI is considered a primary target for future research, and apoptosis may be involved in EBI after experimental SAH.

Methods: We reviewed the published literature about the relationship between SAH induced EBI and apoptosis in PubMed.

Result: Most available information can be obtained from the endovascular filament perforation animal model. After onset of SAH, intracranial pressure is increased and then cerebral blood flow is reduced. Many factors are involved in the mechanism of apoptotic cell death in EBI after SAH. In the neuronal cells, both intrinsic and extrinsic pathways of apoptosis can occur. Some antiapoptotic drugs were studied and demonstrated a protective effect against EBI after SAH. However, apoptosis in EBI after SAH has been little studied and further studies will provide us more beneficial findings.

Conclusions: The study of apoptosis in EBI after experimental SAH may give us new therapies for SAH.

Keywords Apoptosis · Cerebral blood flow · Early brain injury · Intracranial pressure · Subarachnoid hemorrhage

Y. Hasegawa, H. Suzuki, T. Sozen, and O. Altay
Department of Physiology, Loma Linda University School of Medicine, Loma Linda, CA 92354, USA

J.H. Zhang (✉)
Department of Physiology, Loma Linda University School of Medicine, Loma Linda, CA 92354, USA
Department of Neurosurgery, Loma Linda University School of Medicine, Loma Linda, CA 92354, USA
e-mail: johnzhang3910@yahoo.com

Introduction

Subarachnoid hemorrhage (SAH) is associated with high mortality, and 12.4% of patients die suddenly before reaching the hospital [1]. These deaths were mostly due to the initial hemorrhage, and no effective treatment is available for brain injury after the hemorrhage [2]. For survivors, early brain injury (EBI) caused by the initial hemorrhage and delayed ischemic neurologic deficits due to cerebral vasospasm are major causes of the subsequent morbidity and mortality [3]. Although cerebral vasospasm has been studied and treated by a lot of drugs during the past several decades, the outcome is not improved by the reversal of vasospasm [4]. Based on these data, EBI is considered a primary target for future research and may be also an important factor in preventing symptomatic vasospasm because EBI may predispose the brain to ischemic injury due to vasospasm.

Recent studies showed that apoptosis is involved in the pathogenesis of EBI after experimental SAH or in a clinical setting [5, 6]. Therefore, it is thought that an antiapoptotic treatment can be one of the therapeutic candidates for EBI after SAH. In this review, we focus on the relationship between EBI after SAH and apoptotic mechanism in neuronal cells.

Pathophysiology of Early Brain Injury

Most available information about EBI after SAH comes from endovascular filament perforation animal models, which show a high mortality and acute metabolic changes similar to clinical settings [7–9]. Intracranial pressure (ICP) in this model was increased to 40 mmHg immediately after SAH and then decreased to plateau (15–25 mmHg), whereas cerebral perfusion pressure was decreased to 35–40 mmHg from 70 mmHg, cerebral blood flow (CBF) was 20–30% decreased from the baseline after SAH induction, and then

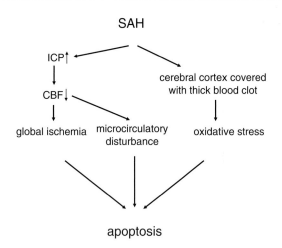

Fig. 1 Apoptotic cascade after subarachnoid hemorrhage. *SAH* subarachnoid hemorrhage, *ICP* intracranial pressure, *CBF* cerebral blood flow

each of the values were gradually recovered [10]. Interestingly, the mortality rate was 100% when CBF was reduced to less than 40% of the baseline for 60 min after SAH, while less CBF reduction resulted in 19% mortality [11].

Many factors, such as global ischemia [12], microcirculatory disturbance [11], and subarachnoid blood toxicity [13] are involved in apoptosis-related mechanisms in EBI after SAH (Fig. 1), whereas distribution of apoptotic cell death is controversial [12, 14]. Although apoptotic cell death detected by TUNEL was seen in both the cortex and subcortex, neuronal cell death in the hippocampus, which is related to global ischemia, might depend on ICP [6, 14]. Blood immediately spreads in the subarachnoid space after SAH, and then the cerebral cortex is covered with a thick blood clot. Hemoglobin is metabolized by neurons and microglia [15], and the released iron induces apoptosis via lipid peroxidation. Thus, subarachnoid blood clotting, which has been linked to cell injury and oxidative stress [13], may cause greater apoptotic cell death in the cerebral cortex compared with the subcortex.

Apoptotic cell death has been reported to occur in neurons [13, 16, 17] and endothelial cells [18–20] in EBI after SAH, and both of them may be correlated with brain edema [21]. In this review, we focus on neuronal cell apoptosis, which consists of the intrinsic and extrinsic pathways [22] (Fig. 2).

Intrinsic Mechanisms of Apoptosis and SAH

Caspase-Dependent Pathway

The intrinsic pathway (mitochondrial pathway), which is mediated by the Bcl-2 family, starts with the increase of outer mitochondrial membrane permeability. The change

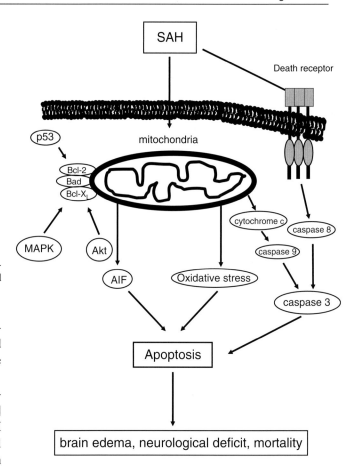

Fig. 2 Schematic representation of the pathway to neuronal apoptosis following subarachnoid hemorrhage. *MAPK* mitogen-activated protein kinase, *AIF* apoptosis-inducing factor

of membrane leads to the leakage of mitochondrial proteins, including cytochrome c. Cytochrome c is translocated from mitochondria to the cytosolic compartment and interacts with apoptotic protease, activating factor-1, forming the apoptosome and leading to caspase-9 activation. Caspase-9, which is an initiator of the cytochrome c-dependent cascade, activates caspase-3, and results in DNA damage [23]. Caspase-3 is well known as one of the effectors of apoptosis, and cleaved caspase-3 was upregulated in the hippocampus and cortex after SAH [12, 24, 25].

It has been reported that some protein kinases might directly interact with mitochondrial proteins in cerebral ischemia, and their role mainly concentrates on the phosphorylation of pro- and anti-apoptotic proteins (Bad, Bax, Bcl-2, Bcl-xL) [26]. Akt (protein kinase B) and mitogen-activated protein kinase (MAPK) were the best studied of them in EBI after SAH. Akt, which is a serine/threonine kinase, is a key antiapoptotic signaling downstream of phosphoinositide 3-kinase (PI3K) in a growth factor mediated signaling cascade. Stimulation of receptor tyrosine kinases or GTP-binding protein-coupled receptors activates Akt via PI3K, and activated Akt modulates many substrates, including Bax, Bad, glycogen synthase kinase-3, apoptosis signal-regulating kinase 1, and caspase-9, which inhibit apoptosis [27]. Moreover, Akt has also been shown to promote cyclic AMP response element-binding protein (CREB) phosphorylation and lead to Bcl-2 induction [28]. Decreased Akt activity is involved in ischemic neuronal cell death, and Akt activation is a principal factor in the prevention of apoptosis via the caspase-dependent pathway in cerebral ischemia [29–31].

Recent studies suggested that Akt might be involved in the mechanism for EBI after SAH, and this conclusion was drawn from using a PI3K inhibitor, which prevented phosphorylation of Akt and increased DNA damage [14, 32]. Moreover, Akt activation by overexpression of copper/zinc-superoxide dismutase (SOD1), which is one of the antioxidant enzymes, attenuated EBI caused by SAH [32]. Timing of Akt phosphorylation after SAH depended on brain regions; Akt were rapidly phosphorylated in the cortex, but it took 24 h to phosphorylate Akt in the hippocampus [14]. Since EBI after SAH may be the most severe in the cortex, it is suggested that Akt phosphorylation depends on the severity of brain injury [14].

The roles of MAPKs are very important in EBI after SAH [33]. MAPK, including extracellular signal-regulated kinase (ERK), c-Jun N-terminal kinase (JNK) and p38, is involved in the survival and apoptotic responses in certain cell death paradigms in cerebral ischemia [34]. These kinases are activated by various stimulants, including vascular endothelial growth factor (VEGF), oxidative stress, and inflammatory cytokines [35–38]. After SAH in a perforation model, these kinases were phosphorylated and induced brain edema, continuous high ICP, and high mortality [33, 39, 40]. Since ERK is activated in response to growth and differentiation factors and might be part of the survival pathway, whether activation of ERK is protective or detrimental to neurons in cerebral ischemia is controversial [41]. In contrast, JNK and p38 are activated in response to inflammatory cytokines and cellular stress, which were highly elevated in the cerebrospinal fluid and in cerebral arteries after SAH [42, 43]. JNK phosphorylates c-Jun, which upregulates apoptotic cascades by inducing expression of the proapoptotic member of Bcl-2 family Hrk/DP5, Bim, and Fas [44, 45]. Phosphorylated JNK and expression of c-Jun were increased after SAH induction and c-Jun mRNA were upregulated in the rat cerebral cortex and hippocampus after SAH [46, 47]. p38 activation by TNF-α and IL-1β was associated with neuronal death, and suppression of p38 activation by Bcl-2 suggested that p38 might be involved in apoptosis [48, 49].

Caspase-Independent Pathway

The caspase-independent component of the intrinsic pathway is carried out by the mitochondria-released apoptosis-inducing factor (AIF), endonuclease G and Bcl-2/adenovirus E1B 19kDa-interacting protein (BNIP3) [50]. AIF, which is the best studied among them, is normally in the mitochondrial intermembrane space and is translocated to the nucleus by some stimulations, inducing large-scale DNA fragmentation and cell apoptosis, which is independent of caspase activity [51]. Nuclear AIF upregulation was reported in cerebral ischemia [52], and the translocation might be triggered by poly (ADP-ribose) polymerase activity [53]. There has not been much reported about AIF expression in EBI after SAH and it is not clear which compartment of AIF expression increases [24].

Oxidative Stress and Early Brain Injury

It is important to hold the balance between reactive oxygen species (ROS) and antioxidants, which control oxidative stress. ROS such as superoxide anion (O^-_2), hydrogen peroxide (H_2O_2), and hydroxyl radical (OH^-) are generated at low levels and play important roles in signaling pathways [54]. Under normal conditions, they are regulated by endogenous antioxidants including SOD, glutathione peroxidase, glutathione, and catalase [55]. Overproduction of ROS and/or inactivation of antioxidants cause tissue injury from oxidative damage [54]. Oxidative stress can play important roles in the pathogenesis of EBI after SAH [56]. Mitochondria disruption, the production of hydroxyl radicals from extravasated hemoglobin, and disruption of the intrinsic antioxidant systems have all been reported in either experimental or human SAH [56–59]. O_2^- production was observed 1 h after SAH, and overexpression of SOD1 inhibited the production and reduced apoptotic cell injury after SAH [32]. The reduction in oxidative stress by SOD1 overexpression attenuated EBI after SAH via activation of Akt [32].

DNA Damage

p53 is a tumor suppressor gene involved in the regulation of apoptosis [60]. Responding to cell damage, p53 upregulates proapoptotic molecules including Bax, p53-upregulated modulator of apoptosis, and Bid, and downregulates antiapoptotic molecules Bcl-2 and Survivin [60]. p53 is upregulated after an

Table 1 Neuronal apoptosis related studies in early brain injury after SAH

Method/animal	Treatment	Neuronal apoptotic pathway	NS	Outcome	References
EP, rat	PP1	p-Erk, VEGF		BE↓	[33]
EP, rat	Z-VAD-FMK	caspase-3	+	BE↓	[12]
EP, rat	Hyperbaric oxygen	VEGF, BNIP3, TUNEL	+	BS↓, NS↑, MT↓	[69]
EP, rat	Hyperbaric oxygen	gp91^{phox}, NADPH oxidase, MDA	+	NS↑	[70]
EP, rat	Pifithrin	p53, cyto c, AIF, TUNEL, caspase-3, -8	+	BE↓, NS↑ MT↓	[62]
EP, rat	SOD1 overexpression	p-Akt, hydroethidine, Cell death assey		MT↓	[32]
EP, rat	SP600125	caspase-3	+	BE↓, NS↑	[40]
EP, rat	Tetramethylpyrazine	TUNEL, caspase-3	+	BE↓, NS↑	[63]
EP, rat	Atorvastatin	TUNEL, caspase-3, -8	+	BE↓, NS↑, MT↓	[24]
EP, rat	Argatroban	Cell death assey	+	BE↓, NS↑	[71]
BSI, rat	Meratonin	MPO, MDA, glutathione	+	BE↓, NS↑	[72]
BSI, rat	N-acetylcysteine	CuZn-SOD, GSH-Px, MDA	+	BE↓, NS↑	[73]
EP, mouse	Ac-YVAD-CMK	p-JNK	+	BE↓, NS↑	[39]
EP, rat	Hypothermia	–	+	NS↑, Weight↑	[10]

EP endovascular perforation, *BSI* blood single injection, *p-ERK* phosphorylated extracellular signal-related kinase, *VEGF* vascular endothelial growth factor, *BNIP3* BCL2/adenovirus E1B 19kDa-interacting protein 3, *TUNEL* terminal deoxynucleotidyl transferase-mediated uridine 5′-triphosphate-biotin nick end-labeling, *NADPH* nicotinamide adenine dinucleotide phosphate, *MDA* malondialdehyde, *cyto c* cytochrome c, *p-Akt* phosphorylated Akt, *MPO* myeloperoxidase, *CuZu-SOD* copper/zinc-superoxide dismutase, *GSH-Px* glutathione peroxidase, *p-JNK* phosphorylated c-Jun N-terminal kinase, *NS* neurological score, *BE* brain edema, *MT* mortality, *BS* brain swelling

ischemia insult and induces mitochondrial damage and activation of caspases [61]. It was reported that in SAH, p53 is one of the key factors in neuronal cell death. p53 was upregulated both at 24 and 72 h after SAH, and p53 inhibitor decreased brain edema and neuronal cell death [24, 62, 63].

Extrinsic Pathway of Apoptosis

The death receptors, which are located on the cell surface, are involved in the extrinsic apoptosis pathway [31]. The receptor ligands expression, including Fas and tumor necrosis factor (TNF), are upregulated after cerebral ischemia [64, 65]. The death receptors can activate caspase-8 or -10, which then directly activate caspase-3 or cause Bid/Bax activation, inducing cytochrome c release [66]. Moreover, forkhead transcriptional factors were activated after cerebral ischemia and then expression of Fas ligand increased, resulting in neuronal cell death [67]. However, little is known regarding the relationship between EBI and death receptors or their ligands, whereas TNF-α were upregulated after SAH [68].

Treatments

Studies of neuronal apoptosis are summarized in Table 1. For evaluating neuronal apoptosis in EBI after SAH, neurological examination should be needed to examine the outcome of neuronal cell injury. These molecular apoptotic pathways in neurons may induce brain edema, neurological deficit, and higher mortality. Previous studies showed that apoptotic related pathway modulation by treatment could improve the outcome in EBI after SAH.

Conclusion

A lot of studies have demonstrated the apoptosis mechanism in cerebral ischemia, whereas relatively few have studied the relationship between apoptosis and SAH, especially in EBI. It would be helpful for us to study the relationship between SAH and another apoptotic mechanism, including autophagy and endoplasmic reticulum stress, which may lead to novel therapies in EBI. Studies regarding EBI after SAH are limited, and further studies are needed for clarifying the exact mechanism. For example, MAPKs, including ERK, JNK, and p38, were reported to induce apoptosis in the brain and cerebral artery after SAH [33], whereas it has reported that ERK phosphorylation induced a beneficial effect on cerebral vasospasm [74]. It is suggested that elevated ERK phosphorylation blocks apoptosis by enhancing the antiapoptotic protein Bcl-2 via CREB activation in cerebral ischemia [41]. The opposite effects may depend on the localization in the brain including neurons, glia, and endothelial cells.

In conclusion, apoptosis may play an important role in EBI after SAH. Further studies regarding apoptosis may lead to the development of new therapies and the improvement of outcome of SAH patients.

Acknowledgments This study was partially supported by grants (NS053407) from the National Institutes of Health to J.H.Z.

Conflict of interest statement We declare that we have no conflict of interest.

References

1. Huang J, van Gelder JM. The probability of sudden death from rupture of intracranial aneurysms: a meta-analysis. Neurosurgery 2002;51:1101–5.
2. O'Hare TH. Subarachnoid hemorrhage: a review. J Emerg Med. 1987;5:135–4
3. Tseng MY, Czosnyka M, Richards H, Pickard JD, Kirkpatrick PJ. Effects of acute treatment with pravastatin on cerebral vasospasm, autoregulation, and delayed ischemic deficits after aneurysmal subarachnoid hemorrhage: a phase II randomized placebo-controlled trial. Stroke 2005;36:1627–32.
4. Schievink WI, Riedinger M, Jhutty TK, Simon P. Racial disparities in subarachnoid hemorrhage mortality: Los Angeles County, California, 1985–1998. Neuroepidemiology 2004;23:299–305.
5. Nau R, Haase S, Bunkowski S, Brück W. Neuronal apoptosis in the dentate gyrus in humans with subarachnoid hemorrhage and cerebral hypoxia. Brain Pathol. 2002;12:329–36.
6. Prunell GF, Mathiesen T, Diemer NH, Svendgaard NA. Experimental subarachnoid hemorrhage: subarachnoid blood volume, mortality rate, neuronal death, cerebral blood flow, and perfusion pressure in three different rat models. Neurosurgery 2003;52:165–75.
7. Bederson JB, Germano IM, Guarino L. Cortical blood flow and cerebral perfusion pressure in a new noncraniotomy model of subarachnoid hemorrhage in the rat. Stroke 1995;26:1086–91.
8. Schwartz AY, Masago A, Sehba FA, Bederson JB. Experimental models of subarachnoid hemorrhage in the rat: a refinement of the endovascular filament model. J Neurosci Methods. 2000;96:161–7.
9. Veelken JA, Laing RJ, Jakubowski J. The Sheffield model of subarachnoid hemorrhage in rats. Stroke 1995;26:1279–83
10. Török E, Klopotowski M, Trabold R, Thal SC, Plesnila N, Schöller K. Mild hypothermia (33 degrees C) reduces intracranial hypertension and improves functional outcome after subarachnoid hemorrhage in rats. Neurosurgery 2009;65:352–9.
11. Bederson JB, Levy AL, Ding WH, Kahn R, DiPerna CA, Jenkins AL III et al. Acute vasoconstriction after subarachnoid hemorrhage. Neurosurgery 1998;42:352–62.
12. Park S, Yamaguchi M, Zhou C, Calvert JW, Tang J, Zhang JH. Neurovascular protection reduces early brain injury after subarachnoid hemorrhage. Stroke 2004;35:2412–7.
13. Matz PG, Copin JC, Chan PH. Cell death after exposure to subarachnoid hemolysate correlates inversely with expression of CuZn-superoxide dismutase. Stroke 2000;31:2450–9.
14. Endo H, Nito C, Kamada H, Yu F, Chan PH. Akt/GSK3beta survival signaling is involved in acute brain injury after subarachnoid hemorrhage in rats. Stroke 2006;37:2140–6.
15. Xi G, Keep RF, Hoff JT. Erythrocytes and delayed brain edema formation following intracerebral hemorrhage in rats. J Neurosurg. 1998;89:991–6.
16. Matz PG, Fujimura M, Chan PH. Subarachnoid hemolysate produces DNA fragmentation in a pattern similar to apoptosis in mouse brain. Brain Res. 2000;858:312–9.
17. Matz PG, Fujimura M, Lewen A, Morita-Fujimura Y, Chan PH. Increased cytochrome c-mediated DNA fragmentation and cell death in manganese-superoxide dismutase-deficient mice after exposure to subarachnoid hemolysate. Stroke 2001;32:506–15.
18. Kimura H, Gules I, Meguro T, Zhang JH. Cytotoxicity of cytokines in cerebral microvascular endothelial cell. Brain Res. 2003; 990:148–56.
19. Meguro T, Klett CP, Chen B, Parent AD, Zhang JH. Role of calcium channels in oxyhemoglobin-induced apoptosis in endothelial cells. J Neurosurg. 2000;93:640–6.
20. Ogihara K, Zubkov AY, Bernanke DH, Lewis AI, Parent AD, Zhang JH. Oxyhemoglobin-induced apoptosis in cultured endothelial cells. J Neurosurg. 1999;91:459–65.
21. Bazán NG, Rodríguez de Turco EB. Membrane lipids in the pathogenesis of brain edema: phospholipids and arachidonic acid, the earliest membrane components changed at the onset of ischemia. Adv Neurol. 1980;28:197–205.
22. Gules I, Satoh M, Nanda A, Zhang JH. Apoptosis, blood-brain barrier, and subarachnoid hemorrhage. Acta Neurochir Suppl. 2003;86:483–7.
23. Chan PH. Mitochondria and neuronal death/survival signaling pathways in cerebral ischemia. Neurochem Res. 2004;29:1943–9.
24. Cheng G, Wei L, Zhi-Dan S, Shi-Guang Z, Xiang-Zhen L. Atorvastatin ameliorates cerebral vasospasm and early brain injury after subarachnoid hemorrhage and inhibits caspase-dependent apoptosis pathway. BMC Neurosci. 2009; doi:10,1186/14712202107.
25. Yan J, Chen C, Hu Q, Yang X, Lei J, Yang L et al., The role of p53 in brain edema after 24 h of experimental subarachnoid hemorrhage in a rat model. Exp Neurol. 2008;214:37–46.
26. Zhang F, Yin W, Chen J. Apoptosis in cerebral ischemia: executional and regulatory signaling mechanisms. Neurol Res. 2004; 26:835–45.
27. Hemmings BA. Akt signaling: linking membrane events to life and death decisions. Science 1997;275:628–30.
28. Pugazhenthi S, Nesterova A, Sable C, Heidenreich KA, Boxer LM, Heasley LE et al. Akt/protein kinase B up-regulates Bcl-2 expression through cAMP-response element-binding protein. J Biol Chem. 2000;275:10761–6.
29. Hasegawa Y, Hamada J, Morioka M, Yano S, Kawano T, Kai Y et al., Neuroprotective effect of postischemic administration of sodium orthovanadate in rats with transient middle cerebral artery occlusion. J Cereb Blood Flow Metab. 2003;23:1040–51.
30. Hasegawa Y, Morioka M, Hasegawa S, Matsumoto J, Kawano T, Kai Y et al. Therapeutic time window and dose dependence of neuroprotective effects of sodium orthovanadate following transient middle cerebral artery occlusion in rats. J Pharmacol Exp Ther. 2006;317:875–81.
31. Shioda N, Ishigami T, Han F, Moriguchi S, Shibuya M, Iwabuchi Y et al. Activation of phosphatidylinositol 3-kinase/protein kinase B pathway by a vanadyl compound mediates its neuroprotective effect in mouse brain ischemia. Neuroscience 2007;148:221–9.
32. Endo H, Nito C, Kamada H, Yu F, Chan PH. Reduction in oxidative stress by superoxide dismutase overexpression attenuates acute brain injury after subarachnoid hemorrhage via activation of Akt/glycogen synthase kinase-3beta survival signaling. J Cereb Blood Flow Metab. 2007;27:975–82.
33. Kusaka G, Ishikawa M, Nanda A, Granger DN, Zhang JH. Signaling pathways for early brain injury after subarachnoid hemorrhage. J Cereb Blood Flow Metab. 2004;24:916–25.
34. Irving EA, Bamford M. Role of mitogen- and stress-activated kinases in ischemic injury. J Cereb Blood Flow Metab. 2002; 22:631–47.
35. Chakraborti S, Chakraborti T. Oxidant-mediated activation of mitogen-activated protein kinases and nuclear transcription factors in the cardiovascular system: a brief overview. Cell Signal. 1988;10:675–83.
36. Chow J, Ogunshola O, Fan SY, Li Y, Ment LR, Madri JA. Astrocyte-derived VEGF mediates survival and tube stabilization of hypoxic brain microvascular endothelial cells in vitro. Brain Res Dev Brain Res. 2001;130:123–32.
37. Parker LC, Luheshi GN, Rothwell NJ, Pinteaux E. IL-1 beta signalling in glial cells in wildtype and IL-1RI deficient mice. Br J Pharmacol. 2002;136:312–20.

38. Sugden PH, Clerk A. "Stress-responsive" mitogen-activated protein kinases (c-Jun N-terminal kinases and p38 mitogen-activated protein kinases) in the myocardium. Circ Res. 1998;83:345–52.
39. Sozen T, Tsuchiyama R, Hasegawa Y, Suzuki H, Jadhav V, Nishizawa S et al., Role of interleukin-1beta in early brain injury after subarachnoid hemorrhage in mice. Stroke 2009;40:2519–25.
40. Yatsushige H, Ostrowski RP, Tsubokawa T, Colohan A, Zhang JH. Role of c-Jun N-terminal kinase in early brain injury after subarachnoid hemorrhage. J Neurosci Res. 2007;85:1436–48.
41. Sawe N, Steinberg G, Zhao H. Dual roles of the MAPK/ERK1/2 cell signaling pathway after stroke. J Neurosci Res. 2008;86:1659–69.
42. Fassbender K, Hodapp B, Rossol S, Bertsch T, Schmeck J, Schütt S et al., Inflammatory cytokines in subarachnoid haemorrhage: association with abnormal blood flow velocities in basal cerebral arteries. J Neurol Neurosurg Psychiatry. 2001;70:534–7.
43. Hirashima Y, Nakamura S, Endo S, Kuwayama N, Naruse Y, Takaku A. Elevation of platelet activating factor, inflammatory cytokines, and coagulation factors in the internal jugular vein of patients with subarachnoid hemorrhage. Neurochem Res. 1997;22:1249–55.
44. Kuan CY, Whitmarsh AJ, Yang DD, Liao G, Schloemer AJ, Dong C et al., A critical role of neural-specific JNK3 for ischemic apoptosis. Proc Natl Acad Sci USA. 2003;100:15184–9.
45. Yuan J, Yankner BA. Apoptosis in the nervous system. Nature 2000;407:802–9.
46. Harada S, Kamiya K, Masago A, Iwata A, Yamada K. Subarachnoid hemorrhage induces c-fos, c-jun and hsp70 mRNA expression in rat brain. Neuroreport 1997;8:3399–404.
47. Kawamura Y, Yamada K, Masago A, Katano H, Matsumoto T, Mase M. Hypothermia modulates induction of hsp70 and c-jun mRNA in the rat brain after subarachnoid hemorrhage. J Neurotrauma. 2000;17:243–50.
48. Cheng A, Chan SL, Milhavet O, Wang S, Mattson MP. p38 MAP kinase mediates nitric oxide-induced apoptosis of neural progenitor cells. J Biol Chem. 2001;276:43320–7.
49. Nito C, Kamada H, Endo H, Niizuma K, Myer DJ, Chan PH. Role of the p38 mitogen-activated protein kinase/cytosolic phospholipase A2 signaling pathway in blood-brain barrier disruption after focal cerebral ischemia and reperfusion. J Cereb Blood Flow Metab. 2008;28:1686–96.
50. Elmore S. Apoptosis: a review of programmed cell death. Toxicol Pathol. 2007;35:495–516.
51. Cho BB, Toledo-Pereyra LH. Caspase-independent programmed cell death following ischemic stroke. J Invest Surg. 2008;21:141–7.
52. Li X, Nemoto M, Xu Z, Yu SW, Shimoji M, Andrabi SA, et al. Influence of duration of focal cerebral ischemia and neuronal nitric oxide synthase on translocation of apoptosis-inducing factor to the nucleus. Neuroscience 2007;144:56–65.
53. Yu SW, Wang H, Poitras MF, Coombs C, Bowers WJ, Federoff HJ et al., Mediation of poly(ADP-ribose) polymerase-1-dependent cell death by apoptosis-inducing factor. Science 2002;297:200–1.
54. Loh KP, Huang SH, De Silva R, Tan BK, Zhu YZ. Oxidative stress: apoptosis in neuronal injury. Curr Alzheimer Res. 2006;3:327–37.
55. Sugawara T, Chan PH. Reactive oxygen radicals and pathogenesis of neuronal death after cerebral ischemia. Antioxid Redox Signal. 2003;5:597–607.
56. Ayer RE, Zhang JH. Oxidative stress in subarachnoid haemorrhage: significance in acute brain injury and vasospasm. Acta Neurochir Suppl. 2008;104:33–41.
57. Asano T. Oxyhemoglobin as the principal cause of cerebral vasospasm: a holistic view of its actions. Crit Rev Neurosurg. 1999;9:303–18.
58. Gaetani P, Lombardi D. Brain damage following subarachnoid hemorrhage: the imbalance between anti-oxidant systems and lipid peroxidative processes. J Neurosurg Sci. 1992;36:1–10.
59. Kaynar MY, Tanriverdi T, Kemerdere R, Atukeren P, Gumustas K. Cerebrospinal fluid superoxide dismutase and serum malondialdehyde levels in patients with aneurysmal subarachnoid hemorrhage: preliminary results. Neurol Res. 2005;27:562–7.
60. Fridman JS, Lowe SW. Control of apoptosis by p53. Oncogene 2003;22:9030–40.
61. Culmsee C, Mattson MP. p53 in neuronal apoptosis. Biochem Biophys Res Commun. 2005;331:761–77.
62. Cahill J, Calvert JW, Marcantonio S, Zhang JH. p53 may play an orchestrating role in apoptotic cell death after experimental subarachnoid hemorrhage. Neurosurgery 2007;60:531–45
63. Gao C, Liu X, Liu W, Shi H, Zhao Z, Chen H et al., Anti-apoptotic and neuroprotective effects of Tetramethylpyrazine following subarachnoid hemorrhage in rats. Auton Neurosci. 2008;141:22–30.
64. Martin-Villalba A, Herr I, Jeremias I, Hahne M, Brandt R, Vogel J et al. CD95 ligand (Fas-L/APO-1L) and tumor necrosis factor-related apoptosis-inducing ligand mediate ischemia-induced apoptosis in neurons. J Neurosci. 1999;19:3809–17.
65. Rosenbaum DM, Gupta G, D'Amore J, Singh M, Weidenheim K, Zhang H et al., Fas (CD95/APO-1) plays a role in the pathophysiology of focal cerebral ischemia. J Neurosci Res. 2000;61: 686–92.
66. Yuan J, Horvitz HR. A first insight into the molecular mechanisms of apoptosis. Cell 2004;116(Suppl):53–6
67. Kawano T, Morioka M, Yano S, Hamada J, Ushio Y, Miyamoto E et al. Decreased akt activity is associated with activation of forkhead transcription factor after transient forebrain ischemia in gerbil hippocampus. J Cereb Blood Flow Metab. 2002;22:926–34.
68. Ma CX, Yin WN, Cai BW, He M, Wu J, Wang JY, et al. Activation of TLR4/NF-kappaB signaling pathway in early brain injury after subarachnoid hemorrhage. Neurol Res. doi:10,1179/016164109x12445616596283.
69. Ostrowski RP, Colohan AR, Zhang JH. Mechanisms of hyperbaric oxygen-induced neuroprotection in a rat model of subarachnoid hemorrhage. J Cereb Blood Flow Metab. 2005;25:554–71.
70. Ostrowski RP, Tang J, Zhang JH. Hyperbaric oxygen suppresses NADPH oxidase in a rat subarachnoid hemorrhage model. Stroke 2006;37:1314–8.
71. Sugawara T, Jadhav V, Ayer R, Chen W, Suzuki H, Zhang JH. Thrombin inhibition by argatroban ameliorates early brain injury and improves neurological outcomes after experimental subarachnoid hemorrhage in rats. Stroke 2009;40:1530–2.
72. Ersahin M, Toklu HZ, Cetinel S, Yüksel M, Yeğen BC, Sener G. Melatonin reduces experimental subarachnoid hemorrhage-induced oxidative brain damage and neurological symptoms. J Pineal Res. 2009;46:324–32.
73. Lu H, Zhang DM, Chen HL, Lin YX, Hang CH, Yin HX, et al. N-acetylcysteine suppresses oxidative stress in experimental rats with subarachnoid hemorrhage. J Clin Neurosci. 2009;16:684–8.
74. Lin CL, Dumont AS, Tsai YJ, Huang JH, Chang KP, Kwan AL, et al. 17beta-estradiol activates adenosine A(2a) receptor after subarachnoid hemorrhage. J Surg Res. doi:10,3171/20093JNS081660.

Early Micro Vascular Changes After Subarachnoid Hemorrhage

Fatima A. Sehba and Victor Friedrich

Abstract During the last decade much effort has been invested in understanding the events that occur early after SAH. It is now widely accepted that these early events not only participate in the early ischemic injury but also set the stage for the pathogenesis of delayed vasospasm. That early cerebral ischemia occurs after SAH is documented in both experimental SAH and in human autopsy studies; however, angiographic evidence for vasoconstriction early after SAH is lacking and the source of early ischemic injury is therefore unclear. Recently, the cerebral microvasculature has been identified as an early target of SAH. Changes in the anatomical structure of cerebral microvessels, sufficient to cause functional deficits, are found early after experimental SAH. These changes may explain cerebral ischemia in human in the absence of angiographic evidence of large vessel vasoconstriction. This paper summarizes known alterations in cerebral microvasculature during the first 48 h after SAH.

Keywords Early brain injury · Microvascular changes · Vasospasm

Introduction

Early events after Subarachnoid hemorrhage (SAH) may not only contribute to ischemic injury at the time of the initial hemorrhage, but also set the stage for the secondary events such as the cerebral vasospasm which occurs 3–7 days later [1]. Early diagnosis and treatment are critical for potential reduction of the mortality after SAH. However, the mechanisms of brain injury during this period remain poorly understood, and few if any specific treatments for them exist.

F.A. Sehba (✉) and V. Friedrich
Departments of Neurosurgery and of Neuroscience, Mount Sinai School of Medicine, New York, NY 10029, USA
e-mail: fatima.sehba@mssm.edu

The events at SAH include elevated Intracranial Pressure (ICP), reduced Cerebral Blood Flow (CBF) and impaired CBF autoregulation [2–6]. *Animal* studies demonstrate that CBF reduction after SAH is accompanied by constriction of cerebral blood vessels ranging from 300 to 500 m in diameter [3, 7]. *In humans*, although acute cerebral ischemia occurs [8–10], cerebral angiography shows little evidence of acute arterial spasm [11, 12], and the source of the early ischemic injury is therefore unclear. However, most investigations of vascular changes after SAH have been directed at the major cerebral vessels [13–15] and changes in small vessels, which might underlie cerebral ischemia in human in the absence of angiographic evidence of vasoconstriction, have been little studied.

More recently, awareness that cerebral microvessels (vessels that are ≤100 μm) may be involved in the pathophysiology of early SAH has increased. More and more investigators are studying the effects of SAH on microvessels vessels in experimental SAH models [16–21] and in human SAH [15, 22, 23]. This paper summarizes their findings. We begin with a brief overview of anatomy of cerebral microvessels emphasizing the difference between cerebral and peripheral microvessels.

Cerebral Microvasculature; Anatomical Architecture

What makes cerebral microvasculature different from the peripheral microvasculature is that it not only serves as a means for blood supply to the brain structures, but is in constant communication with glia and neurons. A cerebral microvessel (≤20 μm) is mainly made up of an endothelial cell layer that is surrounded by the matrix containing basal lamina that in turn is encased by astrocyte end-feets. Together endothelium, basal lamina and astrocyte provide a permeability barrier that limits transmigration of blood elements into the brain parenchyma maintaining the integrity of the vessel [24]. In addition, endothelium also exerts a local control on the vascular tone via secretion and of an array of agents. Basal lamina separates endothelium from circumferential astrocyte end-feet. Basal lamina is a constituent of extracellular matrix (ECM) and is composed of type IV collagen and laminin polymer connected by enactin [25]. Collagen IV constitutes up to 90% of the total protein of the basal lamina and forms a fibrous matrix that confers structural integrity to the vessel wall [26, 27]. Hence, basal lamina plays an important role in maintaining BBB impermeability by regulating tight junctions and provides structural support to the vasculature. The loss of basal lamina is postulated to be the primary cause of many cerebrovascular disorders [28–30].

Cerebral microvessels are sensitive to change in cerebral environment. Hence, occlusive cerebral ischemia elicits a multitude of rapid responses from microvessels. These include breakdown of the primary endothelial cell permeability barrier, expression of endothelial cell-leukocyte adhesion receptors, loss of integrin receptors from endothelial cells and astrocyte and expression of matrix-degrading proteases, resulting in loss of basal lamina matrix components and in increased vascular permeability (for review see [31]).

Alterations in cerebral microvasculature after SAH are studied. It appears that microvascular changes after SAH occur in a more rapidly and dynamic fashion as compared to occlusive stroke. Here, we summarize the changes in cerebral microvessels during the first 48 h after SAH.

Microvascular Injury After SAH

Endothelium

A functional endothelium acts as a barrier for the transvascular migration of blood elements and contributes to the regulation of blood flow via release of vasoactive agents such as Nitric oxide (NO). NO, the major regulator of cerebral blood flow in vessels is synthesized by endothelial nitric oxide synthase (eNOS) which as the name indicates is located on vascular endothelium. A constant supply of NO is needed at the vascular bed to maintain cerebral blood flow. Studies demonstrate that endothelium dependent vasodilation is impaired and vascular response to contractile agents is increased in the early hours after SAH [17, 32–34]. This early change in endothelial response is observed in animal [17, 32–34] as well as in human [32, 35]. In contrast, the capacity of cerebral microvessels to dilate in response to compounds that do not require a functional endothelium remains intact after SAH [17, 18].

A dysfunction of endothelium function is hypothesized to underlie impaired endothelium dependent vasodilation after SAH [17]. Endothelial dysfunction will disrupt NO synthesis and supply promoting unopposed constriction [17]. Decrease in cerebral NO level and microvascular constriction both are found after SAH [18, 36]. Other proposed mechanisms of cerebral NO reduction after SAH are scavenging by hemoglobin or binding with oxygen radicals released oxidative damage to vessel wall or by macrophages during inflammation [36–38].

The dysfunction of endothelium after SAH may result from an injury [17, 39]. We have found interruptions in immunostaining of endothelial specific antigens after SAH. More specifically, staining of endothelial barrier antigen (EBA) and rat endothelial cell antigen-1 (RECA-1) appears interrupted and fragmented within 10 min after SAH and is on its way to recovery 24 h later [18]. Moreover, in many vascular segments endothelium lining appear to be detached from basal lamina layer (Sehba et al. unpublished data). Clower et al. have previously reported corrugation and detachment of endothelial lining of large cerebral vessels in a similar time frame after SAH [39]. Yan et al. examined microvasculature via electron microscope at 24 h after SAH and found broken tight junctions between endothelial cells and widening inter-endothelial spaces [40].

Endothelium injury after SAH might occur via a number of mechanisms. These include; inflammation, oxidative damage, and platelet activation, prolonged vasoconstriction and endothelial cell death [41–44]. Inflammation, observed as expression and activation of various constituents of the inflammatory response, including adhesion molecules, cytokines, and leukocytes, occurs early after SAH [45]. An increase in endothelial expression and CSF levels of adhesion molecules (ICAM-1, VCAM-1 and E-selectin), which contribute to inflammation by promoting adhesion of neutrophils, monocytes, and lymphocytes to the endothelial membrane, is found 24 h after SAH [46–49] and is correlated with development of delayed vasospasm [49, 50]. In humans, an increase in CSF levels of adhesion molecules is observed during the first 72 h after SAH [48]. Activated platelets and leukocytes can also contribute to the endothelial injury after SAH. Activated platelets can disrupt and denude endothelium to make these sites attractive to passing emboli and promote further aggregation [51, 52].

Moreover, platelet activation factor, which promotes platelet activation, accelerates transendothelial migration or diapedesis of leukocytes forming micro lesions in the endothelium [53]. Endothelial injury may also involve cell death. Studies show that apoptotic cell death pathway is active in endothelial cells of large cerebral vessels 24 h after SAH [40, 42, 44, 54, 55]. We have found caspase-3 activation in cerebral microvessels within first 3 h after SAH (Sehba et al. unpublished observation).

Basal Lamina Degradation

Degradation of basal lamina is associated with alterations in vascular tone, increased intravascular pressure and increased microvascular permeability, allowing the extravasation of fluid (edema) and fibrin and erythrocytes as hemorrhage [56]. Basal lamina degradation is noted during occlusive ischemic brain injuries [29, 56–59]. The precise mechanism of dissolution of vascular matrix in cerebral ischemia is not known, but matrix metalloproteinases (MMPs), plasminogen activators (PAs), urokinase (uPA) and serine proteases have been implicated [56, 60]. In brain, MMPs and serine proteases are secreted by microglia, astrocytes and endothelial cells [58]. Among MMPs, gelatinase A (MMP-2) and gelatinase B (MMP-9) can digest the vascular BL [61]. Substrates of MMP-2 and 9 include gelatin, type IV collagen, fibronectin, and elastin [62, 63].

Basal lamina degradation starts early after SAH [19, 55, 64, 65]. Studies demonstrate that the collagen IV loss begins within minutes and is still present at 24 h after SAH [19, 55, 65]. Similarly, a significant reduction in laminin is also found at 24 h after SAH [64]. Degradation of basal lamina after SAH may represent initiation of compensatory, clinically inefficient, angiogenesis in response to hypoxia [66]. In this regards it is important to note that an increase in angiogenic factors (vascular endothelial growth factor (VEGF), soluble tyrosine-kinase receptors sFlt-1and sTie-2 occurs in animal cerebral vessels and in human CSF within the first 24–48 h after SAH [67–69]. Most experimental and human studies associate post SAH increase in VEGF with poor outcome [55, 68–70], however, there are few exceptions [71]. Sun and colleagues report that increased expression of VEGF upon ginko balboa treatment exerts protective effects on secondary cerebral ischemic injury after SAH [71]. Others find that direct or indirect inhibition of inhibition of VEGF expression to be beneficial against ischemic brain injury after SAH [55, 68]. In human, increased VEGF is associated with microvascular injury and in the pathogenesis of delayed vasospasm [69, 70].

Destruction of collagen IV after SAH involves collagenase activity upregulated in microvessels early after SAH [18, 19]. MMP-9 is identified as the major collagenase involved in collagen IV destruction after SAH [19, 40, 64]. As vascular endothelium secretes MMP-9 in response to an injury, the injured endothelium will not only increase luminal level of MMP-9 but also provide it an easy access to collagen IV. Hence, preventing endothelial injury by reducing the extent of ischemia or endothelial cell death after SAH reduces collagen IV destruction after SAH [18, 40, 55]. In addition to vascular endothelium, platelets also represent a rich source of intravascular MMP-9. Platelets express and secrete MMP-2 and 9 upon activation [62, 63, 72]. We have recently found that collagenase activity colocalizes with intraluminal platelet aggregates in microvessels (Sehba et al. unpublished data).

The direct pathological consequence of collagen IV denudation on cerebral microvasculature would be destabilization, increase vascular permeability and edema [56]. Indeed, a marked increase in permeability of cerebral microvessels is documented after SAH [65, 73–75]. Doczi at al., documented increased vascular permeability 3 h after SAH [73]. Recently we have found that microvascular permeability changes are present at 10 min and remain for at least the first 24 h after SAH (Sehba et al. unpublished data). The temporal similarity between endothelium and basal lamina injury and intraluminal platelet aggregation (see below) may imply a causal effect relationship.

Platelet Aggregation

Coagulation disorders, fibrinolysis and homeostatic abnormalities occur early after SAH and are associated with poor early outcome and delayed ischemic deficits [76–79]. Within 5 min after experimental SAH jugular venous blood platelet count decreases and morphological changes associated with activation appear in platelets, indicating sequestration and aggregation in the brain [80]. In major cerebral arteries platelet aggregates appear as early as 2 h after experimental SAH and may last for several weeks [81, 82]. In contrast, in cerebral microvasculature platelet aggregate are found as early as 10 min after experimental SAH and increase with time [20]. The presence of microclots in small arteries is also reported in autopsy specimen of humans who died within 2 days after SAH and is related to intensity of bleed and poor outcome [83].

What promotes massive platelet activation and platelet aggregation after SAH is not clear. Intraluminal aggregation of platelets is a physiological response to several types of acute cerebrovascular injuries [84–86]. After SAH, the initial activation of platelet would be expected at the site of the aneurysm rupture, where coagulation, which stops further bleeding, is normally completed in 1–3 min [87]. The massive appearance of intra-vascular platelet aggregates which follows throughout the brain might be influenced by a number of factors including; the pro-coagulants and vasoconstrictive agents released from the degranulating platelets [41, 88] and the injured endothelium [89], expression of platelet attracting integrin receptors on the endothelium [16], or/and alteration in NO/NOS pathway and cerebral NO level, known to occur early after SAH [90]. Under normal physiology NO, produced either by endothelial cells or by platelets themselves, inhibits platelet adhesion, aggregation, recruitment, and formation of leukocyte-platelet aggregates. Platelets are capable of synthesizing NO in the amount that at rest is comparable to that produced by endothelial cells [91]. Platelet-synthesized NO contributes significantly to the maintenance of vascular tone and blood flow [91]. Platelet NO synthesis is stimulated upon their activation and down regulates further aggregation [92, 93]. Thus, modulation of platelet aggregation by NO is a negative feedback mechanism. After SAH, a decrease in cerebral NO occurs and at the vascular level may involve impaired NO synthesis or its scavenging by free radicals produced during oxidative damage of endothelium or released by macrophages which infiltrate cerebral vessels (see above). Decreased NO at the vascular level will remove this feedback inhibition of platelet aggregation, thus stimulating platelet aggregation.

In microvessels, early platelet aggregation is thought to contribute to the "no-reflow" phenomenon [94], the absence of vascular filling after a period of global cerebral ischemia [95]. Platelets aggregates could in addition alter vessel function in a number of ways. Platelet aggregates can (1) Obstruct the vessel lumen mechanically. (2) Denude microvascular endothelium lining promoting further aggregation [51, 52]. (3) Release vasoconstrictive agents to cause constriction (serotonin, ADP, PDGF etc.) [96–99]. (4) Release enzymes that cause vessel wall injury by degrading important proteins of basal lamina (such as matrix metalloproteinases-2 and 9 (MMP-2 and 9; major collagenases, see below) [19, 20, 100–102].

We have recently found (Sehba at el. unpublished data) that perfusion deficits in microvessels after SAH co localize with luminal platelet aggregates. In addition, we have found destruction of endothelium and basal lamina and increased permeability allowing escape of tracer and luminal platelet aggregates into the brain parenchyma. Active collagenases co localized with the luminal platelet aggregates at the site of vessel injury. The entry of platelet aggregates into the brain parenchyma is not noted in other forms of cerebral ischemia and adds yet another complexity to already complex mechanisms of microvascular and brain injury after SAH.

Conclusion

Microvasculature is an early target of SAH. Within minutes after SAH endothelial damage, basal lamina degradation and luminal aggregation of platelets initiates and continues for at least 24 h. Deficits in microvascular perfusion and permeability, as expected, occur in the similar temporal fashion, implying a causal relationship. A thorough understanding of the early changes in microvasculature after SAH is needed as these changes could be the source of early ischemic injury documented in humans without any angiographic proof of vasoconstriction.

Conflict of interest statement   We declare that we have no conflict of interest.

References

1. Jakobsen M. Role of initial brain ischemia in subarachnoid hemorrhage following aneurysm rupture. A pathophysiological survey. Acta Neurol Scand. 1992;141:1–33.
2. Bederson JB, Germano IM, Guarino L. Cortical blood flow and cerebral perfusion pressure in a new noncraniotomy model of subarachnoid hemorrhage in the rat. Stroke 1995;26:1086–91.
3. Bederson JB, Levy AL, Ding WH, Kahn R, DiPerna CA, Jenkins ALr et al. Acute vasoconstriction after subarachnoid hemorrhage. Neurosurgery 1998;42:352–60.
4. Kamiya K, Kuyama H, Symon L. An experimental study of the acute stage of subarachnoid hemorrhage. J Neurosurg. 1983;59:917–24.
5. Rasmussen G, Hauerberg J, Waldemar G, Gjerris F, Juhler M. Cerebral blood flow autoregulation in experimental subarachnoid haemorrhage in rat. Acta Neurochir. 1992;119:128–33.
6. Travis MA, Hall ED. The effects of chronic two-fold dietary vitamin E supplementation on subarachnoid hemorrhage-induced brain hypoperfusion. Brain Res. 1987;418:366–70.
7. Sehba FA, Ding WH, Chereshnev I, Bederson JB. Effects of S-nitrosoglutathione on acute vasoconstriction and glutamate release after subarachnoid hemorrhage. Stroke 1999;30:1955–61.
8. Hutchinson PJ, O'Connell MT, Al-Rawi PG, Kett-White CR, Gupta AK, Maskell LBet al. Increases in GABA concentrations during cerebral ischaemia: a microdialysis study of extracellular amino acids. J Neurol Neurosurg Psychiatry. 2002;72:99–105.
9. Sarrafzadeh A, Haux D, Sakowitz O, Benndorf G, Herzog H, Kuechler I, et al. Acute focal neurological deficits in aneurysmal subarachnoid hemorrhage: relation of clinical course, CT findings, and metabolite abnormalities monitored with bedside microdialysis. Stroke 2003;34:1382–8.
10. Staub F, Graf R, Gabel P, Kochling M, Klug N, Heiss WD. Multiple interstitial substances measured by microdialysis in patients with subarachnoid hemorrhage. Neurosurgery 2000;47:1106–15; discussion 1115–1106.
11. Grosset DG, Straiton J, McDonald I, Bullock R. Angiographic and Doppler diagnosis of cerebral artery vasospasm following subarachnoid haemorrhage. Br J Neurosurg. 1993;7:291–8.
12. Weir B, Grace M, Hansen J, Rothberg C. Time course of vasospasm in man. J Neurosurg. 1978;48:173–8.
13. Hoelper BM, Hofmann E, Sporleder R, Soldner F, Behr R. Transluminal balloon angioplasty improves brain tissue oxygenation and metabolism in severe vasospasm after aneurysmal subarachnoid hemorrhage: case report. Neurosurgery 2003; 52:970–4; discussion 974–976.
14. Ono S, Date I, Onoda K, Ohmoto T. Time course of the diameter of the major cerebral arteries after subarachnoid hemorrhage using corrosion cast technique. Neurol Res. 2003;25:383–9.
15. Uhl E, Lehmberg J, Steiger HJ, Messmer K. Intraoperative detection of early microvasospasm in patients with subarachnoid hemorrhage by using orthogonal polarization spectral imaging. Neurosurgery 2003;52:1307–15; discussion 1315–1307.
16. Ishikawa M, Kusaka G, Yamaguchi N, Sekizuka E, Nakadate H, Minamitani H, et al. Platelet and leukocyte adhesion in the microvasculature at the cerebral surface immediately after

subarachnoid hemorrhage. Neurosurgery 2009;64:546–53; discussion 553–554.
17. Park KW, Metais C, Dai HB, Comunale ME, Sellke FW. Microvascular endothelial dysfunction and its mechanism in a rat model of subarachnoid hemorrhage. Anesth Analg. 2001;92:990–6.
18. Sehba FA, Makonnen G, Friedrich V, Bederson JB. Acute cerebral vascular injury occurs after subarachnoid hemorrhage and can be prevented by administration of a Nitric Oxide donor. J Neurosurg. 2007;106:321–9.
19. Sehba FA, Mostafa G, Knopman J, Friedrich V Jr, Bederson JB. Acute alterations in Microvascular basal lamina after Subarachnoid Hemorrhage. J Neurosurg. 2004;101:633–40.
20. Sehba FA, Mustafa G, Friedrich V, Bederson JB. Acute microvascular platelet aggregation after Subarachnoid hemorrhage. J Neurosurg. 2005;102:1094–100.
21. Sun BL, Zheng CB, Yang MF, Yuan H, Zhang SM, Wang LX. Dynamic alterations of cerebral pial microcirculation during experimental subarachnoid hemorrhage. Cell Mol Neurobiol. 2009;29:235–41.
22. Critchley GR, Bell BA. Acute cerebral tissue oxygenation changes following experimental subarachnoid hemorrhage. Neurol Res. 2003;25:451–6.
23. Pennings FA, Albrecht KW, Muizelaar JP, Schuurman PR, Bouma GJ. Abnormal responses of the human cerebral microcirculation to papaverin during aneurysm surgery. Stroke 2009;40:317–20.
24. Gregoire N. The blood-brain barrier. J Neuroradiol. 1989;16:238–50.
25. Martinez-Hernandez A, Amenta PS. The basement membrane in pathology. Lab Invest. 1983;48:656–77.
26. Bosman FT, Cleutjens J, Beek C, Havenith M. Basement membrane heterogeneity. Histochem J. 1989;21:629–33.
27. Stanley JR, Woodley DT, Katz SI, Martin GR. Structure and function of basement membrane. J Invest Dermatol. 1982;79: Suppl 1:69s–72s.
28. Hamann GF, Liebetrau M, Martens H, Burggraf D, Kloss CU, Bultemeier G et al. Microvascular Basal lamina injury after experimental focal cerebral ischemia and reperfusion in the rat. J Cereb Blood Flow Metab. 2002;22:526–33.
29. Heo JH, Lucero J, Abumiya T, Koziol JA, Copeland BR, del Zoppo GJ. Matrix metalloproteinases increase very early during experimental focal cerebral ischemia. J Cereb Blood Flow Metab. 1999;19:624–33.
30. Wagner S, Tagaya M, Koziol JA, Quaranta V, del Zoppo GJ. Rapid disruption of an astrocyte interaction with the extracellular matrix mediated by integrin alpha 6 beta 4 during focal cerebral ischemia/reperfusion. Stroke 1997;28:858–65.
31. del Zoppo GJ, Mabuchi T. Cerebral microvessel responses to focal ischemia. J Cereb Blood Flow Metab. 2003;23:879–94.
32. Hatake K, Wakabayashi I, Kakishita E, Hishida S. Impairment of endothelium-dependent relaxation in human basilar artery after subarachnoid hemorrhage. Stroke 1992;23:1111–6; discussion 1116–1117.
33. Hongo K, Kassell NF, Nakagomi T, Sasaki T, Tsukahara T, Ogawa H et al. Subarachnoid hemorrhage inhibition of endothelium-derived relaxing factor in rabbit basilar artery. J Neurosurg. 1988;69:247–53.
34. Nakagomi T, Kassell NF, Sasaki T, Fujiwara S, Lehman RM, Johshita H et al. Effect of subarachnoid hemorrhage on endothelium-dependent vasodilation. J Neurosurg. 1987;66:915–23.
35. Pennings FA, Bouma GJ, Ince C. Direct observation of the human cerebral microcirculation during aneurysm surgery reveals increased arteriolar contractility. Stroke 2004;35:1284–8.
36. Sehba FA, Schwartz AY, Chereshnev I, Bederson JB. Acute decrease in cerebral nitric oxide levels after subarachnoid hemorrhage. J Cereb Blood Flow Metab. 2000;20:604–11.
37. Gryglewski RJ, Palmer RM, Moncada S. Superoxide anion is involved in the breakdown of endothelium-derived vascular relaxing factor. Nature 1986;320:454–6.
38. Pabst MJ, Cummings NP, Hedegaard HB, Johnston RB Jr. Human macrophages may normally be "primed" for a strong oxygen radical response. Adv Exp Med Biol. 1983;166:215–21.
39. Clower BR, Yamamoto Y, Cain L, Haines DE, Smith RR. Endothelial injury following experimental subarachnoid hemorrhage in rats: effects on brain blood flow. Anat Rec. 1994;240:104–14.
40. Yan J, Chen C, Hu Q, Yang X, Lei J, Yang L et al. The role of p53 in brain edema after 24 h of experimental subarachnoid hemorrhage in a rat model. Exp Neurol. 2008;214:37–46.
41. Akopov S, Sercombe R, Seylaz J. Cerebrovascular reactivity: role of endothelium/platelet/leukocyte interactions. Cerebrovasc Brain Metab Rev. 1996;8:11–94.
42. Cahill J, Calvert JW, Solaroglu I, Zhang JH. Vasospasm and p53-induced apoptosis in an experimental model of subarachnoid hemorrhage. Stroke 2006;37:1868–74.
43. Joris I, Majno G. Endothelial changes induced by arterial spasm. Am J Pathol. 1981;102:346–58.
44. Simard JM, Geng Z, Woo SK, Ivanova S, Tosun C, Melnichenko L et al. Glibenclamide reduces inflammation, vasogenic edema, and caspase-3 activation after subarachnoid hemorrhage. J Cereb Blood Flow Metab. 2009;29:317–30.
45. Chaichana[AU3] KL, Pradilla G, Huang J, Tamargo RJ. Role of inflammation (leukocyte-endothelial cell interactions) in vasospasm after subarachnoid hemorrhage. World Neurosurg. 2010;73(1):22–41.
46. Bavbek M, Polin R, Kwan AL, Arthur AS, Kassell NF, Lee KS. Monoclonal antibodies against ICAM-1 and CD18 attenuate cerebral vasospasm after experimental subarachnoid hemorrhage in rabbits. Stroke 1998;29:1930–5; discussion 1935–1936.
47. Handa Y, Kubota T, Kaneko M, Tsuchida A, Kobayashi H, Kawano H. Expression of intercellular adhesion molecule 1 (ICAM-1) on the cerebral artery following subarachnoid haemorrhage in rats. Acta Neurochir (Wien). 1995;132:92–7.
48. Polin RS, Bavbek M, Shaffrey ME, Billups K, Bogaev CA, Kassell NF et al. Detection of soluble E-selectin, ICAM-1, VCAM-1, and L-selectin in the cerebrospinal fluid of patients after subarachnoid hemorrhage. J Neurosurg. 1998;89:559–67.
49. Rothoerl RD, Schebesch KM, Kubitza M, Woertgen C, Brawanski A, Pina AL. ICAM-1 and VCAM-1 expression following aneurysmal subarachnoid hemorrhage and their possible role in the pathophysiology of subsequent ischemic deficits. Cerebrovasc Dis. 2006;22:143–9.
50. Lin CL, Dumont AS, Calisaneller T, Kwan AL, Hwong SL, Lee KS. Monoclonal antibody against E selectin attenuates subarachnoid hemorrhage-induced cerebral vasospasm. Surg Neurol. 2005;64:201–5.
51. Rosenblum WI. Platelet adhesion and aggregation without endothelial denudation or exposure of basal lamina and/or collagen. J Vasc Res. 1997;34:409–17.
52. Said S, Rosenblum WI, Povlishock JT, Nelson GH. Correlations between morphological changes in platelet aggregates and underlying endothelial damage in cerebral microcirculation of mice. Stroke 1993;24:1968–76.
53. Akopov SE, Sercombe R, Seylaz J. Leukocyte-induced endothelial dysfunction in the rabbit basilar artery: modulation by platelet-activating factor. J Lipid Mediat Cell Signal. 1995;11:267–79.
54. Park S, Yamaguchi M, Zhou C, Calvert JW, Tang J, Zhang JH. Neurovascular protection reduces early brain injury after subarachnoid hemorrhage. Stroke 2004;35:2412–7.
55. Yatsushige H, Ostrowski RP, Tsubokawa T, Colohan A, Zhang JH. Role of c-Jun N-terminal kinase in early brain injury after subarachnoid hemorrhage. J Neurosci Res. 2007;85:1436–48.

56. Hamann GF, Okada Y, Fitridge R, del Zoppo GJ. Microvascular basal lamina antigens disappear during cerebral ischemia and reperfusion. Stroke 1995;26:2120–6.
57. Gasche Y, Fujimura M, Morita-Fujimura Y, Copin JC, Kawase M, Massengale J et al. Early appearance of activated matrix metalloproteinase-9 after focal cerebral ischemia in mice: a possible role in blood-brain barrier dysfunction. J Cereb Blood Flow Metab. 1999;19:1020–8.
58. Mun-Bryce S, Rosenberg GA. Matrix metalloproteinases in cerebrovascular disease. J Cereb Blood Flow Metab. 1998;18:1163–72.
59. Zhang ZG, Zhang L, Tsang W, Goussev A, Powers C, Ho K et al. Dynamic platelet accumulation at the site of the occluded middle cerebral artery and in downstream microvessels is associated with loss of microvascular integrity after embolic middle cerebral artery occlusion. Brain Res. 2001;912:181–94.
60. Mignatti P, Rifkin DB. Plasminogen activators and matrix metalloproteinases in angiogenesis. Enzyme Protein. 1996;49:117–37.
61. Rosenberg GA. Matrix metalloproteinases in brain injury. J Neurotrauma. 1995;12:833–42.
62. Clark AW, Krekoski CA, Bou SS, Chapman KR, Edwards DR. Increased gelatinase A (MMP-2) and gelatinase B (MMP-9) activities in human brain after focal ischemia. Neurosci Lett. 1997;238:53–6.
63. Lukes A, Mun-Bryce S, Lukes M, Rosenberg GA. Extracellular matrix degradation by metalloproteinases and central nervous system diseases. Mol Neurobiol. 1999;19:267–84.
64. Guo Z, Sun X, He Z, Jiang Y, Zhang X, Zhang JH. Matrix metalloproteinase-9 potentiates early brain injury after subarach-noid hemorrhage. Neurol Res. 2010 Sep;32(7):715–20.
65. Scholler K, Trinkl A, Klopotowski M, Thal SC, Plesnila N, Trabold R et al. Characterization of microvascular basal lamina damage and blood-brain barrier dysfunction following subarachnoid hemorrhage in rats. Brain Res. 2007;1142:237–46.
66. Josko J, Hendryk S, Jedrzejowska-Szypulka H, Slowinski J, Gwozdz B, Lange D et al. Cerebral angiogenesis after subarachnoid hemorrhage (SAH) and endothelin receptor blockage with BQ-123 antagonist in rats. J Physiol Pharmacol. 2001;52:237–48.
67. Josko J. Cerebral angiogenesis and expression of VEGF after subarachnoid hemorrhage (SAH) in rats. Brain Res. 2003; 981:58–69.
68. Josko J, Gwozdz B, Hendryk S, Jedrzejowska-Szypulka H, Slowinski J, Jochem J. Expression of vascular endothelial growth factor (VEGF) in rat brain after subarachnoid haemorrhage and endothelin receptor blockage with BQ-123. Folia Neuropathol. 2001;39:243–51.
69. Scheufler KM, Drevs J, van Velthoven V, Reusch P, Klisch J, Augustin HG et al. Implications of vascular endothelial growth factor, sFlt-1, and sTie-2 in plasma, serum and cerebrospinal fluid during cerebral ischemia in man. J Cereb Blood Flow Metab. 2003;23:99–110.
70. McGirt MJ, Lynch JR, Blessing R, Warner DS, Friedman AH, Laskowitz DT. Serum von Willebrand factor, matrix metalloproteinase-9, and vascular endothelial growth factor levels predict the onset of cerebral vasospasm after aneurysmal subarachnoid hemorrhage. Neurosurgery 2002;51:1128–34; discussion 1134–1135.
71. Sun BL, Hu DM, Yuan H, Ye WJ, Wang XC, Xia ZL et al. Extract of Ginkgo biloba promotes the expression of VEGF following subarachnoid hemorrhage in rats. Int J Neurosci. 2009;119:995–1005.
72. Sawicki G, Salas E, Murat J, Miszta-Lane H, Radomski MW. Release of gelatinase A during platelet activation mediates aggregation. Nature 1997;386:616–9.
73. Doczi T, Joo F, Adam G, Bozoky B, Szerdahelyi P. Blood-brain barrier damage during the acute stage of subarachnoid hemorrhage, as exemplified by a new animal model. Neurosurgery 1986;18:733–9.
74. Smith SL, Larson PG, Hall ED. A comparison of the effects of tirilazad on subarachnoid hemorrhage-induced blood-brain barrier permeability in male and female rats. J Stroke Cerebrovasc Dis. 1997;6:389–93.
75. Yatsushige H, Calvert JW, Cahill J, Zhang JH. Limited role of inducible nitric oxide synthase in blood-brain barrier function after experimental subarachnoid hemorrhage. J Neurotrauma. 2006;23:1874–82.
76. Antovic J, Bakic M, Zivkovic M, Ilic A, Blomback M. Blood coagulation and fibrinolysis in acute ischaemic and haemorrhagic (intracerebral and subarachnoid haemorrhage) stroke: does decreased plasmin inhibitor indicate increased fibrinolysis in subarachnoid haemorrhage compared to other types of stroke? Scand J Clin Lab Invest. 2002;62:195–9.
77. Ettinger MG. Coagulation abnormalities in subarachnoid hemorrhage. Stroke 1970;1:139–42.
78. Filizzolo F, D'Angelo V, Collice M, Ferrara M, Donati MB, Porta M. Fibrinolytic activity in blood and cerebrospinal fluid in subarachnoid hemorrhage from ruptured intracranial saccular aneurysm before and during EACA treatment. Eur Neurol. 1978; 17:43–7.
79. Nina P, Schisano G, Chiappetta F, Luisa Papa M, Maddaloni E, Brunori A et al. A study of blood coagulation and fibrinolytic system in spontaneous subarachnoid hemorrhage. Correlation with hunt-hess grade and outcome. Surg Neurol. 2001;55: 197–203.
80. Denton IC, Robertson JT, Dugdale M. An assessment of early platelet activity in experimental subarachnoid hemorrhage and middle cerebral artery thrombosis in the cat. Stroke 1971; 2:268–72.
81. Clower BR, Yoshioka J, Honma Y, Smith RR. Pathological changes in cerebral arteries following experimental subarachnoid hemorrhage: role of blood platelets. Anat Rec. 1988;220:161–70.
82. Haining JL, Clower BR, Honma Y, Smith RR. Accumulation of intimal platelets in cerebral arteries following experimental subarachnoid hemorrhage in cats. Stroke 1988;19:898–902.
83. Stein SC, Browne KD, Chen XH, Smith DH, Graham DI. Thromboembolism and delayed cerebral ischemia after subarachnoid hemorrhage: an autopsy study. Neurosurgery 2006;59:781–7; discussion 787–788.
84. Akopov SE, Zhang L, Pearce WJ. Mechanisms of platelet-induced angiospastic reactions: potentiation of calcium sensitivity. Can J Physiol Pharmacol. 1997;75:849–52.
85. Fujimoto T, Suzuki H, Tanoue K, Fukushima Y, Yamazaki H. Autoradiographic observation of platelets in cerebrovascular injuries induced by arachidonic acid and its prevention by ticlopidine. Thromb Haemost. 1988;60:319–23.
86. Umegaki K, Inoue Y, Tomita T. The appearance of platelets at the time of stroke in stroke-prone spontaneously hypertensive rats. Thromb Haemost. 1985;54:764–7.
87. Kapp J, Mahaley MS Jr, Odom GL. Cerebral arterial spasm. 2. Experimental evaluation of mechanical and humoral factors in pathogenesis. J Neurosurg. 1968;29:339–49.
88. Fujimoto T, Suzuki H, Tanoue K, Fukushima Y, Yamazaki H. Cerebrovascular injuries induced by activation of platelets in vivo. Stroke 1985;16:245–50.
89. Andresen J, Shafi NI, Bryan RM Jr. Endothelial influences on cerebrovascular tone. J Appl Physiol. 2006;100:318–27.
90. Sehba FA, Bederson JB. Mechanisms of acute brain injury after subarachnoid hemorrhage. Neurol Res. 2006;28:381–98.
91. Zhou Q, Hellermann GR, Solomonson LP. Nitric oxide release from resting human platelets. Thromb Res. 1995;77:87–96.
92. Moro MA, Russel RJ, Cellek S, Lizasoain I, Su Y, Darley-Usmar VM et al. cGMP mediates the vascular and platelet actions of nitric oxide: confirmation using an inhibitor of the soluble guanylyl cyclase. Proc Natl Acad Sci USA. 1996;93:1480–5.

93. Smith CC, Stanyer L, Cooper MB, Betteridge DJ. Platelet aggregation may not be a prerequisite for collagen-stimulated platelet generation of nitric oxide. Biochim Biophys Acta. 1999;1473:286–92.
94. Abumiya T, Fitridge R, Mazur C, Copeland BR, Koziol JA, Tschopp JF et al. Integrin alpha(IIb)beta(3) inhibitor preserves microvascular patency in experimental acute focal cerebral ischemia. Stroke 2000;31:1402–9; discussion 1409–1410.
95. Ames Ad, Wright RL, Kowada M, Thurston JM, Majno G. Cerebral ischemia. II. The no-reflow phenomenon. Am J Pathol. 1968;52:437–53.
96. del Zoppo GJ. Microvascular responses to cerebral ischemia/inflammation. Ann NY Acad Sci. 1997;823:132–47.
97. Fukami MH, Holmsen H, Kowalska MA, Niewiarowski S. (2001) Platelet secretion. In: Colman RW, Hirsh J, Marder VJ, Clowes AW, George JN editors. Hemostatis and thrombosis basic principles and clinical practice. Phialdelphia: Lippincott Williams & Wilkins, p. 562–73.
98. Okada Y, Copeland BR, Mori E, Tung MM, Thomas WS, del Zoppo GJ. P-selectin and intercellular adhesion molecule-1 expression after focal brain ischemia and reperfusion. Stroke 1994;25:202–11.
99. Reed GL. (2002) Platelet secretion. In: Michelson AD, editor. Platelets. San Diego, CA: Academic press, p. 181–95.
100. Fernandez-Patron C, Martinez-Cuesta MA, Salas E, Sawicki G, Wozniak M, Radomski MW et al. Differential regulation of platelet aggregation by matrix metalloproteinases-9 and -2. Thromb Haemost. 1999;82:1730–5.
101. Rosenberg GA, Estrada EY, Dencoff JE. Matrix metalloproteinases and TIMPs are associated with blood-brain barrier opening after reperfusion in rat brain. Stroke 1998;29:2189–95.
102. Rosenberg GA, Kornfeld M, Estrada E, Kelley RO, Liotta LA, Stetler-Stevenson WG. TIMP-2 reduces proteolytic opening of blood-brain barrier by type IV collagenase. Brain Res. 1992; 576:203–7.

Immunological Response in Early Brain Injury After SAH

Takumi Sozen, Reiko Tsuchiyama, Yu Hasegawa, Hidenori Suzuki, Vikram Jadhav, Shigeru Nishizawa, and John H. Zhang

Abstract This study summarized the role of inflammation in the early brain injury after subarachnoid hemorrhage. Elevation of cytokines, activation of MMPs and phosphorylation of MAPK contributes to neuronal apoptosis and brain edema. Anti-inflammation may be potential strategy for the prevention and suppression of early brain injury after subarachnoid hemorrhage.

Keywords Early brain injury · Immune · Inflammation

Introduction

Subarachnoid hemorrhage (SAH) is a deadly cerebrovascular disorder with high mortality rate; 15% of patients die before reaching the hospital and 30% die within 24 h of onset [1]. The high morbidity and mortality observed with SAH have persisted in spite of recent therapeutic advances [2]. Moreover, patients who survive the initial hemorrhage and overcome the sequelae of cerebral vasospasm frequently experience persistent cognitive deficits, psychosocial impairments, and a decrease in quality of life as a result of early brain injury (EBI) [3]. Recent studies have emphasized the importance of management of EBI to improve outcome after SAH [4].

T. Sozen (✉)
Department of Neurosurgery, University of Occupational and Environmental Health, Japan 1-1, Iseigaoka, Yahata-nishi-ku, Kitakyushu, Fukuoka, 807-8555, Japan
Department of Neurosurgery, University of Occupational and Environmental Health, Japan
e-mail: juzzyns9@yahoo.co.jp

R. Tsuchiyama, Y. Hasegawa, H. Suzuki, and V. Jadhav
Department of Physiology, Loma Linda University of Medicine, Loma Linda, CA 92350, USA

S. Nishizawa
Department of Neurosurgery, University of Occupational and Environmental Health, Japan

J.H. Zhang
Department of Physiology, Loma Linda University of Medicine, Loma Linda, CA 92350, USA
Department of Neurosurgery, Loma Linda University of Medicine, Loma Linda, CA 92350, USA

Cytokine Activity After SAH

Various mechanisms, including inflammation, have been implicated in the pathogenesis of EBI after SAH [4–6]. In clinical settings, many signs associated with EBI such as pyrexia, neutrophilia, and cerebral edema secondary to disruption of the blood–brain barrier (BBB) are believed to be caused by cytokine activity [7]. Elevation of many type of inflammatory cytokines (interleukin (IL)-6 [8], IL-8 [9], tumour necrosis factor (TNF)-α [10], and monocyte chemoattractant protein (MCP)-1 [9]) were reported in the early stage after SAH.

Interleukin-1β

Among many proinflammatory cytokines, IL-1β is considered a key mediator of neural injury in acute central nervous system (CNS) injuries, such as ischemic stroke and brain trauma [11]. IL-1β is also reported to increase in the cerebral cortex [12] and cerebrospinal fluid (CSF) [13] after SAH in both humans and animal models.

Relationship Between IL-1β and Matrix Metalloproteinase (MMP)

The BBB is formed by specialized brain endothelial cells that are interconnected by tight junctions. Tight junctions in the BBB are essential for maintaining the microenvironment [14]. A recent study provides direct evidence that MMPs open the BBB by degrading tight junction proteins [15]. MMPs comprise a family of zinc endopeptidases that can modify several components of the extracellular matrix [16]. In particular, the gelatinases MMP-2 and MMP-9 can degrade neurovascular matrix integrity. IL-1ß plays a pivotal role in the induction of MMP-9 in a variety of acute and chronic inflammatory states and conditions [17, 18].

Relationship Between IL-1β and Mitogen Activated Protein Kinase (MAPK) Signaling Pathways

IL-1β can activate three types of mitogen activated protein kinase (MAPK) signaling pathways, extracellular signal-regulated kinase, p38, and JNK [19, 20].

Anti-Proinflammatory Cytokine Treatment for Ebi After SAH

IL-1β is synthesized as precursor molecules, which are then processed to mature forms by caspase-1, the IL-1β converting enzyme. We examined the effects of N–Ac–Tyr–Val–Ala–Asp–chloromethyl ketone (Ac-YVAD-CMK), a caspase-1 inhibitor that selectively inhibits the cleavage of precursor IL-1β, on EBI in an established endovascular perforation model of SAH in mice. 101 mice were randomly assigned to sham, SAH+ vehicle, and SAH+ Ac-YVAD-CMK groups (6 and 10 mg/kg). Ac-YVAD-CMK or vehicle was administered intraperitoneally 1 h after SAH production by endovascular perforation of the left anterior cerebral artery. EBI was assessed in terms of mortality within 24 h; neurological scores, brain water content at 24 and 72 h; Evans blue dye extravasation and Western blot for IL-1β, c-Jun N-Terminal kinase (JNK), matrix metalloproteinase (MMP)-9 and zonula occludens (ZO)-1 at 24 h after SAH. The high-dose (10 mg/kg), but not low-dose (6 mg/kg) treatment group had significantly improved neurological scores, mortality, brain water content, and Evans blue dye extravasation compared with the vehicle group (Figs. 1 and 2). Although both dosages of Ac-YVAD-CMK attenuated the mature IL-1β induction, only the high-dose treatment significantly inhibited the phosphorylation of JNK, MMP-9 induction and ZO-1 degradation (Figs. 3 and 4).

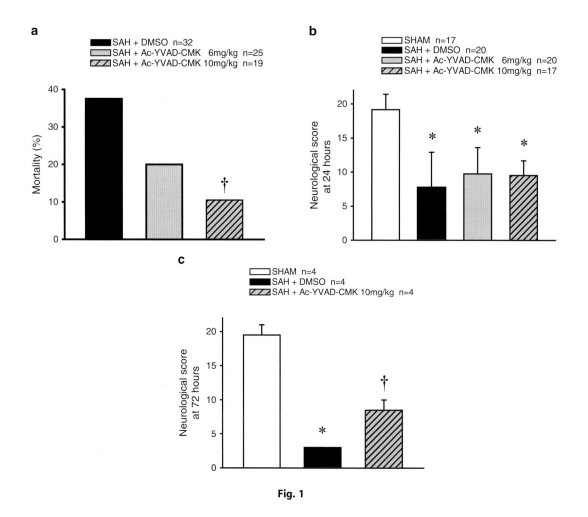

Fig. 1

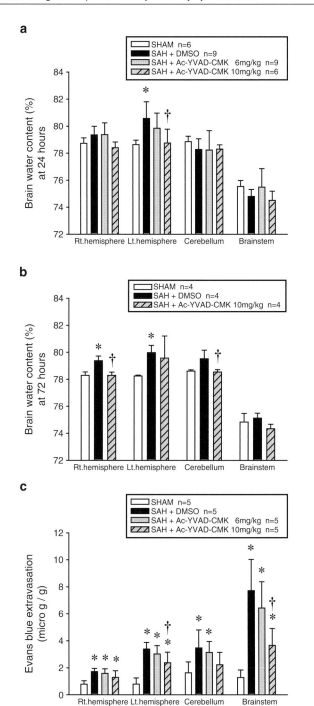

Fig. 2

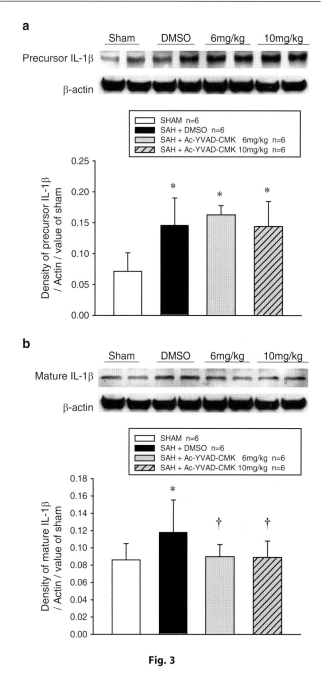

Fig. 3

to 10.5% in a dose-dependent manner. The beneficial effects of Ac-YVAD-CMK resulted, at least in part, from decreased BBB permeability, and consequently reduced brain edema.

We observed that mature IL-1β and MMP-9 were induced, and caspase-1 inhibitor attenuated the increase of MMP-9 and abolished the degradation of ZO-1 in the mouse brain after SAH. These results implicate IL-1ß as a key regulator of brain MMP-9 and as a therapeutic target on EBI following SAH.

Western blotting analysis suggested that mature IL-1β increased expression of MMP-9 as well as phosphorylated

Conclusion

An important observation in this study is the reduction of mortality and improvement of neurological function after Ac-YVAD-CMK treatment. We demonstrated that the intraperitoneal injection of Ac-YVAD-CMK significantly reduced mature IL-1β and attenuated mortality from 37.5

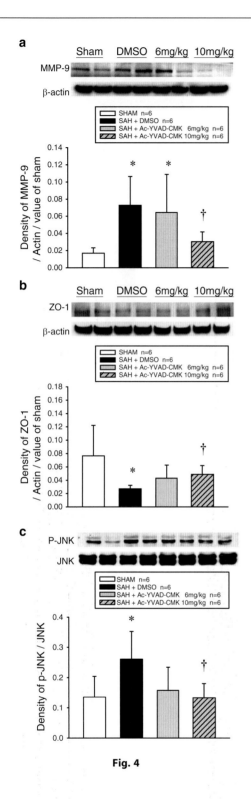

Fig. 4

JNK, which were inhibited by the caspase-1 inhibitor. Our result is consistent with studies showing that MMP-9 secretion may be upregulated by IL-1β via the MAPK signaling pathways [21]. These findings suggest that in SAH, at least, activation of JNK pathway is involved in IL-1β-induced MMP-9 expression. Even though further evidence is needed, it is possible that mature IL-1β activates phosphorylation of JNK which induces MMP-9 level, causing EBI after SAH.

In conclusion, preventing cleavage of precursor IL-1β to its active form by caspase-1 inhibitor could be a new strategy to prevent or attenuate EBI after SAH via neurovascular protection. Future therapies targeting anti-inflammatory response after SAH may help to reduce the development of EBI.

Acknowledgments This study was partially supported by grants (NS053407) from the National Institutes of Health to J.H.Z.

Conflict of interest statement We declare that we have no conflict of interest.

References

1. Broderick JP, Brott T, Tomsick T, Miller R, Huster G. Intracerebral hemorrhage more than twice as common as subarachnoid hemorrhage. J Neurosurg. 1993;78:188–91.
2. Schievink WI, Riedinger M, Jhutty TK, Simon P. Racial disparities in subarachnoid hemorrhage mortality: Los Angeles County, California, 1985–1998. Neuroepidemiology 2004;23:299–305.
3. Hütter BO, Kreitschmann-Andermahr I, Gilsbach JM. Health-related quality of life after aneurysmal subarachnoid hemorrhage: impacts of bleeding severity, computerized tomography findings, surgery, vasospasm, and neurological grade. J Neurosurg. 2001;94:241–51.
4. Cahill J, Calvert JW, Zhang JH. Mechanisms of early brain injury after subarachnoid hemorrhage. J Cereb Blood Flow Metab. 2006; 26:1341–53.
5. Ostrowski RP, Colohan AR, Zhang JH. Molecular mechanisms of early brain injury after subarachnoid hemorrhage. Neurol Res. 2006;28:399–414.
6. Sercombe R, Dinh YR, Gomis P. Cerebrovascular inflammation following subarachnoid hemorrhage. Jpn J Pharmacol. 2002;88: 227–49.
7. McKeating EG, Andrews PJ. Cytokines and adhesion molecules in acute brain injury. Br J Anaesth. 1998;80:77–84.
8. Mathiesen T, Andersson B, Loftenius A, von Holst H. Increased interleukin-6 levels in cerebrospinal fluid following subarachnoid hemorrhage. J Neurosurg. 1993;78:562–7.
9. Gaetani P, Tartara F, Pignatti P, Tancioni F, Rodriguez y Baena R, De Benedetti F. Cisternal CSF levels of cytokines after subarachnoid hemorrhage. Neurol Res. 1998;20:337–42.
10. Mathiesen T, Edner G, Ulfarsson E, Andersson B. Cerebrospinal fluid interleukin-1 receptor antagonist and tumor necrosis factor-alpha following subarachnoid hemorrhage. J Neurosurg. 1997; 87:215–20.
11. Allan SM, Tyrrell PJ, Rothwell NJ. Interleukin-1 and neuronal injury. Nat Rev Immunol. 2005;5:629–40.
12. Prunell GF, Svendgaard NA, Alkass K, Mathiesen T. Inflammation in the brain after experimental subarachnoid hemorrhage. Neurosurgery 2005;56:1082–92.
13. Kwon KY, Jeon BC. Cytokine levels in cerebrospinal fluid and delayed ischemic deficits in patients with aneurysmal subarachnoid hemorrhage. J Korean Med Sci. 2001;16:774–80.
14. Wolburg H, Lippoldt A. Tight junctions of the blood–brain barrier: development, composition and regulation. Vascul Pharmacol. 2002;38:323–37.
15. Yang Y, Estrada EY, Thompson JF, Liu W, Rosenberg GA. Matrix metalloproteinase-mediated disruption of tight junction proteins in

cerebral vessels is reversed by synthetic matrix metalloproteinase inhibitor in focal ischemia in rat. J Cereb Blood Flow Metab. 2007;27:697–709.
16. Yong VW, Power C, Forsyth P, Edwards DR. Metalloproteinases in biology and pathology of the nervous system. Nat Rev Neurosci. 2001;2:502–11.
17. Ruhul Amin AR, Senga T, Oo ML, Thant AA, Hamaguchi M. Secretion of matrix metalloproteinase-9 by the proinflammatory cytokine, IL-1beta: a role for the dual signaling pathways, Akt and Erk. Genes Cells. 2003;8:515–23.
18. Vecil GG, Larsen PH, Corley SM, Herx LM, Besson A, Goodyer CG, et al. Interleukin-1 is a key regulator of matrix metalloproteinase-9 expression in human neurons in culture and following mouse brain trauma in vivo. J Neurosci Res. 2000;61:212–24.
19. Guan Z, Buckman SY, Miller BW, Springer LD, Morrison AR. Interleukin-1beta-induced cyclooxygenase-2 expression requires activation of both c-Jun NH2-terminal kinase and p38 MAPK signal pathways in rat renal mesangial cells. J Biol Chem. 1998;273:28670–6.
20. Larsen CM, Wadt KA, Juhl LF, Andersen HU, Karlsen AE, Su MS, et al. Interleukin-1beta-induced rat pancreatic islet nitric oxide synthesis requires both the p38 and extracellular signal-regulated kinase 1/2 mitogen-activated protein kinases. J Biol Chem. 1998;273:15294–300.
21. Wu CY, Hsieh HL, Jou MJ, Yang CM. Involvement of p42/p44 MAPK, p38 MAPK, JNK and nuclear factor-kappa B in interleukin-1beta-induced matrix metalloproteinase-9 expression in rat brain astrocytes. J Neurochem. 2004;90:1477–88.

Mechanisms of Early Brain Injury After SAH: Matrixmetalloproteinase 9

Zong-duo Guo, Xiao-chuan Sun, and John H. Zhang

Abstract Subarachnoid hemorrhage (SAH) is an important cause of death and disability worldwide. To date, there is not a definitive treatment that completely prevents brain injury after SAH. Recently, early brain injury (EBI) has been pointed out to be the primary cause of mortality in SAH patients. Apoptosis that occurs in neuronal tissues and cerebral vasculature after SAH plays an essential role in EBI. Matrix metalloproteinase 9 (MMP-9) has been found to increase in many cerebral vascular diseases. There have been reports that MMP-9 can mediate apoptosis, which called anoikis in cerebral ischemia models, through cleaving main components of the extracellular matrix (ECM), especially laminin. Therefore, minocycline, which has been found to inhibit MMP-9, may be protective to brain injury after SAH. We based our hypothesis on the fact that SAH possesses some aspects that are similar to those of cerebral ischemia. It is conceivable that MMP-9 may also be involved in the pathological process of EBI after SAH, and minocycline can relieve anoikis and improve EBI after SAH.

Keywords Early brain injury · minocycline · MMPs

Introduction

SAH is a devastating and complicated disease which has a high rate of morbidity and mortality worldwide. Although there have been some advances in treatment for SAH, the rates of morbidity and mortality have not changed in recent years [1, 2]. More and more researchers have pointed out that EBI is the primary cause of mortality in SAH patients [3, 4]. Therefore, the current research is to find whether new agents targeted at MMP-9 can improve EBI.

Early Brain Injury and Apoptosis

The term EBI has recently been coined and refers to the immediate injury to the brain as a whole, involving brain cell death, blood–brain barrier, brain edema, and microvascular dysfunction within the first 72 h of the ictus, secondary to SAH [5]. The etiology of EBI lies with the initial bleed and the complex pathophysiological mechanisms that occur as a result, which predisposes the brain to secondary injury. It has been shown both in clinical and experimental studies that there is a rise in the intracranial pressure (ICP) and a resultant decrease in the cerebral perfusion pressure (CPP) [6]. It is a combination of these factors that results in a global ischemic injury. This ischemic injury is seen as a leading cause of morbidity in patients with SAH [7]. As a result of the global ischemic injury, secondary to raised ICP and decreased CPP as outlined above, apoptosis has been shown to be widespread in the brain after SAH [8]. Thus, it seems clear that an understanding of the apoptotic cascades in relation to SAH is vital to understand and treat SAH patients during EBI in the future.

Apoptosis has been extensively studied in diseases of the central nervous system and has been shown to be an important form of cell death. To date, apoptosis has been studied extensively in stroke and to a limited degree in SAH. Following the global ischemia seen with SAH, apoptosis has been shown to occur in the hippocampus, blood–brain barrier (BBB), and vasculature [9]. There are a number of apoptotic pathways that are believed to play a role in SAH: the death receptor pathway, caspase-dependent and -independent pathways, as well as the mitochondrial pathway.

Z.-d. Guo and X.-c. Sun (✉)
Department of Neurosurgery, the First Affiliated Hospital of Chongqing Medical University, You Yi Road, Chongqing, 400016, People's Republic of China
e-mail: sunxch1445@gmail.com

J.H. Zhang
Department of Neurosurgery, Loma Linda University Medical Center, Loma Linda, CA 92354, USA

But we still need to investigate whether other apoptotic pathways are involved in the pathophysiological process during EBI after SAH.

MMP-9 and Laminin

MMP-9 belongs to a large family of endopeptidases and has been implicated in the pathogenesis of brain injury after ischemia and a number of neurodegenerative disorders [10]. MMP-9 is able to cleave extracellular matrix proteins, especially laminin [11]. Laminins are heterotrimeric molecules that are critical components of the ECM and are known to play an important role in the nervous system [12]. Previously, it had been demonstrated that ECM proteins such as laminins are important for cell survival and prevention of apoptosis, representing a form of cell death known as anoikis, in which cells detach from their matrix [13]. Therefore, the integrity of the laminin matrix in the brain is critical for protecting neurons and vascular endothelial cells. It has been reported that neuronal nitric oxide synthase (NOS) could increase the activity of MMP-9 by S-nitrosylation and lead to laminin cleavage [14]. After various insults, MMP-9 was upregulated and led to anoikis of neurons and endothelial cells because of laminin degradation [15].

Minocycline

Minocycline is a commonly used semi-synthetic tetracycline with anti-inflammatory and anti-apoptotic properties. Several studies have found that minocycline can interfere with MMP-9 activity and is shown to be neuroprotective in cerebral ischemia and in other models of brain injury [16, 17].

The Hypothesis

MMP-9 in the hippocampus of rats after SAH may be involved in the pathological process of EBI through degradating laminin, which led to anoikis in neurons of the hippocampus and vascular endothelial cells in rats. Minocycline, which can inhibit MMP-9, may protect hippocampal neurons and vascular endothelial cells, which results in less damage to neurons and improved neurological functions in EBI after SAH.

Implication of the Hypothesis

Vikman et al. investigated early changes in the cerebral arteries of rats that occur after SAH, and verified the upregulation of MMP-9 [18]. This showed that MMP-9 may be involved in the ECM remodeling processes occurring after SAH. Increased MMP-9 was also found in the microvasculature after acute SAH in rats through intracranial endovascular perforation, which led to an acute loss of ECM from the cerebral microvasculature [19]. This also showed that MMP-9 contributes to blood–brain barrier damage and brain injury by degrading the components of ECM. In SAH patients, it was also found that the serum MMP-9 level increased [20]. Furthermore, research found that a higher MMP-9 level is apparent with vasospasm in SAH patients. Active MMP-9 can degrade the basal lamina of the microvasculature, which leads to brain edema and secondary bleeding [21]. Within the hippocampus, MMP-9 expression is upregulated in both CA pyramidal and dentate granule neurons and astrocytes after global cerebral ischemia [22]. MMP-9 appears to play a deleterious role under the conditions of global ischemia, since both pharmacological inhibition and gene deletion of MMP-9 are neuroprotective in vivo [23, 24]. The mechanisms by which MMP-9 kills neurons is not yet clear, but has been suggested to involve disruption of neuron–ECM interaction, leading to death by anoikis [25]. Recently, research found that MMP-9 degraded the extracellular matrix protein laminin and that this degradation induced neuronal anoikis in a transient focal cerebral ischemia model [13]. Meanwhile, the highly specific gelatinase inhibitor blocked MMP-9 activity, including MMP-9-mediated laminin cleavage, thus rescuing neurons from anoikis. Yamaguchi et al. has found that MMP-9 inhibition can attenuate brain edema and blood–brain barrier disruption in rats after surgically-induced brain injury, which further supports our hypothesis [26]. It was reported recently that delayed treatment with minocycline can inhibit MMP-9 that is elevated after temporary experimental cerebral ischemia [27]. Minocycline has been shown to be neuroprotective. One common pathophysiological mechanism of models of brain ischemic damage is the dysregulation of the proteolytic cascade at the level of the endothelial and microglial cells [28]. Interference of this cascade by minocycline might be the central pathway for these neurovascular protective properties of decreasing tissue injury and also providing functional recovery. Furthermore, because minocycline has been shown to be neuroprotective in different models of brain injury, it is likely to act by multiple mechanisms, with MMP-9 inhibition being a central link for its anti-inflammatory and anti-apoptotic properties in the ischemic cascade and reperfusion [29]. In order to determine the clinical relevance of these findings for subarachnoid hemorrhage treatment, the next step is to determine if the MMP-9 inhibition by minocycline in the model of subarachnoid hemorrhage will result in decreased blood–brain barrier degradation and improved neurological deficits. In addition, the vascular protection properties of minocycline should also be studied after subarachnoid hemorrhage. Lee et al. found that MMP-9 expression increased in intracerebral hemorrhage (ICH), and minocycline could suppress MMP-9 and attenuate ICH [30]. This suggested the therapeutic potential of minocycline in brain protection.

Above all, our understanding of MMP-9's involvement in EBI after SAH has recently been built up. It is possible that targeting MMP-9 in SAH patients can be a highly promising therapeutic approach.

Conflict of interest statement We declare that we have no conflict of interest.

References

1. Schievink WI, Riedinger M, Jhutty TK, Simon P. Racial disparities in subarachnoid hemorrhage mortality: Los Angeles County, California, 1985–1998. Neuroepidemiology 2004;23:299–305.
2. Zhou C, Yamaguchi M, Colohan AR, Zhang JH. Role of p53 and apoptosis in cerebral vasospasm after experimental subarachnoid hemorrhage. J Cereb Blood Flow Metab. 2005;25:572–82.
3. Bederson JB, Germano IM, Guarino L. Cortical blood flow and cerebral perfusion pressure in a new noncraniotomy model of subarachnoid hemorrhage in the rat. Stroke 1995;26:1086–91; discussion 1091–1082.
4. Cahill J, Calvert JW, Zhang JH. Mechanisms of early brain injury after subarachnoid hemorrhage. J Cereb Blood Flow Metab. 2006; 26:1341–53.
5. Kusaka G, Ishikawa M, Nanda A, Granger DN, Zhang JH. Signaling pathways for early brain injury after subarachnoid hemorrhage. J Cereb Blood Flow Metab. 2004;24:916–25.
6. Ostrowski RP, Colohan AR, Zhang JH. Molecular mechanisms of early brain injury after subarachnoid hemorrhage. Neurol Res. 2006;28:399–414.
7. Schubert GA, Thome C. Cerebral blood flow changes in acute subarachnoid hemorrhage. Front Biosci. 2008;13:1594–603.
8. Gao C, Liu X, Liu W, Shi H, Zhao Z, Chen H, et al. Anti-apoptotic and neuroprotective effects of Tetramethylpyrazine following subarachnoid hemorrhage in rats. Auton Neurosci. 2008;141:22–30.
9. Ostrowski RP, Colohan AR, Zhang JH. Mechanisms of hyperbaric oxygen-induced neuroprotection in a rat model of subarachnoid hemorrhage. J Cereb Blood Flow Metab. 2005;25:554–71.
10. Cunningham LA, Wetzel M, Rosenberg GA. Multiple roles for MMPs and TIMPs in cerebral ischemia. Glia 2005;50:329–39.
11. Frisch SM, Francis H. Disruption of epithelial cell-matrix interactions induces apoptosis. J Cell Biol. 1994;124:619–26.
12. Colognato H, ffrench-Constant C, Feltri ML. Human diseases reveal novel roles for neural laminins. Trends Neurosci. 2005;28: 480–6.
13. Gu Z, Cui J, Brown S, Fridman R, Mobashery S, Strongin AY, et al. A highly specific inhibitor of matrix metalloproteinase-9 rescues laminin from proteolysis and neurons from apoptosis in transient focal cerebral ischemia. J Neurosci. 2005;25:6401–8.
14. Harris LK, McCormick J, Cartwright JE, Whitley GS, Dash PR. S-nitrosylation of proteins at the leading edge of migrating trophoblasts by inducible nitric oxide synthase promotes trophoblast invasion. Exp Cell Res. 2008;314:1765–76.
15. Zalewska T, Ziemka-Nalecz M, Sarnowska A, Domanska-Janik K. Transient forebrain ischemia modulates signal transduction from extracellular matrix in gerbil hippocampus. Brain Res. 2003;977:62–9.
16. Stirling DP, Koochesfahani KM, Steeves JD, Tetzlaff W. Minocycline as a neuroprotective agent. Neuroscientist 2005;11:308–22.
17. Sutton TA, Kelly KJ, Mang HE, Plotkin Z, Sandoval RM, Dagher PC. Minocycline reduces renal microvascular leakage in a rat model of ischemic renal injury. Am J Physiol Renal Physiol. 2005;288:F91–7.
18. Vikman P, Beg S, Khurana TS, Hansen-Schwartz J, Edvinsson L. Gene expression and molecular changes in cerebral arteries following subarachnoid hemorrhage in the rat. J Neurosurg. 2006;105:438–44.
19. Sehba FA, Mostafa G, Knopman J, Friedrich V Jr, Bederson JB. Acute alterations in microvascular basal lamina after subarachnoid hemorrhage. J Neurosurg. 2004;101:633–40.
20. Horstmann S, Su Y, Koziol J, Meyding-Lamade U, Nagel S, Wagner S. MMP-2 and MMP-9 levels in peripheral blood after subarachnoid hemorrhage. J Neurol Sci. 2006;251:82–6.
21. Burk J, Burggraf D, Vosko M, Dichgans M, Hamann GF. Protection of cerebral microvasculature after moderate hypothermia following experimental focal cerebral ischemia in mice. Brain Res. 2008;1226:248–55.
22. Lee SR, Tsuji K, Lo EH. Role of matrix metalloproteinases in delayed neuronal damage after transient global cerebral ischemia. J Neurosci. 2004;24:671–8.
23. Copin JC, Gasche Y. Matrix metalloproteinase-9 deficiency has no effect on glial scar formation after transient focal cerebral ischemia in mouse. Brain Res. 2007;1150:167–73.
24. Nagel S, Su Y, Horstmann S, Heiland S, Gardner H, Koziol J, et al. Minocycline and hypothermia for reperfusion injury after focal cerebral ischemia in the rat: effects on BBB breakdown and MMP expression in the acute and subacute phase. Brain Res. 2008;1188:198–206.
25. Gu Z, Kaul M, Yan B, Kridel SJ, Cui J, Strongin A, et al. S-nitrosylation of matrix metalloproteinases: signaling pathway to neuronal cell death. Science 2002;297:1186–90.
26. Yamaguchi M, Jadhav V, Obenaus A, Colohan A, Zhang JH. Matrix metalloproteinase inhibition attenuates brain edema in an in vivo model of surgically-induced brain injury. Neurosurgery 2007;61:1067–75; discussion 1075–1066.
27. Machado LS, Kozak A, Ergul A, Hess DC, Borlongan CV, Fagan SC. Delayed minocycline inhibits ischemia-activated matrix metalloproteinases 2 and 9 after experimental stroke. BMC Neurosci. 2006;7:56.
28. Yenari MA, Xu L, Tang XN, Qiao Y, Giffard RG. Microglia potentiate damage to blood-brain barrier constituents: improvement by minocycline in vivo and in vitro. Stroke 2006;37:1087–93.
29. Xu L, Fagan SC, Waller JL, Edwards D, Borlongan CV, Zheng J, et al. Low dose intravenous minocycline is neuroprotective after middle cerebral artery occlusion-reperfusion in rats. BMC Neurol. 2004;4:7.
30. Lee CZ, Xue Z, Zhu Y, Yang GY, Young WL. Matrix metalloproteinase-9 inhibition attenuates vascular endothelial growth factor-induced intracerebral hemorrhage. Stroke 2007;38:2563–8.

Tyrosine Phosphatase Inhibition Attenuates Early Brain Injury After Subarachnoid Hemorrhage in Rats

Yu Hasegawa, Hidenori Suzuki, Prativa Sherchan, Yan Zhan, Kamil Duris, and John H. Zhang

Abstract *Purpose*: Sodium orthovanadate (SOV) is a representative tyrosine phosphatase inhibitor and has been shown to ameliorate neuronal injury in cerebral ischemia. We hypothesized that tyrosine phosphatase inhibition by SOV might attenuate early brain injury after subarachnoid hemorrhage (SAH) in this study.

Methods: The endovascular perforation model of SAH was produced and animals were randomly assigned to sham-operated rats, saline-treated (vehicle), and 10 mg/kg of SOV-treated SAH rats. Drugs were injected intraperitoneally immediately after SAH induction. Neurological score and brain water content (BWC) were assessed at 24 h after SAH. Cell injury was studied by terminal deoxynucleotidyl transferase-mediated uridine 5′-triphosphate-biotin nick end-labeling (TUNEL) at 24 h after SAH.

Results: Severity of SAH and mortality in SOV-treated rats was similar to that of the saline group. SOV significantly decreased BWC and improved neurological score at 24 h after SAH compared with the saline group. SOV decreased TUNEL-positive cells at 24 h after SAH compared with the saline group.

Conclusions: These data suggest that tyrosine phosphatase inhibition by SOV ameliorates early brain injury after SAH.

Keywords Brain edema · Early brain injury · Sodium orthovanadate · Subarachnoid hemorrhage · Tyrosine phosphatase inhibition

Introduction

Subarachnoid hemorrhage (SAH) is a life-threatening disease. Mortality at 1 month in SAH patients was 45%, of which around 60% occurred within the first 2 days of onset because of the initial bleeding [1]. The major causes of death and disability may be early brain injury and cerebral vasospasm after SAH. Although cerebral vasospasm has been studied and treated by a lot of drugs, the outcome is not improved even if angiographic vasospasm is reversed. Thus, early brain injury, which occurs within 48 h following cerebral aneurysm rupture, has been considered as a new target for improving the outcome of SAH [2].

Sodium orthovanadate (SOV), which is a tyrosine phosphatase inhibitor, was reported to ameliorate ischemic neuronal injury following transient middle cerebral artery occlusion in rats via activation of Akt, which is a key anti-apoptotic factor [4, 5]. In this study, we hypothesized that the tyrosine phosphatase inhibition by SOV might attenuate early brain injury after experimental SAH.

Materials and Methods

Experimental Animals

All experiments were approved by the Institutional Animal Care and Use Committee of Loma Linda University. 30 male Sprague-Dawley rats (Harlan, Indianapolis, Ind) were divided randomly into the following groups: sham-operated group (n = 9), saline-treated SAH group (vehicle; saline group: n = 10), and 10 mg/kg of SOV-treated SAH group (SOV group: n = 11).

Induction of Subarachnoid Hemorrhage

Anesthesia was induced with 5% isoflurane and maintained with 2.5% isoflurane, 30% oxygen, and 70% medical air via a face mask. Mean arterial blood pressure, heart rate, arterial blood gases, and blood glucose levels at pre- and post-operative time points were analyzed via the left femoral artery. The rectal temperature was monitored and kept at 36.5 ± 0.5°C by using a feedback-regulated heating system during surgery.

The SAH model was produced as described previously [8]. Briefly, the left common carotid artery (CCA) was exposed and 4–0 sharpened nylon sutures were advanced to the left internal carotid artery until resistance was felt and perforated to the place. Immediately after surgery, saline or 10 mg/kg of SOV (in saline) were injected intraperitoneally.

SAH Severity

The severity of SAH (n = 9 per group) was evaluated by using the SAH grading scale at the time of sacrifice [9]. Briefly, the basal cistern was divided into six segments. Each segment was allotted a grade from 0 to 3 depending on the amount of subarachnoid blood in the segments. The animals received a total score ranging from 0 to 18 after adding the scores from all six segments.

Measurement of Brain Water Content

Animals were decapitated at 24 h after SAH induction (n = 5). The brains were quickly removed and the left cerebral hemispheres (side of perforation) were cut from the brains. After measuring the weights (wet weight), they were kept in an oven at 105°C for 72 h and weighed again (dry weight). The following formula was used to calculate the percentage of water content: [(wet weight − dry weight)/wet weight] × 100% [8].

Neurological Scoring and Mortality

A 22-point scoring system (higher scores indicate greater function) was used to evaluate the neurological deficit at 24 h after SAH (n = 5 per group) using a modification of the method described by Garcia et al. [3]. Mortality was calculated at 24 h after SAH.

Terminal Deoxynucleotidyl Transferase-Mediated Uridine 5′-Triphosphate-Biotin Nick End-Labeling (TUNEL) Staining

Samples from sham-operated, saline- and SOV-treated rats were used for experiments (n = 4 per group). At 24 h after SAH, the rat brains were fixed by cardiovascular perfusion with phosphate-buffered saline and 10% paraformaldehyde and postfixed in 10% paraformaldehyde followed by 30% sucrose (weight/volume) for 3 days. 10-micron-thick coronal sections at the level of bregma-2 mm were cut on cryostat (Leica Microsystems LM3050S) and mounted on poly-L-lysine-coated slides.

Brain sections were evaluated by TUNEL staining using an in situ cell death detection kit (Roche Inc., Mannheim, Germany). A mixture of FITC-labeled nucleotides and terminal deoxynucleotidyl transferase was applied onto the brain sections for 60 min at 37°C in a dark humidified chamber as previously described [10].

Statistical Analysis

All values are expressed as the mean ± SD. Statistical differences among the various groups were assessed with one-way analysis of variance followed by Scheffe post hoc analysis. Comparisons between two groups were assessed by unpaired *t* test. Differences of P < 0.05 were considered significant.

Results

Mortality

The 24 h mortality rate was as follows: 10% (1 of 10 rats) in the saline group, 18% (2 of 11 rats) in the SOV group. There was no mortality in the sham-operated group. There were no statistical differences among the groups with regard to arterial blood pressure, heart rate, arterial blood gases, and blood glucose levels before and after SAH (data not shown).

SAH Grade

The average SAH grading score was 12 ± 3.1 and 12.4 ± 2.4 in the saline and the SOV groups, respectively, at 24 h after SAH (Fig. 1a).

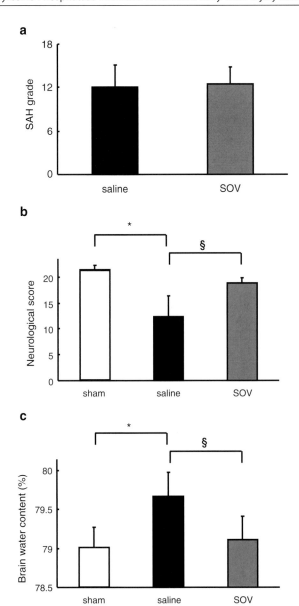

Fig. 1 SAH grade (**a**; n = 9, each group), neurological score (**b**; n = 5, each group), and brain water content in the left cerebral hemisphere (**c**; n = 5, each group) in the saline- or 10 mg/kg of SOV-treated rats, and/or the sham-operated rats at 24 h after SAH induction. Values are the mean ± SD; *$P < 0.05$ vs. sham-operated group; §$P < 0.05$ vs. saline group

Neurological Score and Brain Water Content

Neurological score was decreased and brain water content in the left cerebral hemisphere was significantly increased in the saline group compared with the sham-operated group at 24 h after SAH (Fig. 1b, c). SOV significantly improved the neurological score and brain water content in the left cerebral hemisphere compared with the saline group at 24 h after SAH.

DNA Fragmentation After SAH

Although many TUNEL-positive cells were observed in the saline group in the left temporal basal cortex after SAH, they were markedly decreased in the SOV group (Fig. 2). There were no TUNEL-positive cells in the sham-operated group.

Conclusion

The current study showed that tyrosine phosphatase inhibition by SOV ameliorated early brain injury after SAH. The protective effect might be due to the retention of receptor tyrosine kinase activation caused by SOV. Previously, we demonstrated that SOV had a neuroprotective effect via Akt activation in cerebral ischemia [4, 5]. Therefore, SOV-induced attenuation of early brain injury after SAH might be associated with the anti-apoptotic mechanism.

It was reported that the activation of the tyrosine kinase pathway in the vascular smooth muscle cells caused cerebral vasospasm, and genistein, which is a tyrosine kinase inhibitor, reversed vasospasm, although the effect on neurological outcome has not been studied [12]. Some publications have reported the relationship between receptor tyrosine kinases and early brain injury after SAH. Vascular endothelial growth factor (VEGF), which is one of the receptor tyrosine kinase ligands, increased in the cerebral artery within 24 h

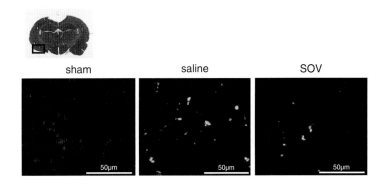

Fig. 2 Evaluation of cell death using TUNEL staining in the saline- or 10 mg/kg of SOV-treated rats, and the sham-operated rats at 24 h after SAH induction (n = 4, respectively)

after SAH and increased permeability of the blood–brain barrier [7]. On the other hand, it has been reported that the VEGF receptors were upregulated in the cortex after SAH and might be an intrinsic protective mechanism in the process of SAH [11]. Moreover, there are many papers about various kinds of receptor tyrosine kinase activation in cerebral ischemia, most of which showed neuroprotective effects [6]. Even though further evidence is needed for clarifying the exact mechanism, the role of receptor tyrosine kinases may be different depending on the type of receptor tyrosine kinase and the localization in the brain including neurons, glia, and endothelial cells.

In conclusion, we suggest that tyrosine phosphatase inhibition by SOV has a protective effect in early brain injury after SAH. Since SOV has been used to treat patients with diabetes mellitus, it may be a good candidate for the treatment of early brain injury after human SAH.

Acknowledgments This study was partially supported by grants (NS053407) from the National Institutes of Health to J.H.Z.

Conflict of interest statement We declare that we have no conflict of interest.

References

1. Broderick JP, Brott TG, Duldner JE, Tomsick T, Leach A. Initial and recurrent bleeding are the major causes of death following subarachnoid hemorrhage. Stroke 1994;25:1342–7.
2. Cahill J, Zhang JH. Subarachnoid hemorrhage: is it time for a new direction? Stroke 2009;40:S86–7.
3. Garcia JH, Liu KF, Ho KL. Neuronal necrosis after middle cerebral artery occlusion in Wistar rats progresses at different time intervals in the caudoputamen and the cortex. Stroke 1995;26:636–42.
4. Hasegawa Y, Hamada J, Morioka M, Yano S, Kawano T, Kai Y, et al. Neuroprotective effect of postischemic administration of sodium orthovanadate in rats with transient middle cerebral artery occlusion. J Cereb Blood Flow Metab. 2003;23:1040–51.
5. Hasegawa Y, Morioka M, Hasegawa S, Matsumoto J, Kawano T, Kai Y, et al. Therapeutic time window and dose dependence of neuroprotective effects of sodium orthovanadate following transient middle cerebral artery occlusion in rats. J Pharmacol Exp Ther. 2006;317:875–81.
6. Kooijman R, Sarre S, Michotte Y, De Keyser J. Insulin-like growth factor I: a potential neuroprotective compound for the treatment of acute ischemic stroke? Stroke 2009;40:83–8.
7. Kusaka G, Ishikawa M, Nanda A, Granger DN, Zhang JH. Signaling pathways for early brain injury after subarachnoid hemorrhage. J Cereb Blood Flow Metab. 2004;24:916–25.
8. Sozen T, Tsuchiyama R, Hasegawa Y, Suzuki H, Jadhav V, Nishizawa S, et al. Role of interleukin-1beta in early brain injury after subarachnoid hemorrhage in mice. Stroke 2009;40:2519–25.
9. Sugawara T, Ayer R, Jadhav V, Zhang JH. A new grading system evaluating bleeding scale in filament perforation subarachnoid hemorrhage rat model. J Neurosci Methods. 2008;167:327–34.
10. Sun Y, Zhou C, Polk P, Nanda A, Zhang JH. Mechanisms of erythropoietin-induced brain protection in neonatal hypoxia-ischemia rat model. J Cereb Blood Flow Metab. 2004;24:259–70.
11. Sun BL, Xia ZL, Hu DM, Niu JZ, Yuan H, Ye WJ, et al. Expression of the receptors of VEGF and the influence of extract of Ginkgo biloba after cisternal injection of autologus arterial hemolysate in rats. Clin Hemorheol Microcirc. 2006;34:117–24.
12. Tani E, Matsumoto T. Continuous elevation of intracellular Ca^{2+} is essential for the development of cerebral vasospasm. Curr Vasc Pharmacol. 2004;2:13–21.

Protection of Minocycline on Early Brain Injury After Subarachnoid Hemorrhage in Rats

Zong-duo Guo, Hai-tao Wu, Xiao-chuan Sun, Xiao-dong Zhang, and John H. Zhang

Abstract Minocycline has been shown to be neuroprotective in cerebral ischemia and in other models of brain injury. Our goal is to observe the protection of minocycline on EBI after SAH and the mechanism. 48 adult male SD rats were randomly divided into four groups: the sham-operated group, SAH group, vehicle group (SAH + normal sodium), and minocycline group (SAH + minocycline). The SAH model was induced by injecting 300 μl of autologous arterial blood into the prechiasmatic cistern. Expressions of MMP-9 in the hippocampus were examined at 24 h by western blot and zymography. Western blot and zymography showed that the expression of total and active MMP-9 increased dramatically at 24 h after SAH compared with that of the sham group ($P < 0.01$). The clinical assessments got a lower score than that of the sham-operated group. After treated with minocycline, the expression of MMP-9 decreased significantly ($P < 0.01$ vs. vehicle group), and the clinical assessments improved. We conclude that minocycline can protect EBI after SAH, which may be related to the mechanism of inhibiting the expression of MMP-9 in the hippocampus.

Keywords Early brain injury · Matrix metalloproteinase 9 · Minocycline · Subarachnoid hemorrhage

Introduction

Subarachnoid hemorrhage (SAH) is a deadly stroke which has a high rate of morbidity and mortality worldwide. Although there have been some advances in treatment for SAH, the rates of morbidity and mortality have not changed in recent years [1]. More and more researchers have pointed out that early brain injury (EBI) is the primary cause of mortality in SAH patients [2]. We have also found that matrix metalloproteinase 9 (MMP-9) is involved in the pathological process of EBI after SAH [3]. Minocycline is a commonly used semi-synthetic tetracycline with anti-inflammatory and anti-apoptotic properties [4]. Some researchers have found that minocycline could inhibit MMP-9 expression, shown to be neuroprotective in many models of brain injury [5, 6]. Therefore, the current research is to find whether minocycline can improve EBI by inhibiting MMP-9 after SAH.

Materials and Methods

Experimental Groups

Forty-eight male Sprague-Dawley rats between 250 and 300 g were randomly assigned to four groups with 15 animals in each group: sham operated, SAH, SAH treated with vehicle, and SAH treated with minocycline groups. Rats were euthanized and brain samples were collected for MMP-9 expression and TUNEL staining. This protocol was evaluated and approved by the Animal Care and Use Committee at Chongqing Medical University in Chongqing, China.

Antibodies and Reagents

Gelatin was purchased from Sigma. MMP-9 mouse monoclonal antibody was purchased from Lab Vision Corporation.

SAH Rat Model

SAH induction was performed as reported previously with slight modifications [7]. Briefly, rats were anesthetized with

Table 1 Clinical Assessment

Category	Behavior	Score
Appetite	Finished meal	0
	Left meal unfinished	1
	Scarcely ate	2
Activity	Walk and reach at least three corners of the cage	0
	Walk with some stimulation	1
	Almost always lying down	2
Deficits	No deficits	0
	Unstable walk	1
	Impossible to walk	2

chloral hydrate (40 mg/kg IP). Animals were intubated, and respiration was maintained with a small animal respirator (Harvard Apparatus). Rectal temperature was maintained at 37°C with a heating pad. At either side of the skull, 3 mm from the midline and 5 mm anteriorly from the bregma, holes were drilled through the skull bone down to dura mater without perforation. Finally, a PE ten canula was introduced about 10 mm from the hole; 250 µL blood was withdrawn from the femoral artery and injected intracranially through the canula at a pressure equal to the mean arterial blood pressure (80–100 mmHg). Subsequently, the canula was removed and incisions closed. Minocycline (45 mg/kg body weight) was injected intraperitoneally at 30 min and 12 h after SAH induction. In the vehicle group, rats underwent SAH induction and were treated with the same volume of vehicle (DMSO in saline). In the sham group, rats were treated by the same protocol as described above except that no blood was injected after the canula was introduced.

Clinical Assessment

Three behavioral examinations were performed at 24 h after SAH using the scoring system reported by Yamaguchi et al. to record appetite, activity, and neurological deficits [8].

Preparation of Tissue Extracts

At 24 h after SAH, rats (n = 5 in each group) were deeply anesthetized. The brains were removed quickly, and hippocampi were dissected and frozen immediately in liquid nitrogen, stored at 80°C. Sham operated control rats were killed at the same time. Brain tissue extracts were prepared as previously described [9]. Briefly, brain samples were homogenized in lysis buffer on ice. After centrifugation, supernatant was collected, and total protein concentrations were determined using the Coomassie Brilliant Blue Method.

Gelatin Zymogram

Activity of MMP-9 was examined by gelatin zymography as described previously [10]. Prepared protein samples were loaded and separated by 10% Tris–glycine gel with 0.1% gelatin as substrate. After separation by electrophoresis, the gel was renatured and then incubated with developing buffer at 37°C for 24 h. After developing, the gel was stained with 0.5% Coomassie Blue R-250 for 30 min and then destained appropriately.

Western Blot

Western blot analysis was performed as described previously [10]. Briefly, equal amounts of protein were loaded in each lane of SDS–PAGE, electrophoresed, and transferred to a nitrocellulose membrane. The membrane was blocked with MMP-9 mouse monoclonal antibody and probed with anti-mouse IgG-horseradish peroxidase conjugated antibody. Densitometry analysis was performed with the ChemiDoc detection system (Bio-Rad) and Quantity One software (Bio-Rad).

Statistics

Data were expressed as mean ± SD. Statistical differences between individual groups were analyzed using 1-way ANOVA. P value of < 0.05 was considered statistically significant.

Results

Behavior Scores Assessment

The behavior scores for appetite, activity, and neurological deficit are shown in Fig. 1. The appetite score in the minocycline group was better than those in SAH and SAH+ DMSO groups at 24 h (P < 0.05; Fig. 1). No statistical difference was found between the SAH group and the vehicle group (P > 0.05). The activity of rats in the minocycline group was significantly better than those in the vehicle group (P < 0.05), and decreased to a level similar to that of the sham-operated group (P > 0.05). On the contrary, most rats did not have neurological deficits, and no significant difference was observed among the groups (P > 0.05).

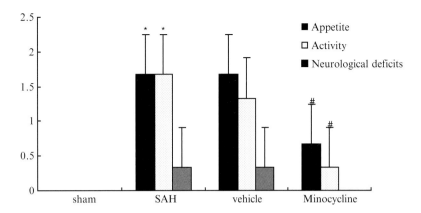

Fig. 1 Clinical assessment scores for appetite, activity, and neurological deficit. The appetite and activity of rats in minocycline group was significantly better than those in other groups at 24 h. No differences in neurological deficit were observed (P > 0.05). (*P < 0.05 vs. sham group, #P < 0.05 vs. SAH group)

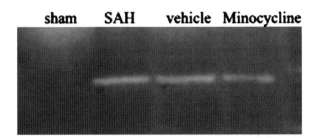

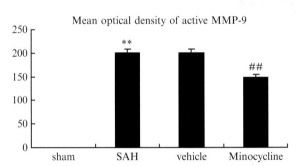

Fig. 2 Representative bands for active MMP-9 by zymography. Active MMP-9 was reduced significantly by minocycline treatment, but still higher than that of sham group. (**P < 0.01 vs. sham group, ##P < 0.01 vs. SAH group)

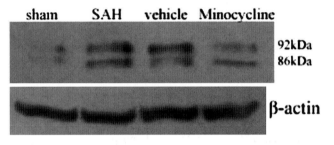

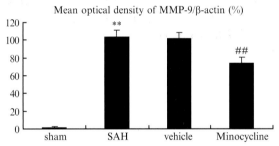

Fig. 3 Representative bands for total MMP-9 and β-actin by western blot. Total MMP-9 increased significantly at 24 h after SAH, and decreased by minocycline treatment. (**P < 0.01 vs. sham group, ##P < 0.01 vs. SAH group)

Evaluation of MMP-9 Protein

The protein level of MMP-9 in the rat hippocampus was evaluated using gelatin zymography. At 24 h after SAH, significantly increased activity of MMP-9 was found in the hippocampus of the SAH group as compared to that of the sham operated group (P < 0.01, Fig. 2). The densitometric analysis revealed that minocycline treatment significantly reduced the gelatin activity of MMP-9 (P < 0.01 vs. vehicle). The protein level of total MMP-9 was examined in the hippocampus by western blot. Quantification showed increased expression of MMP-9 in hippocampus at 24 h after SAH (P < 0.01 vs. sham, Fig. 3). Minocycline significantly reduced the SAH-induced increase in MMP-9 total protein concentration (P < 0.01 vs. vehicle).

Conclusion

In the previous study, we have observed that MMP-9 was activated in the early phase after SAH and inhibition of MMP-9 decreased the anoikis of neurons, reduced brain edema, and improved behavioral and activities of rats [3]. In the present study, we found minocycline could improve behavioral activities and decreased neuronal death by inhibiting MMP-9 expression.

It has been verified that the upregulation of MMP-9 in the cerebral arteries of rats after SAH [11]. After acute SAH, MMP-9 expression was increased in the microvasculature, which led to an acute loss of ECM from the cerebral microvasculature [12]. It has been shown that MMP-9 contributes to blood brain barrier damage and brain injury by degrading the components of ECM. Furthermore, research found that a higher MMP-9 level is apparent with vasospasm in SAH patients. Within the hippocampus, MMP-9 expression is upregulated in CA pyramidal after global cerebral ischemia [13]. MMP-9 appears to play a deleterious role under conditions of global ischemia, since both pharmacological inhibition and gene deletion of MMP-9 are neuroprotective in vivo [14, 15]. It was reported that treatment with minocycline can inhibit MMP-9 after temporary experimental cerebral ischemia [16]. Minocycline has been shown to be neuroprotective [17]. Because minocycline has been shown to be neuroprotective in different models of brain injury, it is likely to act by multiple mechanisms, with MMP-9 inhibition being a central link for its anti-inflammatory and anti-apoptotic properties [18]. Lee et al. found that MMP-9 expression increased in intracerebral hemorrhage (ICH) and minocycline could suppress MMP-9 and attenuate ICH [5]. This suggested the therapeutic potential of minocycline in brain protection.

In summary, our study has shown that MMP-9 inhibition by minocycline may reduce EBI after SAH. The role of minocycline in SAH treatment should be given more attention.

Conflict of interest statement We declare that we have no conflict of interest.

References

1. Schievink WI, Riedinger M, Jhutty TK, Simon P. Racial disparities in subarachnoid hemorrhage mortality: Los Angeles County, California, 1985–1998. Neuroepidemiology 2004;23:299–305.
2. Pluta RM, Hansen-Schwartz J, Dreier J, Vajkoczy P, Macdonald RL, Nishizawa S, et al. Cerebral vasospasm following subarachnoid hemorrhage: time for a new world of thought. Neurol Res. 2009;31:151–8.
3. Guo Z, Sun X, He Z, Jiang Y, Zhang X, Zhang JH. Matrix metalloproteinase-9 potentiates early brain injury after subarachnoid hemorrhage. Neurol Res. 2009;15:2.
4. Zemke D, Majid A. The potential of minocycline for neuroprotection in human neurologic disease. Clin Neuropharmacol. 2004;27:293–8.
5. Lee CZ, Xue Z, Zhu Y, Yang GY, Young WL. Matrix metalloproteinase-9 inhibition attenuates vascular endothelial growth factor-induced intracerebral hemorrhage. Stroke 2007;38:2563–8.
6. Sutton TA, Kelly KJ, Mang HE, Plotkin Z, Sandoval RM, Dagher PC. Minocycline reduces renal microvascular leakage in a rat model of ischemic renal injury. Am J Physiol Renal Physiol. 2005;288:F91–7.
7. Prunell GF, Mathiesen T, Diemer NH, Svendgaard NA. Experimental subarachnoid hemorrhage: subarachnoid blood volume, mortality rate, neuronal death, cerebral blood flow, and perfusion pressure in three different rat models. Neurosurgery 2003;52:165–75; discussion 175–166.
8. Yamaguchi M, Zhou C, Nanda A, Zhang JH. Ras protein contributes to cerebral vasospasm in a canine double-hemorrhage model. Stroke 2004;35:1750–5.
9. Kawakita K, Kawai N, Kuroda Y, Yasashita S, Nagao S. Expression of matrix metalloproteinase-9 in thrombin-induced brain edema formation in rats. J Stroke Cerebrovasc Dis. 2006;15:88–95.
10. Sifringer M, Stefovska V, Zentner I, Hansen B, Stepulak A, Knaute C, et al. The role of matrix metalloproteinases in infant traumatic brain injury. Neurobiol Dis. 2007;25:526–35.
11. Vikman P, Beg S, Khurana TS, Hansen-Schwartz J, Edvinsson L. Gene expression and molecular changes in cerebral arteries following subarachnoid hemorrhage in the rat. J Neurosurg. 2006;105:438–44.
12. Sehba FA, Mostafa G, Knopman J, Friedrich V Jr, Bederson JB. Acute alterations in microvascular basal lamina after subarachnoid hemorrhage. J Neurosurg. 2004;101:633–40.
13. Lee SR, Tsuji K, Lo EH. Role of matrix metalloproteinases in delayed neuronal damage after transient global cerebral ischemia. J Neurosci. 2004;24:671–8.
14. Copin JC, Gasche Y. Matrix metalloproteinase-9 deficiency has no effect on glial scar formation after transient focal cerebral ischemia in mouse. Brain Res. 2007;1150:167–73.
15. Nagel S, Su Y, Horstmann S, Heiland S, Gardner H, Koziol J, et al. Minocycline and hypothermia for reperfusion injury after focal cerebral ischemia in the rat: effects on BBB breakdown and MMP expression in the acute and subacute phase. Brain Res. 2008;1188:198–206.
16. Machado LS, Kozak A, Ergul A, Hess DC, Borlongan CV, Fagan SC. Delayed minocycline inhibits ischemia-activated matrix metalloproteinases 2 and 9 after experimental stroke. BMC Neurosci. 2006;7:56.
17. Stirling DP, Koochesfahani KM, Steeves JD, Tetzlaff W. Minocycline as a neuroprotective agent. Neuroscientist 2005;11:308–22.
18. Xu L, Fagan SC, Waller JL, Edwards D, Borlongan CV, Zheng J, et al. Low dose intravenous minocycline is neuroprotective after middle cerebral artery occlusion-reperfusion in rats. BMC Neurol. 2004;4:7.

Role of Osteopontin in Early Brain Injury After Subarachnoid Hemorrhage in Rats

Hidenori Suzuki, Robert Ayer, Takashi Sugawara, Wanqiu Chen, Takumi Sozen, Yu Hasegawa, Kenji Kanamaru, and John H. Zhang

Abstract *Background*: Subarachnoid hemorrhage (SAH)-induced early brain injury (EBI) contributes to delayed ischemic neurological deficits, one of whose key pathologic manifestation is the blood–brain barrier (BBB) disruption. Although post-SAH BBB breakdown is a self-repairable phenomenon, the molecular pathways are unknown. We determined the role of osteopontin (OPN), a pleiotropic extracellular matrix glycoprotein, in the post-SAH BBB disruption in rats.

Method: First, we produced the endovascular perforation model of SAH and studied if OPN is induced in the brain after SAH. Secondly, we examined the effects of blockage of endogenous OPN induction on neurological impairments and BBB disruption. Thirdly, we evaluated the effects of exogenous OPN on neurological impairments, brain edema and BBB disruption, and the related protein expression levels.

Findings: OPN was significantly induced and peaked at 72 h after SAH, in the recovery phase of EBI. OPN small interfering RNA significantly aggravated neurological impairment and BBB disruption 72 h after SAH. Exogenous OPN significantly prevented neurological impairment, brain edema and BBB disruption associated with the deactivation of nuclear factor-κB activity, the inhibition of matrix metalloproteinase (MMP)-9 induction and tissue inhibitor of MMP-1 reduction, and the consequent preservation of cerebral microvessel basal lamina protein laminin and tight junction protein zona occludens-1.

Conclusions: These findings suggest the protective effects of OPN against BBB disruption after SAH, a finding which should provide a novel therapeutic approach for post-SAH EBI.

Keywords Blood–brain barrier · Brain injury · Osteopontin · Subarachnoid hemorrhage

Introduction

Osteopontin (OPN) is a secreted pleiotropic extracellular matrix glycoprotein that is involved in both physiological and pathological processes in a wide range of tissue [1]. In the central nervous system (CNS), OPN has been most extensively studied in multiple sclerosis, and its corresponding animal model, experimental autoimmune encephalomyelitis, where it is strongly implicated in the exacerbation of disease activity through the promotion of T-cell survival [2]. However, there is compelling evidence that OPN can, in a variety of situations, help cells survive an otherwise lethal insult [3]. OPN is induced in response to tissue injuries or inflammation, and may play a role in the maintenance of tissue homeostasis and the induction of tissue repair or remodeling [3]. Although the precise function of OPN in the CNS remains unknown, its induced expression has been demonstrated in activated microglia and reactive astrocytes after focal ischemic stroke [4]. The absence of endogenous OPN did not change the infarct size after transient [5] or permanent [6] focal cerebral ischemia, but increased delayed retrograde degeneration of the ipsilateral thalamus associated with pronounced microglia activation and inflammatory gene expression [6]. On the other hand, the administration of recombinant OPN (r-OPN) markedly reduced the infarct size via anti-apoptotic actions [5]. We therefore hypothesized that OPN might act as an intrinsic protective mechanism against early brain injury (EBI), and evaluated the functional significance of OPN in EBI after SAH.

H. Suzuki, T. Sugawara, W. Chen, T. Sozen, and Y. Hasegawa
Department of Physiology, Loma Linda University School of Medicine, Loma Linda, CA 92354, USA

R. Ayer and J.H. Zhang (✉)
Department of Physiology, Loma Linda University School of Medicine, Loma Linda, CA 92354, USA
Department of Neurosurgery, Loma Linda University of Medicine, Loma Linda, CA 92354, USA
e-mail: johnzhang3910@yahoo.com

K. Kanamaru
Department of Neurosurgery, Suzuka Kaisei Hospital, Suzuka, Japan

Materials and Methods

All protocols were evaluated and approved by the Institutional Animal Care and Use Committee of Loma Linda University.

Experimental Model of SAH and Study Protocol

A total of 163 male adult Sprague-Dawley rats (300–370 g, Harlan, Indianapolis, IN) were used. The endovascular perforation model of SAH was produced as previously described [7, 8]. First, 22 rats were randomly assigned to one of four groups: Pre-SAH (n = 4), 24-h SAH (n = 6), 72-h SAH (n = 6), and 120-h (n = 6) SAH groups. Pre-SAH rats were healthy controls, and 24-, 72- and 120-h SAH rats were sacrificed at 24, 72 and 120 h post-SAH, respectively. Neurological scores, severity of SAH and OPN expression levels were evaluated. Secondly, 28 SAH rats were treated with OPN small interfering RNA (siRNA; n = 14) or negative control siRNA (n = 14). Neurological scores were evaluated prior to and after SAH at each interval of 24 h until the sacrifice. Surviving rats were sacrificed at 72 h post-SAH, and the severity of SAH, OPN expression levels and BBB permeability were assessed. Sham-operated rats also received OPN siRNA or a sham intracerebroventricular injection and subsequently underwent the same assessments (n = 3, respectively). Thirdly, 107 rats were divided into three groups: sham-operated rats treated with vehicle (n = 23), and SAH rats treated with vehicle (n = 45) or r-OPN (n = 39). Surviving rats were sacrificed at 24 or 72 h post-surgery. In addition to neurological evaluation, the brain water content measurements and Western blot analyses were performed at 24 h and BBB permeability was determined at 24 and 72 h post-surgery.

Neurological Scoring and SAH Grading

Neurological scores and the severity of SAH were evaluated in a blinded fashion as previously described [7].

Intracerebroventricular Infusion of siRNA or r-OPN

Drugs or siRNA were administered by an intracerebroventricular infusion as previously reported [9]. OPN siRNA (sense, 5′-CUAUCAAGGUCAUCCCAGU[dT][dT]-3′, and antisense, 5′-ACUGGGAUGACCUUGAUAG[dT][dT]-3′; Sigma-Aldrich, St. Louis, MO) or irrevelant control siRNA (Dharmacon/Thermo Fisher Scientific, Lafayette, CO) at 500 pmol/1 μL in sterile phosphate-buffered saline was injected at a rate of 0.5 μL/min at 24 h before the SAH production or sham-operation. Sterile saline vehicle (1 μL) or mouse r-OPN (0.1 μg in 1 μL; EMD Chemicals, La Jolla, CA) was infused at a rate of 0.1 μL/min irrespective of the animal's body weight at 1 h before the animal model production. In rats having a sham intracerebroventricular infusion, a burr hole was perforated on the skull at the same position, but neither needle insertion nor drug infusion was received.

Brain Water Content and BBB Permeability

Brains were divided into the right and left cerebral hemispheres, brain stem and cerebellum, and water content or Evans blue extravasation was measured as previously described [10].

Western Blot Analyses

Western blot analysis was performed using the following primary antibodies as described previously [10]: mouse anti-OPN, rabbit anti-IκB-α, goat anti-phospho-IκB-α, goat anti-phospho-IκB kinase (IKK)α/β, goat anti-β-Actin (a loading control) antibodies (Santa Cruz Biotechnology, Santa Cruz, CA), goat anti-interleukin (IL)-1β antibody (BioVision, Mountain View, CA), rabbit anti-zona occludens (ZO)-1 antibody (Invitrogen, Carlsbad, CA), rabbit anti-matrix metalloproteinase (MMP)-9, mouse anti-tissue inhibitor of MMP (TIMP)-1 antibodies (Millipore, Temecula, CA), and mouse anti-laminin antibody (EMD Chemicals, La Jolla, CA).

Statistics

All values were expressed as mean ± SD. Unpaired t test, chi-square test and repeated-measures ANOVA with Scheffe correction were used as appropriate. $P < 0.05$ was considered statistically significant.

Results

OPN Expression Levels in the Brain After SAH

Subarachnoid blood was cleared from the basal cisterns as time passed, but significant hemorrhage remained even at 120 h post-SAH. Neurological deficits peaked at 48 h and began to recover 72 h post-SAH. OPN was significantly induced in the bilateral cerebral hemispheres, cerebellum and brain stem and peaked at 72 h post-SAH.

Effects of Endogenous OPN Inhibition

OPN inhibition resulted in significantly worse neurological scores and BBB breakdown at 72 h post-SAH (Fig. 1). OPN siRNA treatment did not affect neurological scores and Evans blue extravasation in the sham-operated rats (n = 3).

Effects of r-OPN

Mild SAH rats (SAH grading score of 9 or less at 24 h or 6 or less at 72 h post-SAH) treated with vehicle did not significantly increase Evans blue extravasation in comparison with sham-operated rats. Thus, further analysis was performed on severe SAH rats (SAH grading score of 10 or more at 24 h or 7 or more at 72 h post-SAH).

r-OPN significantly prevented neurological impairment, BBB disruption and brain edema compared with the control SAH groups at 24 (and 72) h post-SAH (Fig. 2a–c). Western blot analyses (Fig. 2d) showed that SAH significantly increased active MMP-9 expression and decreased TIMP-1 expression, which were significantly inhibited by r-OPN. The degradation of laminin and ZO-1 was also significantly suppressed by r-OPN. Active IL-1β levels were significantly elevated in SAH rats, but was not suppressed by r-OPN. Post-SAH activation of NF-κB as assessed by increased phosphorylation of IKKα/β and IκB-α along with a degradation of IκB-α was significantly inhibited by r-OPN. Interestingly, r-OPN treatment decreased endogenous OPN expression levels in the brain. This finding may reflect the decreased brain damage after the r-OPN treatment, or suggest the existence of an endogenous negative feedback system being influenced by the presence of r-OPN.

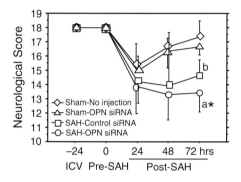

Fig. 1 Effects of OPN siRNA on neurological score ICV, intracerebroventricular infusion; ANOVA, *$P < 0.05$ vs. SAH rats treated with control siRNA; $^{a}P < 0.0001$, $^{b}P < 0.0025$ vs. sham-operated rats; error bar, standard deviation

Conclusion

The present study demonstrated that OPN was induced during initial recovery from EBI in a rat model of SAH; and that the blockage of endogenous OPN expression predisposed the brain to greater injury. Moreover, pre-SAH administration of exogenous OPN significantly prevented EBI as measured by neurological impairment, brain edema, and

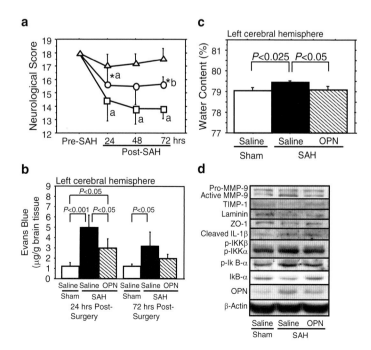

Fig. 2 Effects of r-OPN on neurological score (**a**), Evans blue extravasation (**b**), brain water content (**c**) and protein expression levels on Western blots (**d**) in the left cerebral hemisphere *Triangle*, sham-operated rats; *square*, SAH rats treated with vehicle; *circle*, SAH rats treated with r-OPN; ANOVA, *$P < 0.05$ vs. SAH+vehicle rats; $^{a}P < 0.005$, $^{b}P < 0.05$ vs. sham-operated rats; error bar, standard deviation

BBB disruption. This protection was provided by OPN-mediated deactivation of NF-κB activity, thereby improving the balance between proteolytic (MMP-9) and matrix stabilizing factors (TIMP-1). These findings suggest that OPN may represent a naturally occurring protective factor against EBI after SAH.

A key pathologic manifestation of EBI after SAH is BBB disruption, leading to vasogenic edema. BBB dysfunction may allow greater influx of blood-borne cells and substances into brain parenchyma, thus amplifying inflammation, causing further parenchymal damage and edema formation [11]. However, post-SAH BBB breakdown is a transient phenomenon and a functional recovery may ensue. Sehba et al. [12] reported that even an acute loss of collagen IV from the cerebral microvasculature due to MMP-9 induction recovered within 48 h after SAH in an endovascular puncture model of rats. A clarification of the intrinsic mechanisms to reverse BBB disruption may lead to a novel therapeutic approach for the treatment of EBI.

A balanced interaction between MMP-9 and TIMP-1 may determine the severity of BBB disruption and neuronal apoptosis after insults [13]. The activation of NF-κB has been detected in the cerebral cortices adjacent to SAH [11], and is known to directly regulate the transcription of MMP-9 and TIMP-1 in addition to orchestrating the inflammatory cascade [14, 15]. OPN alone has no effect on MMP-9 and NF-κB activity in various non-tumor culture cells [16, 17]. However, there are several studies demonstrating OPN's role as an inhibitor of MMP-9 and NF-κB activity in the presence of pro-inflammatory cytokine, IL-1β [16, 17]. Our data also demonstrate OPN's role as an inhibitor of MMP-9 and NF-κB activity in the presence of IL-1β elevation following SAH. IL-1β-induced MMP-9 secretion from astrocytes is critically dependant on NF-κB signaling pathways [18].

It has been reported that IL-1β induces OPN up-regulation [1]. However, our study showed that r-OPN treatment decreased endogenous OPN induction irrespective of IL-1β levels. To explain these findings we propose the presence of a mechanism in which IL-1β-induced NF-κB activity regulates itself through OPN negative feedback in a process that is all downstream of IL-1β [17]. SAH-induced IL-1β stimulates NF-κB activity which in turn induces endogenous OPN and MMP-9 activity through divergent pathways. OPN expression levels negatively feedback on NF-κB, thereby having an inhibitory influence on MMP-9 which is downstream of NF-κB. This mechanism demonstrates how r-OPN influences endogenous OPN levels as well as providing neuroprotection against NF-κB-dependent MMP-9 induction and EBI following SAH (Fig. 3).

Most molecular targets for therapy have biphasic roles in stroke pathophysiology: signals that mediate cell death during the acute stage of stroke might promote repair during the recovery phase [19]. Approaches to augment endogenous

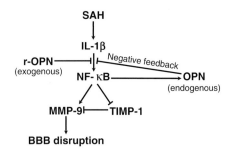

Fig. 3 Possible mechanisms showing the relationships between SAH-induced BBB disruption and protective effects of OPN against it. Post-SAH IL-1β-induced NF-κB activation may cause BBB disruption, while NF-κB may induce endogenous OPN which feedback regulates NF-κB

protective pathways might be more likely to succeed than those that aim to block targets that are detrimental to recovery. OPN is potentially one of these therapies, and our findings warrant more research.

Acknowledgments This study was partially supported by grants (NS053407) from the National Institutes of Health to J.H.Z.

Conflict of interest statement We declare that we have no conflict of interest.

References

1. Mazzali M, Kipari T, Ophascharoensuk V, Wesson JA, Johnson R, Hughes J. Osteopontin. A molecule for all seasons. Q J Med. 2002;95:3–13.
2. Chabas D, Baranzini SE, Mitchell D, Bernard CCA, Rittling SR, Denhardt DT, et al. The influence of the proinflammatory cytokine, osteopontin, on autoimmune demyelinating disease. Science 2001;294:1731–5.
3. Denhardt DT, Noda M, O'Regan AW, Pavlin D, Berman JS. Osteopontin as a means to cope with environmental insults: regulation of inflammation, tissue remodeling, and cell survival. J Clin Invest. 2001;107:1055–61.
4. Kang W-S, Choi J-S, Shin Y-J, Kim H-Y, Cha J-H, Lee J-Y, et al. Differential regulation of osteopontin receptors, CD44 and the $α_v$ and $β_3$ integrin subunits, in the rat hippocampus following transient forebrain ischemia. Brain Res. 2008;1228:208–16.
5. Meller R, Stevens SL, Minami M, Cameron JA, King S, Rosenzweig H, et al. Neuroprotection by osteopontin in stroke. J Cereb Blood Flow Metab. 2005;25:217–25.
6. Schroeter M, Zickler P, Denhardt DT, Hartung HP, Jander S. Increased thalamic neurodegeneration following ischaemic cortical stroke in osteopontin-deficient mice. Brain 2006;129:1426–37.
7. Sugwara T, Ayer R, Jadhav V, Zhang JH. A new grading system evaluating bleeding scale in filament perforation subarachnoid hemorrhage rat model. J Neurosci Methods. 2007;167:327–34.
8. Ayer RE, Sugawara T, Chen W, Tong W, Zhang JH. Melatonin decreases mortality following severe subarachnoid hemorrhage. J Pineal Res. 2008;44:197–204.
9. Allen RM, Uban KA, Atwood EM, Albeck DS, Yamamoto DJ. Continuous intracerebroventricular infusion of the competitive NMDA receptor antagonist, LY235959, facilitates escalation of

cocaine self-administration and increases break point for cocaine in Sprague-Dawley rats. Pharmacol Biochem Behav. 2007;88: 82–8.
10. Yatsushige H, Ostrowski RP, Tsubokawa T, Colohan A, Zhang JH. Role of c-Jun N-terminal kinase in early brain injury after subarachnoid hemorrhage. J Neurosci Res. 2007;85:1436–48.
11. Simard JM, Geng Z, Woo SK, Ivanova S, Tosun C, Melnichenko L, et al. Glibenclamide reduces inflammation, vasogenic edema, and caspase-3 activation after subarachnoid hemorrhage. J Cereb Blood Flow Metab. 2009;29:317–30.
12. Sehba FA, Mostafa G, Knopman J, Friedrich Jr. V., Bederson JB. Acute alterations in microvascular basal lamina after subarachnoid hemorrhage. J Neurosurg. 2004;101:633–40.
13. Fujimoto M, Takagi Y, Aoki T, Hayase M, Marumo T, Gomi M, et al. Tissue inhibitor of metalloproteinases protect blood-brain barrier disruption in focal cerebral ischemia. J Cereb Blood Flow Metab. 2008;28:1674–85.
14. Bond M, Chase AJ, Baker AH, Newby AC. Inhibition of transcription factor NF-κB reduces matrix metalloproteinase-1, -3 and -9 production by vascular smooth muscle cells. Cardiovasc Res. 2001;50:556–65.
15. Trescher K, Bernecker O, Fellner B, Gyongyosi M, Schafer R, Aharinejad S, et al. Inflammation and postinfarct remodeling: overexpression of IκB prevents ventricular dilation via increasing TIMP levels. Cardiovasc Res. 2006;69:746–54.
16. Xie Z, Singh M, Singh K. Differential regulation of matrix metalloproteinase-2 and -9 expression and activity in adult rat cardiac fibroblasts in response to interleukin-1β. J Biol Chem. 279:39513–9.
17. Arafat HA, Katakam AK, Chipitsyna G, Gong Q, Vancha AR, Gabbeta J, et al. Osteopontin protects the islets and β-cells from interleukin-1β-mediated cytotoxicity through negative feedback regulation of nitric oxide. Endocrinology 2007;148:575–84.
18. Wu CY, Hsieh HL, Jou MJ, Yang CM. Involvement of p42/p44 MAPK, p38 MAPK, JNK and nuclear factor-kappa B in interleukin-1beta-induced matrix metalloproteinase-9 expression in rat brain astrocytes. J Neurochem. 2004;90:1477–88.
19. Lo EH. A new penumbra: transitioning from injury into repair after stroke. Nat Med. 2008;14:497–500.

Matrix Metalloproteinase 9 Inhibition Reduces Early Brain Injury in Cortex After Subarachnoid Hemorrhage

Zong-duo Guo, Xiao-dong Zhang, Hai-tao Wu, Bin Lin, Xiao-chuan Sun, and John H. Zhang

Abstract This study investigated the role of matrix metalloproteinase-9 (MMP-9) in early brain injury (EBI) after subarachnoid hemorrhage (SAH). Sprague-Dawley male rats (n = 30) between 250 and 300 g were used. SAH was produced by injecting autologous arterial blood into the prechiasmatic cistern. SB-3CT, a selective MMP-9 inhibitor, was injected intraperitoneally after SAH induction. MMP-9 protein expression was measured by western blot; laminin expression and neuronal cells in the cerebral cortex were studied by immunohistochemistry and TUNEL staining at 24 h after SAH. MMP-9 expression was increased after SAH and decreased by SB-3CT inhibition at 24 h after SAH ($P < 0.01$). Laminin, the substrate of MMP-9, was decreased at 24 h after SAH, and SB-3CT prevented laminin degradation. The number of TUNEL-positive neurons in cerebral cortex was increased after SAH and decreased by SB-3CT ($P < 0.01$). MMP-9 may be involved in EBI after SAH and inhibition of MMP-9 may reduce EBI in cerebral cortex.

Keywords Cell death · Early brain injury · Matrix metalloproteinase-9 · Subarachnoid hemorrhage

Introduction

Subarachnoid hemorrhage (SAH) is an important cause of death and disability of cerebrovascular diseases worldwide. The mortality of SAH is related mostly to the initial bleeding brain injury or called early brain injury (EBI) [1]. The major features of EBI include neuronal apoptosis, which contributes to the poor outcomes of SAH [9].

MMP-9 is able to cleave main components of extracellular matrix (ECM), especially laminin [3]. Activation of MMP-9, especially via laminin, may lead to apoptosis-like cell death, called anoikis in ischemic brain injury [3]. Selective inhibition of MMP-9 by SB-3CT may rescue laminin from proteolysis to prevent neuronal cell death [3]. In this study, we employed SB-3CT to investigate the role of MMP-9 in EBI after SAH in rats.

Subjects and Methods

This protocol was evaluated and approved by the Animal Care and Use Committee at Chongqing Medical University in Chongqing, China.

Subjects

30 male Sprague-Dawley rats between 250 and 300 g were randomly assigned to four groups with 15 animals in each group: sham operated, SAH, SAH treated with vehicle (SAH + DMSO), and SAH treated with SB-3CT (SAH + SB 3CT) groups. Rats were euthanized and brain samples were collected for MMP-9 expression, TUNEL staining and immunohistochemistry.

SAH Rat Model

SAH induction was performed as reported previously [4]. Briefly, rats were anesthetized with chloral hydrate (40 mg/kg IP). At either side of the skull, 3 mm from the midline and

5 mm anteriorly from the bregma, holes were drilled through the skull bone down to dura mater without perforation. Finally, a PE 10 canula was introduced about 10 mm from the hole; 250 μL blood was withdrawn from the femoral artery and injected intracranially through the canula at a pressure equal to the mean arterial blood pressure (80–100 mmHg). Subsequently, the canula was removed and incisions closed. MMP-9 inhibitor SB-3CT (25 mg/kg body weight) was injected intraperitoneally as a suspension in a vehicle solution (10% DMSO diluted in normal saline) at 2 and 5 h after SAH induction. In the vehicle group, rats underwent SAH induction and were treated with the same volume of vehicle (DMSO in saline). In the sham group, rats were treated by the same protocol as described above except that no blood was injected after the canula was introduced.

Antibodies and Reagents

MMP-9 mouse monoclonal antibody was purchased from Santa Cruz. Rabbit polyclonal antibody against laminin was purchased from Lab Vision Corporation. The TUNEL apoptosis assay kit was purchased from Roche Diagnostics.

Histology

At 24 h after SAH, rats were anesthetized and intracardially perfused with ice-cold PBS, pH 7.4, followed by 4% paraformaldehyde in PBS, pH 7.4 (n = 5 in each group). Brain were removed and immersed with 4% paraformaldehyde in PBS overnight at 4°C. Coronal sections (5 m thick) were prepared using Sham-operated control mice with a microtome.

For immunohistochemistry, brain sections were incubated overnight at 4°C with primary antibody rabbit polyclonal antibody against laminin (1:200). Sections were then incubated with goat anti-rabbit biotinylated secondary antibody and placed in avidin-biotin-peroxidase complex enzyme. Slides were visualized by incubation with 3, 3′-diaminobenzidine (DAB). Negative control sections received identical treatment except for the primary antibody. TUNEL staining was conducted according to the protocol of the manufacturer (Roche Diagnostics) as described. Briefly, brain sections were deparaffinaged, permeabilized, treated with 0.3% H_2O_2, and incubated with 150 U/mL terminal transferase and 2 ml biotin-16-dUTP for 1 h at 37°C. DNA degradation was visualized using DAB.

Preparation of Tissue Extracts

At 24 h after SAH, rats (n = 5 in each group) were deeply anesthetized and then the brains were removed quickly and cerebral cortexes were dissected and frozen immediately in liquid nitrogen, and stored at 80°C. Sham operated control rats were killed at the same time. Brain tissue extracts were prepared as previously described [5]. Briefly, brain samples were homogenized in lysis buffer on ice. After centrifugation, supernatant was collected, and total protein concentrations were determined using the Coomassie Brilliant Blue Method.

Western Blot

Briefly, equal amounts of protein were loaded in each lane of SDS-PAGE, electrophoresed, and transferred to a nitrocellulose membrane. The membrane was blocked with MMP-9 mouse monoclonal antibody and probed with anti-mouse IgG-horseradish peroxidase conjugated antibody. Densitometry analysis was performed with the ChemiDoc detection system (Bio-Rad) and Quantity One software (Bio-Rad).

Statistics

Data were expressed as mean ± SD. Statistical differences between individual groups were analyzed using 1-way ANOVA. P value < 0.05 was considered statistically significant.

Results

Laminin and TUNEL Staining

In SAH group, laminin in cerebral cortexes was detected to decrease compared with that of the sham operated group at 24 h (Fig. 1a, b). Treatment with SB-3CT succeeded in preventing degradation of laminin (Fig. 1d). Meanwhile, the number of neuronal death increased significantly compared with the sham operated group at 24 h after SAH (Fig. 1e, f). SB-3CT significantly attenuated the neuronal death compared with the vehicle group (Fig. 1g, h)

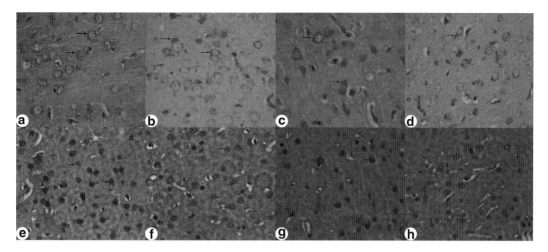

Fig. 1 Normal laminin staining (*arrow*) was shown in cerebral cortex in sham-operated rats (**a**, *arrow*). Significantly decreased laminin staining (*arrow*) was observed in cerebral cortex at 24 h after SAH (**b**). SB-3CT treatment (**c**) increased the laminin staining (*arrow*) compared with vehicle (**d**, *arrow*). Normal cortical neurons (*arrow*) were observed in sham rats (**e**). Positive staining of TUNEL (*arrow*) was found in cerebral cortex at 24 h after SAH (**f**). The number of TUNEL-positive neurons (*arrow*) decreased to a lesser degree in SB-3CT treated group (**g**) than those in vehicle group (**h**)

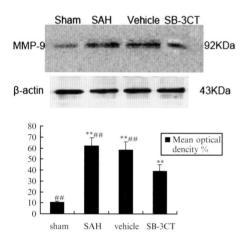

Fig. 2 Representative bands for MMP-9 protein are shown at 24 h after SAH (**a**). MMP-9 expression was reduced significantly by SB-3CT treatment (##$P < 0.01$ vs. SB-3CT, B), but still higher than that of sham group (**$P < 0.01$ vs. sham, **b**)

Western Blot of MMP-9 Expression

Protein expression of MMP-9 in the rat cerebral cortex was evaluated using western blot. At 24 h after SAH, significantly increased expression of MMP-9 was found in the cerebral cortex of SAH group as compared to that of the sham operated group ($P < 0.01$, Fig. 2a, b). The densitometric analysis revealed that SB-3CT treatment significantly reduced the protein expression of MMP-9 ($P < 0.01$ vs. vehicle).

Conclusion

In previous study, we examined the protein expression of MMP-9 and laminin, and cell death was also observed. Results showed that MMP-9 was probably involved in the pathophysiological events of early brain injury after SAH, through degrading laminin, which lead to neuronal death of the hippocampus [4]. But further study is still required to examine the relationship between MMP-9 and SAH.

In the present study, we have observed that MMP-9 was activated in the early phase after SAH in rats. Activation of MMP-9 resulted in the degradation of laminin which may contribute to cortical neuronal cell death (anoikis). SB-3CT, the inhibitor of MMP-9, decreased the anoikis of neurons. All of these observations further support our hypothesis that MMP-9 activation contributes to early brain injury after SAH.

We observed neuronal death in cerebral cortex at 24 h after SAH accompanied by the degradation of laminin. The reduction of laminin matches the increase of MMP-9, supporting their causal relationship. Prevention of MMP-9 activation by SB-3CT preserved laminin and probably resulted in the reduction of TUNEL positive staining in cortical neurons.

It is known that laminins are important for cell survival and laminin prevents the occurrence of a form of cell death known as anoikis, in which cells detach from their matrix [7]. Matrix loss renders the neurons sensitive to neuronal death. Therefore, prevention of laminin degradation by inhibition of the proteases (such as MMP-9) may lead to neuronal survival [6]. Neuronal cell death, or in some cases apoptosis, have been extensively studied in diseases of the central nervous system [2, 10]. It was reported that apoptosis may play an essential role in the pathophysiology of early brain injury after SAH [8]. In previous studies, we have found that inhibition of MMP-9 could decrease neuronal apoptosis in the hippocampus. In this study, the degradation of laminin decreased and neuronal death reduced after SAB-3CT treatment in the cerebral cortex.

In summary, this study demonstrated that increased MMP-9 expression may lead to laminin degradation and neuronal anoikis in the cortex after SAH. Inhibition of MMP-9 at the early stage of SAH may play an important role in preventing or reducing EBI after SAH.

Conflict of interest statement We declare that we have no conflict of interest.

References

1. Cahill J, Calvert JW, Zhang JH. Mechanisms of early brain injury after subarachnoid hemorrhage. J Cereb Blood Flow Metab. 2006;26:1341–53.
2. Cai J, Kang Z, Liu WW, Luo X, Qiang S, Zhang JH, et al. Hydrogen therapy reduces apoptosis in neonatal hypoxia-ischemia rat model. Neurosci Lett. 2008;441:167–72.
3. Gu Z, Cui J, Brown S, Fridman R, Mobashery S, Strongin AY, et al. A highly specific inhibitor of matrix metalloproteinase-9 rescues laminin from proteolysis and neurons from apoptosis in transient focal cerebral ischemia. J Neurosci. 2005;25:6401–08.
4. Guo Z, Sun X, He Z, Jiang Y, Zhang X, Zhang JH. Matrix metalloproteinase-9 potentiates early brain injury after subarachnoid hemorrhage. Neurol Res. 2009.
5. Kawakita K, Kawai N, Kuroda Y, Yasashita S, Nagao S. Expression of matrix metalloproteinase-9 in thrombin-induced brain edema formation in rats. J Stroke Cerebrovasc Dis. 2006;15:88–95.
6. Lee KJ, Jang YH, Lee H, Yoo HS, Lee SR. PPARgamma agonist pioglitazone reduces [corrected] neuronal cell damage after transient global cerebral ischemia through matrix metalloproteinase inhibition. Eur J Neurosci. 2008;27:334–42.
7. Miner JH, Yurchenco PD. Laminin functions in tissue morphogenesis. Annu Rev Cell Dev Biol. 2004;20:255–84.
8. Ostrowski RP, Colohan AR, Zhang JH. Molecular mechanisms of early brain injury after subarachnoid hemorrhage. Neurol Res. 2006;28:399–414.
9. Schubert GA, Poli S, Schilling L, Heiland S, Thome C. Hypothermia reduces cytotoxic edema and metabolic alterations during the acute phase of massive SAH: a diffusion-weighted imaging and spectroscopy study in rats. J Neurotrauma. 2008;25:841–52.
10. Sen O, Caner H, Aydin MV, Ozen O, Atalay B, Altinors N, et al. The effect of mexiletine on the level of lipid peroxidation and apoptosis of endothelium following experimental subarachnoid hemorrhage. Neurol Res. 2006;28:859–63.

Section IV: Nitric Oxide & Cortical Spreading Depolarization After Subarachnoid Hemorrhage

Nitric Oxide Synthase Inhibitors and Cerebral Vasospasm

C.S. Jung

Abstract L-arginine is a source of nitric oxide (NO) that is cleaved from the terminal guanidino nitrogen atom by nitric oxide synthase (NOS). NO evokes, because of its free radical properties and affinity to heme, ferrous iron and cysteine, a wide spectrum of physiological and pathophysiological effects. For many years, different exogenous NOS inhibitors were used to elucidate the role of NOS and NO in health and disease. Later, endogenous NOS inhibitors, as asymmetric dimethylarginine (ADMA) were discovered. Endogenous inhibitors as ADMA are produced by post-translational methylation of L-arginine which is catalyzed by a family of protein *N*-methyltransferases (PRMT), using *S*-adenosylmethionine as a methyl group donor. ADMA is eliminated by dimethylarginine dimethylaminohydrolases (DDAH I or II). ADMA hydrolysis increases NOS activity and NO production. Furthermore, L-citrulline, a by-product of ADMA hydrolysis as well as of NO production by NOS, can in turn inhibit DDAH. Therefore, endogenous inhibition of NOS can be modified via different ways (1) changing the availability of L-arginine and/or of L-citrulline; (2) stimulating or inhibiting DDAH activity; (3) modifying methylation via regulating availability of adenosylmethionine; or (4) modifying PRMT activity. Research elucidating the role of NOS inhibitors in respect of delayed cerebral vasospasm after subarachnoid hemorrhage is summarized.

Keywords Endogenous NOS inhibitor · ADMA · L-NMMA · Vasospasm · Subarachnoid hemorrhage

C.S. Jung
Department of Neurosurgery, Ruprecht-Karls-University Heidelberg,
Im Neuenheimer Feld 400, 69120 Heidelberg, Germany
e-mail: Carla.Jung@med.uni-heidelberg.de

Introduction

Since the first cases of aneurismal subarachnoid hemorrhage (aSAH) were diagnosed, significant progress has been made in the understanding of the pathophysiology and treatment of aSAH and delayed cerebral vasospasm. However, morbidity and mortality following SAH remain high. Although, cerebral vasospasm, delayed cerebral neurological deficits (DIND) and ischemia remain the major causes for morbidity and mortality, they also represent the most promising treatable factors affecting outcome after aneurismal subarachnoid hemorrhage [1].

NO and NOS-Pathway in Vasospasm

NO is a powerful vasodilator and plays a major role in regulating cerebrovascular tone and brain perfusion [2–4]. Although, a few controversial reports exist, many studies reported decreased NO metabolite levels after SAH [5]. NO is synthesized by a family of nitric oxide synthases (NOS) and is derived from the terminal guanidino nitrogen atoms of L-arginine yielding L-citrulline as a by-product [6]. NO diffuses across the endothelial cell membrane and activates soluble guanylate cyclase, leading to smooth muscle relaxation and vasodilation [7]. NO production is regulated by negative feedback between NO and NOS [8] and can be influenced by exogenous and endogenous NOS-inhibitors [9]. After SAH neuronal NOS (nNOS) immunoreactivity was reported to be decreased in perivascular nerves of cerebral vessels [3]. Observations on endothelial NOS (eNOS) expression after SAH were controversial. Park et al. observed reduction of eNOS protein in rats 20 minutes after SAH [10] while others described uneffected and unchanged eNOS protein expression at the time of highest vasospasm incidence [11, 12]. In a primate model of delayed cerebral vasospasm eNOS immunoreactivity and mRNA remained unchanged or increased [3, 7]. Furthermore, spastic cerebral vessels lost their ability to dilate in response to intracarotid acetylcholine application [13], similar to endothelium-denuded arteries in vitro [14], although they maintained the ability to dilate when exposed to intracarotid infusion of exogenous NO or NO donors [15, 16], suggesting dysfunction of eNOS in the intima of spastic arteries after SAH. There is growing evidence that this NOS dysfunction due to decreased availability of NO and cerebral vasospasm are associated with increased levels of the endogenous NOS-inhibitor ADMA [17–19].

Endogenous NOS Inhibitor Production and Hydrolysis

Endogenous NOS-inhibitors belong to a family of free methyl-arginines: mono methylated L-arginine (L-NMMA), asymmetric methylated L-arginine (ADMA) and symmetric methylated L-arginine (SDMA) [20]. The role of SDMA is unknown, but L-NMMA and ADMA are proven competitive NOS inhibitors [9]. They are produced by post-translational methylation of L-arginine residues by protein arginine methyltransferases (PRMT) [21, 22]. Seven genes encoding for 7 different PRMT enzymes (PRMT1–7) were discovered, which can each be assigned to one of two different PRMT enzyme activities (Type I and Type II) according to their substrate specificity and catalytic activities [21, 22]: Type I PRMTs (PRMT1,2,3,4 and 6) are predominantly responsible for asymmetrical di-methylation, producing L-NMMA and ADMA, while type II PRMTs (PRMT5 and 7) catalyse SDMA. Both types of PRMT use S-adenosylmethionine as principal methyl group donor [23]. L-NMMA and ADMA are metabolized to L-citrulline by dimethylarginine dimethylamine hydrolases (DDAH1 and 2): DDAH1 predominates in tissues which express nNOS, whereas, DDAH2 is mainly found in tissues containing eNOS [9, 24].

ADMA and L-NMMA and Vasospasm

ADMA and L-NMMA are effective competitive inhibitors of NOS. ADMA is synthesized and released by endothelial cells in amounts that are sufficient to inhibit NO production by competing with the enzyme substrate L-arginine [25, 26]. ADMA seems to be equipotent with L-NMMA, however its concentration in plasma is higher [27]. L-NMMA intravenously infused in healthy volunteers showed in high doses a reduction of cerebral blood flow associated with an increase in mean arterial pressure [28], while, low doses had no effect [29]. ADMA lead already in sub-pressor doses to increased vascular stiffness and decreased cerebral blood flow and – perfusion [30]. ADMA in concentrations of 1–300 µM causes a dose dependent inhibition of NO-synthesis. A concentration of 5 µM inhibited isolated NOS, increased the tone of rat aortic rings, and raised blood pressure of anesthetized guinea pigs [31]. Treatment of cerebral arteries, from several species, including humans, with ADMA and L-NMMA caused concentration- and endothelium-dependent constriction of cerebral arteries comparable to vasospasm after SAH [32, 33]. In a primate model of delayed cerebral vasospasm after subarachnoid hemorrhage, ADMA was detected in CSF and serum of control animals and in animals after SAH. While ADMA levels in the serum remained unchanged, ADMA levels in CSF increased after SAH and were correlated with the degree of cerebral vasospasm [17]. Furthermore, ADMA CSF levels followed the time-course of development and resolution of cerebral vasospasm in primates. The increase of ADMA in CSF was negatively correlated with NO-metabolite levels [17]. Furthermore, ADMA CSF levels were associated with decreased DDAH2 expression in vasospastic arteries, while PRMT remained unchanged [17]. Experimental findings were further supported by similar observations made in patients after SAH [18, 19]. Patients who developed cerebral vasospasm showed increased levels of ADMA in CSF [18, 19], which closely followed the time course of the development and resolution of cerebral vasospasm and were correlated with the degree of arteriographic vasospasm [18]. ADMA levels in patients after SAH were negatively correlated with nitrite levels [18]. Furthermore, a decrease of the L-arginine/ADMA ratio was observed and interpreted as a sign of impaired NO production after SAH being responsible for a simultaneous decrease of NO-metabolites in CSF [19]. The cause of ADMA increase in CSF is unclear. Two major mechanisms may produce ADMA elevation (1) increased methylation of protein-bound L-arginine by up-regulation of PRMT and (2) decreased hydrolysis of ADMA by DDAH. PRMT upregulation or overexpression could not be observed in spastic arteries after SAH, which makes PRMT unlikely to be the major cause for ADMA changes in vasospasm [17]. Osanai et al., observed in an experimental shear stress model that at a shear stress of 15 dyne/cm^2 ADMA was increased up to 1.7-fold, with a parallel enhanced gene expression of PRMT I. Shear stress at higher magnitudes of 25 dyne/cm^2 changed the gene expression pattern from PRMTI to DDAH facilitating the degradation of ADMA, thus returning ADMA to normal baseline levels [34]. After experimental SAH a reduced DDAH activity was observed [17]. Comparable to these findings a decreased SDMA/ADMA ratio, as an indirect indicator of decreased DDAH activity, was reported during SAH in patients [19]. Pharmacological blockage of DDAH increases ADMA levels in endothelial cells leading to inhibition of NO-mediated relaxation [9] and endothelial dysfunction [35]. Thus, it is likely that changes in DDAH activity or DDAH dysfunction play a role in ADMA increase after SAH and in cerebral vasospasm.

Therapeutic Approaches

Potential targets for therapeutic approaches and modification of the endogenous inhibition of NOS and NO-production can be in principle, any step of the ADMA/L-NMMA methylation– and hydrolysation cycle and several agents have been proposed to decrease ADMA levels in vitro and in vivo.

Statins

Statins were reported to decrease ADMA plasma levels. Therefore, Probucol, a statin that preserved eNOS function by reducing ADMA serum levels in rats [36] was examined in a blinded, placebo-controlled experiment to evaluate its effect on vasospasm after SAH. However, Probucol failed to inhibit ADMA increases and to prevent vasospasm in primates [37].

L-Arginine

L-arginine, the substrate for NOS and NO-production, can reverse the competitive inhibition of NOS by ADMA or L-NMMA. In biological systems however, the stoichiometry was reported to vary from a 1:1 ratio, requiring an excess of L-arginine to reverse NOS inhibition [9]. Intravenous L-arginine infusion decreased ADMA and improved endothelial function in patients with angina pectoris [38]. In several experimental studies L-arginine and NO donors reduced total cerebral infarct volume in permanent and transient models of ischemia [39]. Furthermore, exogenous intracisternal administration of L-arginine lead to dilation of preconstricted arteries in several SAH models [40, 41]. In primates after SAH, an increase in cerebral blood flow was observed after infusion of L-arginine however vasospasm was not prevented [42]. Nevertheless, these observations support the hypothesis, that increased concentrations and/or availability of L-arginine may help to overcome competitive inhibition of eNOS by endogenous NOS inhibitors and prevent development of vasospasm after SAH.

PRMT and S-Adenosylmethionine

L-arginine methylation by PRMT is the initial step in the endogenous formation of L-NMMA and ADMA [21, 22]. In vitro, upregulation of PRMT mRNA expression was observed in association with raised ADMA levels in models of shear stress [34]. However, no increase in PRMT expression was observed in arteries in spasm after SAH [17]. Elevation of S-adenosylmethionine stimulates PRMT activity and production of ADMA [43]. Therefore, lowering S-adenosylmethionine levels and reducing substrate availability might be another therapeutic approach. However, post-translational methylation of L-arginine residues is an universal biological process affecting hundreds of proteins [21] and the effects of this process remain in most cases unknown. Therefore, targeting PRMT or S-adenosylmethionine and reducing methylation processes at this stage is difficult and may imply unforeseen complications [44].

DDAH

The major pathway of ADMA metabolism is hydrolysis by DDAH [9, 24]. Decreased activity of DDAH was observed in patients after SAH [19] and attenuated expression of DDAH2 was described in spastic arteries [17]. Therefore, it seems likely that changes in DDAH activity or DDAH dysfunction play a role in ADMA increase in the setting of cerebral vasospasm after SAH. In DDAH-1 deficient mice, plasma and tissue levels of ADMA were increased [45], whereas overexpression of DDAH-1 in transgenic mice produced a marked decrease in ADMA levels, selectively affecting endothelium-mediated vascular responses without altering endothelium-independent responses [46]. Although, various pharmacological agents have been shown to reduce plasma ADMA levels, no specific drug is yet available that can increase degradation of ADMA by DDAH, lowering ADMA levels.

Conflict of interest statement I declare that I have no conflict of interest.

References

1. van Gijn J, Rinkel GJ. Subarachnoid haemorrhage: diagnosis, causes and management. Brain 2001;124:249–78.
2. Iadecola C, Zhang F, Xu X. Role of nitric oxide synthase-containing vascular nerves in cerebrovasodilation elicited from cerebellum. Am J Physiol. 1993;264:R738–46.
3. Pluta RM, Thompson JG, Dawson TM, Snyder SH, Book RJ, Oldfield EH. Loss of nitric oxide synthase immunoreactivity in cerebral vasospasm. J Neurosurg. 1996;84:648–54.

4. Toda N, Tanaka T, Ayajiki K, Okamura T. Cerebral vasodilatation induced by stimulation of the pterygopalatine ganglion and greater petrosal nerve in anesthetized monkeys. Neuroscience 2000;96:393–8.
5. Hirose H, Ide K, Sasaki T, Takahashi R, Kobayashi M, Ikemoto F, et al. The role of endothelin and nitric oxide in modulation of normal and spastic cerebral vascular tone in the dog. Eur J Pharmacol. 1995;277:77–87.
6. Hibbs JB, Jr., Taintor RR, Vavrin Z, Rachlin EM. Nitric oxide: a cytotoxic activated macrophage effector molecule. Biochem Biophys Res Commun. 1988;157:87–94.
7. Sobey CG, Faraci FM. Subarachnoid haemorrhage: what happens to the cerebral arteries? Clin Exp Pharmacol Physiol. 1998;25: 867–76.
8. Ignarro LJ. Nitric oxide as a unique signaling molecule in the vascular system: a historical overview. J Physiol Pharmacol. 2002;53:503–14.
9. McAllister RJ, Parry H, Kimoto M, Ogawa T, Russell RJ, Hodson H, et al. Regulation of nitric oxide synthesis by dimethylarginine dimethylaminohydrolase. Br J Pharmacol. 1996;119:1533–40.
10. Park KW, Metais C, Dai HB, Comunale ME, Sellke FW. Microvascular endothelial dysfunction and its mechanism in a rat model of subarachnoid hemorrhage. Anesth Analg. 2001;92:990–6.
11. Hino A, Tokuyama Y, Weir B, Takeda J, Yanc H, Bell GI, et al. Changes in endothelial nitric oxide synthase mRNA during vasospasm after subarachnoid hemorrhage in monkeys. Neurosurgery 1996;39:562–7; discussion 567–568.
12. Kasuya H, Weir BK, Nakane M, Pollock JS, John L, Marton LS, et al. Nitric oxide synthase and guanylate cyclase levels in canine basilar artery after subarachnoid hemorrhage. J Neurosurg. 1995;82:250–5.
13. Iuliano BA, Pluta RM, Jung C, Oldfield EH. Endothelial dysfunction in a primate model of cerebral vasospasm. J Neurosurg. 2004;100:287–94.
14. Furchgott RF, Zawadzki JV. The obligatory role of endothelial cells in the relaxation of arterial smooth muscle by acetylcholine. Nature 1980;288:373–6.
15. Afshar JK, Pluta RM, Boock RJ, Thompson BG, Oldfield EH. Effect of intracarotid nitric oxide on primate cerebral vasospasm after subarachnoid hemorrhage. J Neurosurg. 1995;83:118–22.
16. Pluta RM, Oldfield EH, Boock RJ. Reversal and prevention of cerebral vasospasm by intracarotid infusions of nitric oxide donors in a primate model of subarachnoid hemorrhage. J Neurosurg. 1997;87:746–51.
17. Jung CS, Iulianc B, Harvey-White J, Espey M, Oldfield EH, Pluta PM. Association between cerebrospinal fluid levels of asymmetric dimethyl-L-arginine, an endogenous inhibitor of endothelial nitric oxide synthase, and cerebral vasospasm in a primate model of subarachnoid hemorrhage. J Neurosurg. 2004;101:836–42.
18. Jung CS, Oldfield EH, Harvey-Wuik J, Espey MG, Zimmermann M, Seifert V, et al. Association of an endogenous inhibitor of nitric oxide synthase with cerebral vasospasm in patients with aneurysmal subarachnoid hemorrhage. J Neurosurg. 2007;107:945–50.
19. Marhus-Lobeuholter J, Sulyok E, Creikr E, Buki A, Kohl J, Firsching R. Determination of cerebrospinal fluid concentrations of arginine and dimethylarginines in patients with subarachnoid haemorrhage. J Neurosci Methods. 2007;164:155–60.
20. Kakimoto Y, Akazawa S. Isolation and identification of N-G,N-G- and N-G,N'-G-dimethyl-arginine, N-epsilon-mono-, di-, and trimethyllysine, and glucosylgalactosyl- and galactosyl-delta-hydroxylysine from human urine. J Biol Chem. 1970;245:5751–8.
21. Boisvert FM, Cote J, Boulanger MC, Richard S. A proteomic analysis of arginine-methylated protein complexes. Mol Cell Proteomics. 2003;2:1319–30.
22. Tang J, Frankel A, Cook RJ, Kim S, Paik WK, Williams KR, et al. PRMT1 is the predominant type I protein arginine methyltransferase in mammalian cells. J Biol Chem. 2000;275:7723–30.
23. Boger RH, Sydow K, Borlak J, Thum T, Lenzen H, Schubert B, et al. LDL cholesterol upregulates synthesis of asymmetrical dimethylarginine in human endothelial cells: involvement of S-adenosylmethionine-dependent methyltransferases. Circ Res. 2000;87:99–105.
24. Leiper JM, Santa Maria J, Chubb A, MacAllister RJ, Charles IG, Whitley GS, et al. Identification of two human dimethylarginine dimethylaminohydrolases with distinct tissue distributions and homology with microbial arginine deiminases. Biochem J. 1999;343 Pt 1:209–14.
25. Chardonnel AJ, Cui H, Samouilov A, Johnson AW, Kearns P, Tsai AL, et al. Evidence for the pathophysiological role of endogenous methylarginines in regulation of endothelial NO production and vascular function. J Biol Chem. 2007;282:879–87.
26. McDermott JR. Studies on the catabolism of Ng-methylarginine, Ng, Ng-dimethylarginine and Ng, Ng-dimethylarginine in the rabbit. Biochem J. 1976;154:179–84.
27. Vallance P. Importance of asymmetrical dimethylarginine in cardiovascular risk. Lancet 2001;358:2096–7.
28. Kamper AM, Spilt A, de Craen AJ, van Buchem MA, Westendorp RG, Blauw GJ. Basal cerebral blood flow is dependent on the nitric oxide pathway in elderly but not in young healthy men. Exp Gerontol. 2004;39:1245–8.
29. White RP, Hindley C, Bloomfield PM, Cunningham VJ, Valiance P, Brooks DJ, et al. The effect of the nitric oxide synthase inhibitor L-NMMA on basal CBF and vasoneuronal coupling in man: a PET study. J Cereb Blood Flow Metab. 1999;19:673–8.
30. Kielstein JT, Donnerstag F, Gasper S, Menne J, Kielstein A, Martens-Lobenhoffer J, et al. ADMA increases arterial stiffness and decreases cerebral blood flow in humans. Stroke 2006;37:2024–9.
31. Vallance P, Leone A, Calver A, Collier J, Moncada S. Accumulation of an endogenous inhibitor of nitric oxide synthesis in chronic renal failure. Lancet 1992;339:572–5.
32. Faraci FM, Brian JE, Jr., Heistad DD. Response of cerebral blood vessels to an endogenous inhibitor of nitric oxide synthase. Am J Physiol. 1995;269:H1522–7.
33. Segarra G, Medina P, Ballester RM, Lluch P, Aldasoro M, Vila JM, et al. Effects of some guanidino compounds on human cerebral arteries. Stroke 1999;30:2206–10; discussion 2210–2211.
34. Osanai T, Saitoh M, Sasaki S, Tomita H, Matsunaga T, Okumura K. Effect of shear stress on asymmetric dimethylarginine release from vascular endothelial cells. Hypertension 2003;42:985–90.
35. Ito A, Tsao PS, Adimoolam S, Kimoto M, Ogawa T, Cooke JP. Novel mechanism for endothelial dysfunction: dysregulation of dimethylarginine dimethylaminohydrolase. Circulation 1999; 99:3092–5.
36. Jiang JL, Li NS, Li YJ, Deng HW. Probucol preserves endothelial function by reduction of the endogenous nitric oxide synthase inhibitor level. Br J Pharmacol. 2002;135:1175–82.
37. Pluta RM, Jung CS, Harvey-White J, Whitehead A, Shilad S, Espey MG, et al. In vitro and in vivo effects of probucol on hydrolysis of asymmetric dimethyl L-arginine and vasospasm in primates. J Neurosurg. 2005;103:731–8.
38. Piatti P, Fragasso G, Monti LD, Setola E, Lucotti P, Fermo I, et al. (2003) Acute intravenous L-arginine infusion decreases endothelin-1 levels and improves endothelial function in patients with angina pectoris and normal coronary arteriograms: correlation with asymmetric dimethylarginine levels. Circulation 2001;107:429–36.
39. Willmot M, Gray L, Gibson C, Murphy S, Bath PM. A systematic review of nitric oxide donors and L-arginine in experimental stroke; effects on infarct size and cerebral blood flow. Nitric Oxide 2005;12:141–9.
40. Goksel HM, Ozum U, Oztoprak I. The therapeutic effect of continuous intracisternal L-Arginine infusion on experimental cerebral vasospasm. Acta Neurochir (Wien). 2001;143:277–85.
41. Kajita Y, Suzuki Y, Oyama H, Tanatawa T, Takayasu M, Shibuya M, et al. Combined effect of L-arginine and superoxide

dismutase on the spastic basilar artery after subarachnoid hemorrhage in dogs. J Neurosurg. 1994;80:476–83.
42. Pluta RM, Afshar JK, Thompson BG, Book RJ, Harvey-White J, Oldfield EH. Increased cerebral blood flow but no reversal or prevention of vasospasm in response to L-arginine infusion after subarachnoid hemorrhage. J Neurosurg. 2000;92:121–6.
43. Lentz SR, Rodionov RN, Dayal S. Hyperhomocysteinemia, endothelial dysfunction, and cardiovascular risk: the potential role of ADMA. Atheroscler Suppl. 2003;4:61–5.
44. Maas R. Pharmacotherapies and their influence on asymmetric dimethylargine (ADMA). Vasc Med. 2005;10 Suppl 1:S49–57.
45. Leiper J, Nandi M, Torondel B, Murray-Rust J, Malaki M, O'Hara B, et al. Disruption of methylarginine metabolism impairs vascular homeostasis. Nat Med. 2007;13:198–203.
46. Dayoub H, Achan V, Adimoolam S, Jacob J, Stuehliuger MC, Wang BY, et al. Dimethylarginine dimethylaminohydrolase regulates nitric oxide synthesis: genetic and physiological evidence. Circulation 2003;108:3042–7.

The Role of Nitric Oxide Donors in Treating Cerebral Vasospasm After Subarachnoid Hemorrhage

Ali R. Fathi, Kamran D. Bakhtian, and Ryszard M. Pluta

Abstract Reduced intra- and perivascular availability of nitric oxide (NO) significantly contributes to the multifactorial pathophysiology of cerebral vasospasm after aneurysmal subarachnoid hemorrhage (SAH). The short half-life of NO demands its therapeutic substitution via NO donors. Classic NO donors such as sodium nitroprusside and nitroglycerin cannot be used as routine therapeutics because of serious side effects. Thus, a new generation of NO donors has been the subject of experimental investigations to avoid the drawbacks of the classic drugs. The purpose of this paper is to review the characteristics of different NO donors with regard to their promise and potential consequences in treating cerebral vasospasm. Additional novel concepts to increase NO concentrations, such as the activation of endothelial nitric oxide synthase (eNOS), are discussed.

Keywords Cerebral vasospasm · DIND · Nitric oxide · NO Donors · Subarachnoid hemorrhage

Introduction

The high morbidity and mortality rate (30%) after aneurysmal subarachnoid hemorrhage (SAH) results predominantly from cerebral vasospasm and delayed ischemic neurological deficits (DIND) [1]. The multifactorial nature of DIND pathophysiology is a major impediment in developing successful treatments and improving patient outcome. The pathophysiology associated with DIND includes re-bleeding, peri-hemorrhage ischemia, increased intracranial pressure, blood-brain barrier dysfunction, cortical spreading ischemia, and macro- and microcirculatory embolism and spasm [2]. Additionally, cerebral vasospasm itself as part of the complex pathophysiology has multiple causal factors. One such factor is deprivation of nitric oxide (NO) in the vicinity of brain vessels as a result of nitric oxide synthase (NOS) dysfunction [3] and scavenging of NO by deoxyhemoglobin [4]. Considerable research has been carried out to enhance the perivascular NO concentration after SAH and to prevent or reverse vasospasm. The positive effect of NO donors on vessel diameter is known; however, their impact on overall outcome is still uncertain.

Sodium nitroprusside (SNP) and nitroglycerin (GTN) are the only NO donors which have been clinically studied with limited success. The chemical properties and adverse effects of both drugs preclude them from routine clinical application and have led to research aimed at discovering newer classes of NO donors.

The purpose of this paper is to provide an overview of the ongoing research with this new generation of NO donors and to discuss their pharmacologic properties relating to the treatment of cerebral vasospasm.

A.R. Fathi
Surgical Neurology Branch, National Institute of Neurological Disorders and Stroke, National Institutes of Health, 10 Center Drive, Bldg 10, Room 3D20, SNB/NINDS/NIH, Bethesda, MD, USA
Department of Neurosurgery, Kantonsspital Aarau AG, Aarau, Switzerland

K.D. Bakhtian and R.M. Pluta (✉)
Surgical Neurology Branch, National Institute of Neurological Disorders and Stroke, National Institutes of Health, 10 Center Drive, Bldg 10, Room 3D20, SNB/NINDS/NIH, Bethesda, MD, USA
e-mail: rysiek@ninds.nih.gov

Classic NO Donors

Sodium Nitroprusside

Early animal studies with SNP demonstrated effective vasodilation of cerebral vessels [5]. In early human studies to treat vasospasm, intravenous SNP led to serious side effects, predominantly hypotension and brain edema [6]. Thus, intrathecal administration was introduced in several experimental

[7] and clinical studies to bypass the systemic side effects [8, 9]. The results of these studies indicated a positive effect on vessel diameter in the majority of cases. However, due to side effects such as nausea, vomiting, migraine headaches, cardiac arrhythmia, and uncontrolled increases in cerebral blood flow (CBF), this treatment modality was not routinely used clinically. Additionally, another serious side effect of SNP is cyanide poisoning [10].

Nitroglycerin

GTN is an NO donor widely used to treat angina pectoris. Preclinical studies in primates have been successful in reversing vasospasm via intravenous administration [11]. Transdermal administration in humans has resulted in improved transcranial Doppler (TCD) velocity and CBF [12]. Improved clinical outcome and reduced DIND occurrence [13] have been causally related to GTN administration. In all studies, systemic hypotension was the major side effect of the treatment and disqualified the systemic use of GTN. Systemic administration should also be avoided due to the development of drug tolerance as well as the occurrence of the hypertensive rebound phenomenon after cessation of treatment.

In a single-SAH model study in rabbits, continuous intrathecal administration of GTN showed positive effects on vessel diameter without systemic hypotension [14]. However, the safety and efficacy of intrathecal use in humans has not yet been evaluated.

New Generation of NO Donors

The aforementioned properties and shortcomings associated with the classic NO donors prompted the search for a new generation of NO donors to treat cerebral vasospasm. To date, a variety of chemical compounds are available as NO donors. The main difference between the compounds is the mechanism of NO release. Table 1 shows the new generation of NO donors, which have been tested in animal studies

Table 1 New generation of NO donors used in experimental therapies for cerebral vasospasm in animals

NONOates
S-Nitrosothiols
Sodium nitrite
Fungal-derived NO
Hydroxylamine
NO gas
Sydnonimines

for their potential to treat cerebral vasospasm after SAH. Presently, only one of these drugs, sodium nitrite, is tested in a clinical trial.

NONOates

NONOates (diazeniumdiolates) are water-soluble compounds characterized by their ability to spontaneously release NO at physiological pH levels [15]. They have proven to be reliable sources of NO both in vitro and in vivo. Their half-lives and rates of NO release are pharmacologically predictable making them useful to treat cerebral vasospasm. Animal studies have been conducted to evaluate NONOates for their capacity to prevent and reverse cerebral vasospasm. These vascular effects were analyzed in vivo [16–18]. With the exception of one study [16], all others revealed a significant relaxation of constricted vessels.

Systemic hypotension was reported in only one of the studies [16]; all studies reported neither drug tolerance nor resistance following up to 8 days of intrathecal or intracarotid administration.

The main concern in using NONOates is the possibility of carcinogenesis, as it has been reported that NONOates can convert to *N*-nitrosopyrrolidines, which are known to be hepatocarcinogens in an experimental setting [15].

S-Nitrosothiols

Like NONOates, *S*-nitrosothiols have a chemically predictable half-life depending on the R-group. Animal studies have shown promising results in preventing and reversing vasospasm. Sehba et al. investigated intravenous [19] and intraarterial [20] administration of S-nitrosoglutathione (GSNO) in rats and reported siginificant relaxation of the cerebral arteries. Moreover, GSNO preserved both formation of collagen IV and endothelial barrier antigen in the vessel wall and thickening of the vessel wall [19, 20]. In these studies, no changes in mean arterial blood pressure, intracranial pressure, or uncontrolled CBF increases occurred. However, Kiris et al. observed hypotension [21]. There was no report of drug tolerance and no evaluation in clinical trials has been conducted.

Sodium Nitrite

Sodium nitrite has been used as a color fixative and preservative in food since ancient times. In 1953, Furchgott and

Bhadrakom proved sodium nitrite to be a direct vasodilator using rabbit aorta rings [22]. The first description of sodium nitrate-induced vasorelaxation of cerebral arteries was in 1974 by Toda [23]. Others confirmed this effect and postulated the theory that such an effect is mediated by the conversion of oxyhemoglobin to methemoglobin [24]. Decreased cerebrospinal fluid (CSF) nitrite levels during cerebral vasospasm after SAH confirm the hypothesis that decreased NO availability contributes to cerebral vasospasm [25]. Recently it was discovered that deoxyhemoglobin acts under acidic conditions as a nitrite reductase enzyme; as a result, this NO donor becomes a selective on-demand source, releasing NO into the subarachnoid space after SAH [3]. Intravenous sodium nitrite is very effective in preventing [25] and reversing [26] cerebral vasospasm by enhancing local CSF levels of NO without developing tolerance in a primate model of SAH. Relevant hypotension was not observed in any of the studies. A Phase I safety and toxicity study in healthy human volunteers showed that therapeutic dosages of intravenous sodium nitrite infusions are safe and there is no risk of systemic hypotension (manuscript submitted).

Along with NONOates the carcinogenic potential of nitrites has to be kept in mind for future investigations. Animal studies have reported higher risks of cancer after long-term administration [27]. However, oncogenic effects of nitrite were only observed after long-term exposure over many months and with higher concentrations [28]. The maximum treatment period for vasospasm would only range from 3–4 weeks.

Intrathecal and intraarterial administration of sodium nitrite to treat SAH has not been evaluated thus far. Oral administration is also a viable route since the bioactivity of sodium nitrite after oral intake is 97% [29].

Other New Generation NO Donors

Other NO donors include fungal-derived compounds, hydroxylamine, direct NO gas, and 3-morpholinosydnonimine (SIN-1). Each of these drugs has been evaluated in animal models of SAH [30–33]. Thus far, the only reported side effect is hypotension [30]. Initial reports are promising but translation into clinical evaluation is premature given the present state of knowledge regarding these compounds.

Other Biochemical Potentials to Enhance NO Concentration

NO donors bypass dysfunctional NOS to enhance NO concentration leading to cGMP-mediated vasodilation. Another future approach to reconstitute this pathway and deliver NO without NO donors is activation of endothelial nitric oxide synthase (eNOS) (Fig. 1).

Asymmetric dimethyl-L-arginine (ADMA) is known to inhibit eNOS and increased ADMA levels are associated with the development of vasospasm in a primate model of SAH [34]. Knowing this, inhibition of ADMA production might be beneficial.

NOS activity, particularly endothelial NOS, is regulated by enzyme phosphorylation at different sites [35]. eNOS is activated by kinase phosphorylation at serine residue 1177 and induces NO production [36]. Thus, activation of protein kinases and inhibition of the dephosphorylating phosphatases provide another therapeutic possibility to enhance NO availability [37].

An additional novel experimental approach to treat cerebral vasospasm is provided by erythropoietin (EPO). Animal

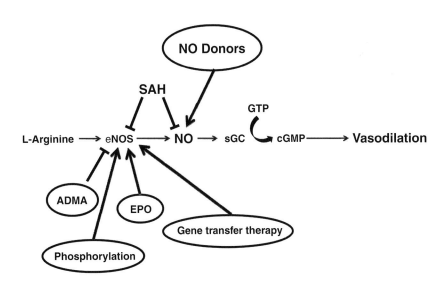

Fig. 1 Pathway of NO production via eNOS and possible therapeutic targets: SAH impairs eNOS activity and reduces NO concentrations perivascularly. NO donors reconstitute NO concentration via direct NO release while inhibition of ADMA, eNOS phosphorylation, EPO and gene transfer therapy all increase eNOS activity. (*eNOS* endothelial nitric oxide synthase, *SAH* subarachnoid hemorrhage, *NO* nitric oxide, *sGC* soluble guanylyl cyclase, *GTP* guanosine triphosphate, *cGMP* cyclic guanosine monophosphate, *ADMA* asymmetric dimethyl-L-arginine, *EPO* erythropoietin)

experiments and initial human studies indicate that there are beneficial effects of EPO treatment after SAH [38]. EPO's molecular mechanism of neuroprotection and vasodilation is thought to involve enhancement of the NO pathway via phosphorylation of eNOS [39, 40].

Finally, preliminary results suggest that eNOS gene transfer therapy increases NO production [41]. This approach is likely to gain more interest once the safety and feasibility of gene transfer has been established in clinical trials.

Conclusion

In the multimodal approach to treating vasospasm, enhancement of NO either via direct administration of a new generation of NO donors or activation of the eNOS pathways will serve as important pharmacological tools.

Acknowledgements Dr. Ali Reza Fathi was supported by a grant from the Swiss National Science Foundation (PBSKP3-123454). This research was partially supported by the Intramural Research Program of the National Institute of Neurological Disorders and Stroke at the NIH.

Conflict of interest statement We declare that we have no conflict of interest.

References

1. Pluta RM, Hansen-Schwartz J, Dreier J, Vajkoczy P, Macdonald RL, Nishizawa S, et al. Cerebral vasospasm following subarachnoid hemorrhage: time for a new world of thought. Neurol Res. 2009;31:151–58.
2. Macdonald RL, Pluta RM, Zhang JH. Cerebral vasospasm after subarachnoid hemorrhage: the emerging revolution. Nat Clin Pract Neurol. 2007;3:256–63.
3. Pluta RM. Dysfunction of nitric oxide synthases as a cause and therapeutic target in delayed cerebral vasospasm after SAH. Neurol Res. 2006;28:730–37.
4. Macdonald RL, Weir BK. A review of hemoglobin and the pathogenesis of cerebral vasospasm. Stroke 1991;22:971–82.
5. Allen GS, Gross CJ. Cerebral arterial spasm. Part 7: In vitro effects of alpha adrenergic agents on canine arteries from six anatomical sites and six blocking agents on serotonin-induced contractions of the canine basilar artery. Surg Neurol. 1976;6:63–70.
6. Allen GS. Cerebral arterial spasm. Part 8: The treatment of delayed cerebral arterial spasm in human beings. Surg Neurol. 1976;6: 71–80.
7. Egemen N, Turker RK, Sanlidilek U, Zorlutuna A, Bilgic S, Baskaya M, et al. The effect of intrathecal sodium nitroprusside on severe chronic vasospasm. Neurol Res. 1993;15:310–15.
8. Raabe A, Zimmermann M, Setzer M, Vatter H, Berkefeld J, Seifert V. Effect of intraventricular sodium nitroprusside on cerebral hemodynamics and oxygenation in poor-grade aneurysm patients with severe, medically refractory vasospasm. Neurosurgery 2002;50:1006–13; discussion 1013–1004.
9. Thomas JE, Rosenwasser RH, Armonda RA, Harrop J, Mitchell W, Galaria I. Safety of intrathecal sodium nitroprusside for the treatment and prevention of refractory cerebral vasospasm and ischemia in humans. Stroke 1999;30:1409–16.
10. Ram Z, Spiegelman R, Findler G, Hadani M. Delayed postoperative neurological deterioration from prolonged sodium nitroprusside administration. Case report. J Neurosurg. 1989;71:605–7.
11. Nakao K, Murata H, Kanamaru K, Waga S. Effects of nitroglycerin on vasospasm and cyclic nucleotides in a primate model of subarachnoid hemorrhage. Stroke 1996;27:1882–87; discussion 1887–1888.
12. Reinert M, Wiest R, Barth L, Andres R, Ozdoba C, Seiler R. Transdermal nitroglycerin in patients with subarachnoid hemorrhage. Neurol Res. 2004;26:435–39.
13. Tanaka Y, Masuzawa T, Saito M, Yamada T, Ebihara A, Iwasa H, et al. Combined administration of Fasudil hydrochloride and nitroglycerin for treatment of cerebral vasospasm. Acta Neurochir Suppl. 2001;77:205–7.
14. Marbacher S, Neuschmelting V, Graupner T, Jakob SM, Fandino J. Prevention of delayed cerebral vasospasm by continuous intrathecal infusion of glyceroltrinitrate and nimodipine in the rabbit model in vivo. Intensive Care Med. 2008;34:932–38.
15. Keefer LK. Progress toward clinical application of the nitric oxide-releasing diazeniumdiolates. Annu Rev Pharmacol Toxicol. 2003; 43:585–607.
16. Aihara Y, Jahromi BS, Yassari R, Sayama T, Macdonald RL. Effects of a nitric oxide donor on and correlation of changes in cyclic nucleotide levels with experimental vasospasm. Neurosurgery 2003;52:661–7; discussion 666–667.
17. Clatterbuck RE, Gailloud P, Tierney T, Clatterbuck VM, Murphy KJ, Tamargo RJ. Controlled release of a nitric oxide donor for the prevention of delayed cerebral vasospasm following experimental subarachnoid hemorrhage in nonhuman primates. J Neurosurg. 2005;103:745–51.
18. Pluta RM, Oldfield EH, Boock RJ. Reversal and prevention of cerebral vasospasm by intracarotid infusions of nitric oxide donors in a primate model of subarachnoid hemorrhage. J Neurosurg. 1997;87:746–51.
19. Sehba FA, Friedrich V, Jr., Makonnen G, Bederson JB. Acute cerebral vascular injury after subarachnoid hemorrhage and its prevention by administration of a nitric oxide donor. J Neurosurg. 2007;106:321–29.
20. Sehba FA, Ding WH, Chereshnev I, Bederson JB. Effects of S-nitrosoglutathione on acute vasoconstriction and glutamate release after subarachnoid hemorrhage. Stroke 1999;30:1955–61.
21. Kiris T, Karasu A, Yavuz C, Erdem T, Unal F, Hepgul K, et al. Reversal of cerebral vasospasm by the nitric oxide donor SNAP in an experimental model of subarachnoid haemorrhage. Acta Neurochir (Wien). 1999;141:1323–28; discussion 1328–1329.
22. Furchgott RF, Bhadrakom S. Reactions of strips of rabbit aorta to epinephrine, isopropylarterenol, sodium nitrite and other drugs. J Pharmacol Exp Ther. 1953;108:129–43.
23. Toda N. The action of vasodilating drugs on isolated basilar, coronary and mesenteric arteries of the dog. J Pharmacol Exp Ther. 1974;191:139–46.
24. Sonobe M, Suzuki J. Vasospasmogenic substance produced following subarachnoid hemorrhage, and its fate. Neurol Med-Chir. 1978;18 II:29–37.
25. Pluta RM, Dejam A, Grimes G, Gladwin MT, Oldfield EH. Nitrite infusions to prevent delayed cerebral vasospasm in a primate model of subarachnoid hemorrhage. JAMA 2005;293:1477–84.
26. Fathi AR, Pluta RM, Qi M, Bakhtian KD, Lonser RR. Short-lasting intravenous sodium nitrite ameliorates cerebral vasospasm in a primate model of SAH. The 10th International Conference on Cerebral Vasospasm Chongqing, China; 2009.

27. Soderberg LS. Increased tumor growth in mice exposed to inhaled isobutyl nitrite. Toxicol Lett. 1999104:35–41.
28. Hord NG, Tang Y, Bryan NS. Food sources of nitrates and nitrites: the physiologic context for potential health benefits. Am J Clin Nutr. 2009;90:1–10.
29. Hunault CC, van Velzen AG, Sips AJ, Schothorst RC, Meulenbelt J. Bioavailability of sodium nitrite from an aqueous solution in healthy adults. Toxicol Lett. 2009;190:48–53.
30. Afshar JK, Pluta RM, Boock RJ, Thompson BG, Oldfield EH. Effect of intracarotid nitric oxide on primate cerebral vasospasm after subarachnoid hemorrhage. J Neurosurg. 1995;83:118–22.
31. Islam MS, Ohkuma H, Kimura M, Suzuki S. In vitro effects of new generation fungal derived nitric oxide donors on rabbit basilar artery. Neurol Med Chir (Tokyo). 2003;43:175–80; discussion 180.
32. Ryba MS, Gordon-Krajcer W, Walski M, Chalimoniuk M, Chrapusta SJ. Hydroxylamine attenuates the effects of simulated subarachnoid hemorrhage in the rat brain and improves neurological outcome. Brain Res. 1999;850:225–33.
33. Yamamoto S, Nishizawa S, Yokoyama T, Ryu H, Uemura K. Subarachnoid hemorrhage impairs cerebral blood flow response to nitric oxide but not to cyclic GMP in large cerebral arteries. Brain Res. 1997;757:1–9.
34. Jung CS, Iuliano BA, Harvey-White J, Espey MG, Oldfield EH, Pluta RM. Association between cerebrospinal fluid levels of asymmetric dimethyl-l-arginine, an endogenous inhibitor of endothelial nitric oxide synthase, and cerebral vasospasm in a primate model of subarachnoid hemorrhage. J Neurosurg. 2004;101:836–42.
35. Mount PF, Kemp BE, Power DA. Regulation of endothelial and myocardial NO synthesis by multi-site eNOS phosphorylation. J Mol Cell Cardiol. 2007;42:271–79.
36. Fulton D, Gratton JP, Sessa WC. Post-translational control of endothelial nitric oxide synthase: why isn't calcium/calmodulin enough? J Pharmacol Exp Ther. 2001;299:818–24.
37. Fathi AR, Zhuang Z, Xia J, Lu J, Merrill M, Cleary S, et al. Inhibition of protein phosphatase 2A stimulates endothelial nitric oxide synthase in human umbilical vein endothelial and renal carcinoma cell line The 10th International Conference on Cerebral Vasospasm Chongqing, China; 2009.
38. Tseng MY, Hutchinson PJ, Richards HK, Czosnyka M, Pickard JD, Erber WN, et al. Acute systemic erythropoietin therapy to reduce delayed ischemic deficits following aneurysmal subarachnoid hemorrhage: a Phase II randomized, double-blind, placebo-controlled trial. Clinical article. J Neurosurg. 2009;111:171–80.
39. Grasso G, Passalacqua M, Sfacteria A, Conti A, Morabito A, Mazzullo G, et al. Does administration of recombinant human erythropoietin attenuate the increase of S-100 protein observed in cerebrospinal fluid after experimental subarachnoid hemorrhage? J Neurosurg. 2002;96:565–70.
40. Santhanam AV, Katusic ZS. Erythropoietin and cerebral vascular protection: role of nitric oxide. Acta Pharmacol Sin. 2006;27:1389–94.
41. Onoue H, Tsutsui M, Smith L, Stelter A, O'Brien T, Katusic ZS. Expression and function of recombinant endothelial nitric oxide synthase gene in canine basilar artery after experimental subarachnoid hemorrhage. Stroke 1998;29:1959–65; discussion 1965–1956.

Nitric Oxide in Early Brain Injury After Subarachnoid Hemorrhage

Fatima A. Sehba and Joshua B. Bederson

Abstract Nitric Oxide (NO) is the major regulator of cerebral blood flow. In addition, it inhibits platelet adherence and aggregation, reduces adherence of leukocytes to the endothelium, and suppresses vessel injury. NO is produced on demand by nitric oxide synthase and has a very short half life. Hence maintenance of its cerebral level is crucial for normal vascular physiology. Time dependent alterations in cerebral NO level and the enzymes responsible for its synthesis are found after subarachnoid hemorrhage (SAH). Cerebral NO level decreases, recovers and increases within the first 24 h after SAH. Each change in cerebral NO level elicits a different pathological response form already compromised brain. These response range from constriction, platelet aggregation and vascular injury that occurs during the early hours and delayed occurring vasospasm, neuronal and axonal damage. This review summarizes the underlying mechanism and the consequence of alteration in cerebral NO level on brain during the first 72 h after SAH.

Keywords Early brain injury · Nitric oxide · Vasospasm

Introduction

SAH accounts for 10% of annual stroke cases and kills nearly 50% of patients within 30 days. Brain injury after SAH is biphasic in nature; early ischemic injury at the time of the initial hemorrhage, followed by delayed vasospasm and ischemia that develops three to seven days later. It is believed that early diagnosis and treatment is critical for potential reduction of the mortality rate after SAH. However, the mechanisms of brain injury during this period

F.A. Sehba (✉) and J.B. Bederson
Departments of Neurosurgery and of Neuroscience, Mount Sinai School of Medicine, New York, NY 10029, USA
e-mail: fatima.sehba@mssm.edu

remain poorly understood, and few if any specific treatments for them exist.

Experimental studies [1, 2] as well as autopsies performed on the brains of patients who expired early after SAH [3] demonstrate extensive ischemic damage. Cerebral blood flow (CBF) is acutely decreased after SAH. Many investigators believe this decrease is a passive event caused by profound reductions in cerebral perfusion pressure (CPP) upon elevation of intracranial pressure (ICP) during aneurysm rupture [4–6]. Others have postulated the contribution of additional interrelated processes that reduce CBF and cause ischemia. These include release of vasoactive substances during erythrocyte lysis [7], platelet aggregation [8, 9], and lipid peroxidation [10, 11], unopposed sympathetic activity [12], and alterations in the nitric oxide/nitric oxide synthase (NO/NOS) pathways [13–15] etc.

This paper discusses the role of Nitric oxide pathway in early brain injury after SAH.

Nitric Oxide

NO plays an important role in vascular pharmacology, immunology, toxicology, and neurobiology [16–21]. It is produced from L-arginine by Nitric oxide synthase (NOS) [22, 23] by its three isozymes, neuronal (nNOS), endothelial (eNOS), and inducible-NOS (iNOS) [24]. e and nNOS are constitutive isoenzymes and responsible of the basal NO levels under normal physiology. These isoforms function transiently and depend on intracellular calcium levels. iNOS in contrast is inducible by immune responses of the organism (View Record in Scopus Cited By in Scopus (367) [25]). It is generally accepted that eNOS derived NO is important for vascular function in terms of regulation of vascular tone and blood pressure, for effects on smooth muscle cell proliferation, for responses to vessel injury, inhibition of adherence and aggregations of platelets and adherence of leukocytes to the endothelium [25].

Cerebral ischemia profoundly affects the NO biosynthetic pathway, increasing NOS activity and gene expression [26]. Within an hour of onset of occlusive cerebral ischemia, *e* and *n* NOS are up-regulated in microvessels and parenchyma, respectively [27, 28] and 6–12 h later iNOS expression is increased in reactive astrocytes and neutrophils infiltrating ischemic brain [29, 30]. The initial increased NO availability immediately after ischemia is considered beneficial as it can inhibit further decreases in blood flow [26, 31] and adhesion of platelets and leukocytes to microvessels [32, 33]. Later, when vascular effects of NO are no longer beneficial, large amounts of NO produced by nNOS containing neurons or iNOS in non-neuronal cells are damaging [26, 31].

A number of studies show that NO/NOS pathway is pathologically altered after SAH, contributing to early ischemic injury [13–15] and pathogeneses of delayed vasospasm [34–41]. It appears that the nature of role that NO plays in ischemic brain changes with time after SAH [42]. Hence present review discusses the role of NO in brain injury with respect to the time elapse after the initial bleed. A time period of 72 h is discussed and is divided into three phases based on literature search and data obtained in our laboratory that suggests a *triphasic* alteration in NO levels after SAH. Since in typical clinical scenario there is usually a delay before patients reach critical care units after SAH most of the information discussed in Phase I and II comes from animal studies. Phase III, however, is studied in both humans and animals.

Phase I (0–60 min After SAH)

Phase I is the period during which cerebral NO level is acutely decrease. This decrease, studied as reduction in major NO metabolites (nitrate and nitrite) occurs within 10 min after SAH in both hemispheres and all brain regions, reiterating the global aspect of brain injury after SAH [15].

It should be noted that decrease in NO after SAH is in contrast to occlusive ischemic stroke where an increase in cerebral NO is reported [27, 28, 43–47]. Hence, the decreased NO availability during Phase I makes SAH unique as compared to other forms of cerebral ischemia [27, 44, 45]. The cause of decrease in cerebral NO level may include scavenging by hemoglobin [20, 34, 48], binding with free radicals [49], consumption by vascular neutrophils [50], etc.

Over all NOS activity is studied and is found to be unchanged during phase I [51]. However, as this study used an in vitro assay that relies on conversion on tritiated arginine into citrulline, an endogenous inhibition of these enzymes, such as by asymmetric dimethyl-arginine (ADMA) can not be ruled out [52]. Protein expression of NOS isozymes is also studied during phase I and n and iNOS are found increased while eNOS is decreased [51]. Expression of eNOS mRNA increase during phase I, however, as eNOS protein remains decreased probably due to impaired translation or decreased stability of newly synthesized protein product after SAH [53, 54]. The decrease in eNOS in cerebral vessels after SAH is in contrast to occlusive stroke where an increase in eNOS is found. The absence of change in NOS activity at a time when n and iNOS protein is increased might be related to the decrease in eNOS protein at this time. eNOS decrease will create a local NO deficiency in the cerebral vessels promoting constriction and adhesion of platelet and leukocytes to the endothelium [1, 55]. It is also interesting to note that animals that are either pretreated or given multiple statins (increases eNOS protein expression) treatment extending from phase I to III develop little delayed vasospasm after SAH [56, 57]. That, this observation could not be repeated in clinical SAH may represent delay in initiation of this therapy due to reasons mentioned above [58, 59].

Large and small cerebral vessels are constricted and CBF is reduced in phase I after SAH. A number of studies show that NO dependent vasodilation is impaired after SAH, however, the capacity of arteries to dilate and recover CBF in response to an NO donor remains intact [14, 49, 53]. Hence use of an NO donor during phase I dilates cerebral vessels, attenuates CBF reductions [14, 53]. In contrast, NOS inhibition fails to effect CBF till the very end (60 min) of phase I, indicating NO probably due to its deficiency plays little role in arterial tone at this time [13].

Other early vascular events during phase I include; intraluminal platelet aggregation, loss of endothelial barrier antigen (EBA: a marker of blood brain barrier integrity in rats), activation of vascular collagenases (such as matrix metalloproteinase-9), and destruction of collagen IV (the major protein of basal lamina) leading to increased permeability. Use of NO donor in phase I decreases activation of vascular collagenases and EBA and collagen IV destruction [60].

Taken together, these findings show that reductions in cerebral NO level in phase I play a major role in brain injury during the early hours after SAH.

Phase II (1–6 h After SAH)

Phase II is defined by recovery of cerebral NO level to baseline. In most of the brain regions NO recovery is complete by 3 h after SAH. [15] The mechanism of NO recovery may involve saturation of scavenging mechanisms or increased synthesis. Both neuronal and inducible NOS are increased during phase II, while eNOS protein level is recovering towards the basal levels [54]. Cerebral vessels remain constricted and CBF remains reduced during this phase [60, 61] and NOS inhibitors at this time deceases but

NO donors elicit little effect on CBF ([13];and personal observation). Hence, it appears that although NOS is active at this time, NO produced is un able to recover CBF, probably due to additional vasoconstrictive mechanisms that are in play at this time [10, 62–64]. Because NO availability is presumably already increasing during this period, pharmacological interventions that further increase NO availability would be expected to gradually loose effectiveness during phase II marking an end to the therapeutic window of NO donor administration.

Phase III (6–72 h After SAH)

Phase III is defined by an increase in cerebral NO levels above baseline. In addition to animal data, clinical data is also available for the 24–72 h of phase III. Both animal [65] and human [41, 66] studies report an increase in NO levels at 24 h after SAH. Moreover, in humans cerebral NO level remain increased for at least 3 days after SAH [35, 37, 38] and decrease 6–7 days later [67]. The source of increased NO during phase III involves increased expression of NOS, especially iNOS [51, 68, 69]. Arterial diameter [56] and response to NO donors remains reduced at this phase, possibly due to alteration in cGMP pathways [70]. The large amount of NO produced during phase III is considered destructive for the already compromised brain. Phase III increase in NO level has been linked to oxidative damage of cell membranes [71], axonal degeneration [72], pathogenesis of delayed vasospasm and to the poor clinical presentation [35, 37, 38, 41].

NO, as a free radical by it self and in the form of peroxynitrate formed by its interaction with super oxide can cause oxidative damage [73, 74]. Putative mechanisms of this neurotoxicity involve lipid peroxidation of cell membranes, causing pathological changes in the endothelium and smooth muscle cell structures [75], DNA and mitochondrial damage activation of poly(ADP-ribose) synthase with subsequent depletion of NAD^+ and ATP [76] leading to necrosis and apoptosis [26, 43]. Axonal degeneration probably involves NO-mediated ion fluxes in sodium, potassium, and calcium channels [72]. The mechanisms proposed in NO role in cerebral vasospasm after SAH involve oxidative injury of the endothelium and inflammation, [35, 37, 38, 41]. Yet another mechanism of NO linked vasospasm may be that although over all NO in increased in phase III, amount of NO available to arteries in reduced. A decrease in eNOS protein and eNOS activity linked to cerebral vasospasm is reported 7 days after SAH [52, 77]. We have found recovery of eNOS protein to the basal levels at 24 h after SAH, however, if eNOS activity is altered during phase III is not known [54].

Conclusion

Three phases of alterations in cerebral NO levels can be identified during the first 72 h after SAH. Each phase elicits a different response form the injured brain and contributes differently to the pathophysiology of SAH. A thorough understanding of each phase is required so that they can be taken in account while designing effective therapies against early cerebral injury after SAH. It is very likely that ultimate treatment design is individualized depending upon the time a patient reaches a heath care unit.

Conflict of interest statement We declare that we have no conflict of interest.

References

1. Bederson JB, Levy AL, Ding WH, Kahn R, DiPerna CA, Jenkins AL 3rd, Vallabhajosyula P. Acute vasoconstriction after subarachnoid hemorrhage. Neurosurgery. 1998;42:352–60.
2. Gewirtz RJ, Dhillon HS, Goes SE, DeAtley SM, Scheff SW. Lactate and free fatty acids after subarachnoid hemorrhage. Brain Res. 1999;840:84–91.
3. Stoltenburg-Didinger G, Schwartz K. Brain lesions secondary to subarachnoid hemorrhage due to ruptured aneurysms. In: Cervos-Navarro J, Ferst R, editors. Stroke and microcirculation. New York: Raven Press; 1987. p. 471–80.
4. Fisher CM. Clinical syndromes in cerebral thrombosis, hypertensive hemorrhage, and ruptured saccular aneurysm. Clin Neurosurg. 1975;22:117–47.
5. Nornes H. The role of intracranial pressure in the arrest of hemorrhage in patients with ruptured intracranial aneurysm. J Neurosurg. 1973;39:226–34.
6. Nornes H. Cerebral arterial flow dynamics during aneurysm haemorrhage. Acta Neurochir. 1978;41:39–48.
7. Guan YY, Weir BK, Marton LS, Macdonald RL, Zhang H. Effects of erythrocyte lysate of different incubation times on intracellular free calcium in rat basilar artery smooth-muscle cells. J Neurosurg. 1998;89:1007–14.
8. Clower BR, Yoshioka J, Honma T, Smith R. Blood platelets and early intimal changes in cerebral arteries following experimental subarachnoid hemorrhage. In: Wilkins RL, editor. Cerebral vasospasm. New York: Ravens Press; 1988. p. 335–41.
9. Schumacher MA, Alksne JF. Mechanisms of whole blood-induced cerebral arterial contraction. Neurosurgery 1981;9:275–82.
10. Hall ED, Travis MA. Effects of the nonglucocorticoid 21-aminosteroid U74006F on acute cerebral hypoperfusion following experimental subarachnoid hemorrhage. Exp Neurol. 1988;102:244–48.
11. Travis MA, Hall ED. The effects of chronic two-fold dietary vitamin E supplementation on subarachnoid hemorrhage-induced brain hypoperfusion. Brain Res. 1987;418:366–70.
12. Furuichi S, Endo S, Haji A, Takeda R, Nisijima M, Takaku A. Related changes in sympathetic activity, cerebral blood flow and intracranial pressure, and effect of an alpha-blocker in experimental subarachnoid haemorrhage. Acta Neurochir. 1999;141:415–23.
13. Schwartz AY, Sehba FA, Bederson JB. Decreased nitric oxide availability contributes to acute cerebral ischemia after subarachnoid hemorrhage. Neurosurgery 2000;47:208–14; discussion 214–205.

14. Sehba FA, Ding WH, Chereshnev I, Bederson JB. Effects of S-nitrosoglutathione on acute vasoconstriction and glutamate release after subarachnoid hemorrhage. Stroke 1999;30:1955–61.
15. Sehba FA, Schwartz AY, Chereshnev I, Bederson JB. Acute decrease in cerebral nitric oxide levels after subarachnoid hemorrhage. J Cereb Blood Flow Metab. 2000;20:604–11.
16. Knight JA. Review: Free radicals, antioxidants, and the immune system. Ann Clin Lab Sci. 2000;30:145–58.
17. Rubbo H, Darley-Usmar V, Freeman BA. Nitric oxide regulation of tissue free radical injury. Chem Res Toxicol. 1996;9:809–20.
18. Szabo C. Physiological and pathophysiological roles of nitric oxide in the central nervous system. Brain Res Bull. 1996;41:131–41.
19. Troncy E, Francoeur M, Blaise G. Inhaled nitric oxide: clinical applications, indications, and toxicology. Can J Anaesth. 1997;44:973–88.
20. Watkins LD. Nitric oxide and cerebral blood flow: an update. Cerebrovasc Brain Metab Rev. 1995;7:324–37.
21. Yun HY, Dawson VL, Dawson TM. Neurobiology of nitric oxide. Crit Rev Neurobiol. 1996;10:291–316.
22. Palmer RM, Ashton DS, Moncada S. Vascular endothelial cells synthesize nitric oxide from L-arginine. Nature 1988;333:664–66.
23. Palmer RM, Ferrige AG, Moncada S. Nitric oxide release accounts for the biological activity of endothelium-derived relaxing factor. Nature 1987;327:524–26.
24. Nathan C, Xie QW. Nitric oxide synthases: roles, tolls, and controls. Cell 1994;78:915–18.
25. Cooke JP, Dzau VJ. Nitric oxide synthase: role in the genesis of vascular disease. Annu Rev Med. 1997;48:489–509.
26. Iadecola C. Bright and dark sides of nitric oxide in ischemic brain injury. Trends Neurosci. 1997;20:132–39.
27. Kader A, Frazzini VI, Solomon RA, Trifiletti RR. Nitric oxide production during focal cerebral ischemia in rats. Stroke 1993;24:1709–16.
28. Zhang ZG, Chopp M, Gautam S, Zaloga C, Zhang RL, Schmidt HH, et al. Upregulation of neuronal nitric oxide synthase and mRNA, and selective sparing of nitric oxide synthase-containing neurons after focal cerebral ischemia in rat. Brain Res. 1994;654:85–95.
29. Iadecola C, Zhang F, Casey R, Clark HB, Ross ME. Inducible nitric oxide synthase gene expression in vascular cells after transient focal cerebral ischemia. Stroke 1996;27:1373–80.
30. Iadecola C, Zhang F, Xu S, Casey R, Ross ME. Inducible nitric oxide synthase gene expression in brain following cerebral ischemia. J Cereb Blood Flow Metab. 1995;15:378–84.
31. Bolanos JP, Almeida A. Roles of nitric oxide in brain hypoxia-ischemia. Biochim Biophys Acta. 1999;1411:415–36.
32. Daughters K, Waxman K, Nguyen H. Increasing nitric oxide production improves survival in experimental hemorrhagic shock. Resuscitation 1996;31:141–44.
33. Kosaka H. Nitric oxide and hemoglobin interactions in the vasculature. Biochim Biophys Acta. 1999;1411:370–77.
34. Afshar JK, Pluta RM, Boock RJ, Thompson BG, Oldfield EH. Effect of intracarotid nitric oxide on primate cerebral vasospasm after subarachnoid hemorrhage. J Neurosurg. 1995;83:118–22.
35. Durmaz R, Ozkara E, Kanbak G, Arslan O, Dokumacioğlu A, Kartkaya K, et al. Nitric oxide level and adenosine deaminase activity in cerebrospinal fluid of patients with subarachnoid hemorrhage. Turk Neurosurg. 2008;18:157–64.
36. Edwards DH, Byrne JV, Griffith TM. The effect of chronic subarachnoid hemorrhage on basal endothelium-derived relaxing factor activity in intrathecal cerebral arteries. J Neurosurg. 1992;76:830–37.
37. Khaldi A, Zauner A, Reinert M, Woodward JJ, Bullock MR. Measurement of nitric oxide and brain tissue oxygen tension in patients after severe subarachnoid hemorrhage. Neurosurgery 2001;49:33–8; discussion 38–40.
38. Ng WH, Moochhala S, Yeo TT, Ong PL, Ng PY. Nitric oxide and subarachnoid hemorrhage: elevated level in cerebrospinal fluid and their implications. Neurosurgery 2001;49:622–26; discussion 626–627.
39. Pluta RM, Oldfield EH, Boock RJ. Reversal and prevention of cerebral vasospasm by intracarotid infusions of nitric oxide donors in a primate model of subarachnoid hemorrhage. J Neurosurg. 1997;87:746–51.
40. Suzuki Y, Kajita Y, Oyama H, Tanazawa T, Takayasu M, Shibuya M, et al. Dysfunction of nitric oxide in the spastic basilar arteries after subarachnoid hemorrhage. J Auton Nerv Syst. 1994;49 Suppl:S83–7.
41. Woszczyk A, Deinsberger W, Boker DK. Nitric oxide metabolites in cisternal CSF correlate with cerebral vasospasm in patients with a subarachnoid haemorrhage. Acta Neurochir (Wien). 2003;145:257–64.
42. Sehba FA, Bederson JB. Mechanisms of acute brain injury after subarachnoid hemorrhage. Neurol Res. 2006;28:381–98.
43. Higuchi Y, Hattori H, Hattori R, Furusho K. Increased neurons containing neuronal nitric oxide synthase in the brain of a hypoxic-ischemic neonatal rat model. Brain Dev. 1996;18:369–75.
44. Kumura E, Kosaka H, Shiga T, Yoshimine T, Hayakawa T. Elevation of plasma nitric oxide end products during focal ischemia and reperfusion in the rat. J Cereb Blood Flow Meteb. 1994;14:487–91.
45. Malinski T, Bailey F, Zhang ZG, Chopp M. Nitric oxide measured by a porphyrinic microsensor in rat brain after transient middle cerebral artery occlusion. J Cereb Blood Flow Metab. 1993;13:355–58.
46. Shibata M, Araki N, Hamada J, Sasaki T, Shimazu K, Fukuuchi Y. Brain nitrite production during global ischemia and reperfusion: an in vivo microdialysis study. Brain Res. 1996;734:86–90.
47. Zhang ZG, Chopp M, Bailey F, Malinski T. Nitric oxide changes in the rat brain after transient middle cerebral artery occlusion. J Neurol Sci. 1995;128:22–7.
48. Kajita Y, Suzuki Y, Oyama H, Tanazawa T, Takayasu M, Shibuya M, Sugita K. Combined effect of L-arginine and superoxide dismutase on the spastic basilar artery after subarachnoid hemorrhage in dogs. J Neurosurg. 1994;80:476–83.
49. Sobey CG, Faraci FM. Subarachnoid haemorrhage: what happens to the cerebral arteries? Clin Exp Pharmacol Physiol. 1998;25:867–76.
50. Provencio JJ, Vora N. Subarachnoid hemorrhage and inflammation: bench to bedside and back. Semin Neurol. 2005;25:435–44.
51. Sehba FA, Chereshnev I, Maayani S, Friedrich V, Jr., Bederson JB. Nitric oxide synthase in acute alteration of Nitric oxide levels after subarachnoid hemorrhage. Neurosurgery 2004;55:671–77; discussion 677–678.
52. Pluta RM. Dysfunction of nitric oxide synthases as a cause and therapeutic target in delayed cerebral vasospasm after SAH. Acta Neurochir Suppl. 2008;104:139–47.
53. Park KW, Metais C, Dai HB, Comunale ME, Sellke FW. Microvascular endothelial dysfunction and its mechanism in a rat model of subarachnoid hemorrhage. Anesth Analg. 2001;92:990–96.
54. Sehba FA, Flores R, Muller A, Friedrich V, Bederson JB. Early decrease in cerebral endothelial nitric oxide synthase occurs after subarachnoid hemorrhage. Annu Stroke Conf. 2007;172:P527.
55. Sehba FA, Mustafa G, Friedrich V, Bederson JB. Acute microvascular platelet aggregation after subarachnoid hemorrhage. J Neurosurg. 2005;102:1094–100.
56. McGirt MJ, Pradilla G, Legnani FG, Thai QA, Recinos PF, Tamargo RJ, et al. Systemic administration of simvastatin after the onset of experimental subarachnoid hemorrhage attenuates cerebral vasospasm. Neurosurgery 2006;58:945–51; discussion 945–951.
57. Sugawara T, Ayer R, Jadhav V, Chen W, Tsubokawa T, Zhang JH. Simvastatin attenuation of cerebral vasospasm after subarachnoid

58. Kern M, Lam MM, Knuckey NW, Lind CR. Statins may not protect against vasospasm in subarachnoid haemorrhage. J Clin Neurosci. 2009;16:527–30.
59. McGirt MJ, Garces Ambrossi GL, Huang J, Tamargo RJ. Simvastatin for the prevention of symptomatic cerebral vasospasm following aneurysmal subarachnoid hemorrhage: a single-institution prospective cohort study. J Neurosurg. 2009;110:968–74.
60. Sehba FA, Makonnen G, Friedrich V, Bederson JB. Acute cerebral vascular injury occurs after subarachnoid hemorrhage and can be prevented by administration of a nitric oxide donor. J Neurosurg. 2007;106:321–29.
61. Sun BL, Zheng CB, Yang MF, Yuan H, Zhang SM, Wang LX. Dynamic alterations of cerebral pial microcirculation during experimental subarachnoid hemorrhage. Cell Mol Neurobiol. 2009;29:235–41.
62. Asano T, Sano K. Pathogenetic role of no-reflow phenomenon in experimental subarachnoid hemorrhage in dogs. J Neurosurg. 1977;46:454–66.
63. Clower BR, Yoshioka J, Honma Y, Smith RR. Pathological changes in cerebral arteries following experimental subarachnoid hemorrhage: role of blood platelets. Anat Rec. 1988;220:161–70.
64. Schubert GA, Schilling L, Thome C. Clazosentan, an endothelin receptor antagonist, prevents early hypoperfusion during the acute phase of massive experimental subarachnoid hemorrhage: a laser Doppler flowmetry study in rats. J Neurosurg. 2008;109:1134–40.
65. Yatsushige H, Calvert JW, Cahill J, Zhang JH. Limited role of inducible nitric oxide synthase in blood-brain barrier function after experimental subarachnoid hemorrhage. J Neurotrauma. 2006;23:1874–82.
66. Suzuki M, Asahara H, Endo S, Inada K, Doi M, Kuroda K, et al. Increased levels of nitrite/nitrate in the cerebrospinal fluid of patients with subarachnoid hemorrhage. Neurosurg Rev. 1999;22:96–8.
67. Jung CS, Iuliano BA, Harvey-White J, Espey MG, Oldfield EH, Pluta RM. Association between cerebrospinal fluid levels of asymmetric dimethyl-L-arginine, an endogenous inhibitor of endothelial nitric oxide synthase, and cerebral vasospasm in a primate model of subarachnoid hemorrhage. J Neurosurg. 2004;101:836–42.
68. Seidel B, Stanarius A, Wolf G. Differential expression of neuronal and endothelial nitric oxide synthase in blood vessels of the rat brain. Neurosci Lett. 1997;239:109–12.
69. Vikman P, Beg S, Khurana TS, Hansen-Schwartz J, Edvinsson L. Gene expression and molecular changes in cerebral arteries following subarachnoid hemorrhage in the rat. J Neurosurg. 2006;105:438–44.
70. Yamamoto S, Nishizawa S, Yokoyama T, Ryu H, Uemura K. Subarachnoid hemorrhage impairs cerebral blood flow response to nitric oxide but not to cyclic GMP in large cerebral arteries. Brain Res. 1997;757:1–9.
71. Ayer RE, Zhang JH. Oxidative stress in subarachnoid haemorrhage: significance in acute brain injury and vasospasm. Acta Neurochir Suppl. 2008;104:33–41.
72. Petzold A, Rejdak K, Belli A, Sen J, Keir G, Kitchen N, et al. Axonal pathology in subarachnoid and intracerebral hemorrhage. J Neurotrauma. 2005;22:407–14.
73. Eliasson MJ, Huang Z, Ferrante RJ, Sasamata M, Molliver ME, Snyder SH, Moskowitz MA. Neuronal nitric oxide synthase activation and peroxynitrite formation in ischemic stroke linked to neural damage. J Neurosci. 1999;19:5910–918.
74. Forman LJ, Liu P, Nagele RG, Yin K, Wong PY. Augmentation of nitric oxide, superoxide, and peroxynitrite production during cerebral ischemia and reperfusion in the rat. Neurochem Res. 1998;23:141–48.
75. Beckman JS, Beckman TW, Chen J, Marshall PA, Freeman BA. Apparent hydroxyl radical production by peroxynitrite: implications for endothelial injury from nitric oxide and superoxide. Proc Natl Acad Sci USA. 1990;87:1620–24.
76. Leist M, Nicotera P. Apoptosis, excitotoxicity, and neuropathology. Exp Cell Res. 1998;239:183–201.
77. Pluta RM, Thompson BG, Dawson TM, Snyder SH, Boock RJ, Oldfield EH. Loss of nitric oxide synthase immunoreactivity in cerebral vasospasm. J Neurosurg. 1996;84:648–54.

Nitric Oxide Related Pathophysiological Changes Following Subarachnoid Haemorrhage

Mohammed Sabri, Jinglu Ai, and R. Loch Macdonald

Abstract Subarachnoid hemorrhage (SAH) comprises only about 7% of all strokes worldwide but is associated with severe mortality and morbidity. SAH is associated with a number of secondary pathologies, such as: transient cerebral vasospasm, delayed ischemic neuronal deficit (DIND), cortical spreading depression, microcirculatory modifications, microthrombosis and ischemic complications. Available data demonstrate that there are complix interactions among these secondary complications, and NO plays an important role among the interactions. NO has been implicated to be a crucial molecule in eliminating vasospasm, facilitating neuroprotection, anti-microthrombosis, cerebral ischemic tolerance and promoting endothelial cell function. Therefore, therapeutic agent targeting a key component in the pathopyhysiology of SAH such as NO and its related enzymes would be favorable for future development of SAH drugs. Alternatively, because of the complex nature of the secondary complications after SAH, agents with multiple efficacies on these complications, or the combination of several agents such as NO donors, oxide radical scavengers and neuroprotectants might be more desirable.

Keywords eNOS · Microthrombosis · Nitric oxide (NO) · Oxidative stress · Subarachnoid hemorrhage (SAH)

Introduction

Subarachnoid hemorrhage (SAH) comprises only about 7% of all strokes worldwide but is associated with severe mortality and morbidity [1]. SAH is the spontaneous bleeding into the subarachnoid space due to a traumatic hit to the head or rupture of intracranial aneurysms. SAH is associated with a number of secondary pathologies, such as: transient cerebral vasospasm, delayed ischemic neuronal deficit (DIND), cortical spreading depression, microcirculatory modifications, microthrombosis and ischemic complications [2, 3] (Fig. 1). Several molecular theories behind the onset of vasospasm, DIND and microthrombosis have been proposed, among which, the nitric oxide (NO)-based hypothesis is getting recognized. NO is produced by endothelial nitric oxide synthase (eNOS) in endothelium cells, and regulates vascular tone and dilatation for focal blood flow control [4]. NO has been implicated to be a crucial molecule in the brain, facilitating neuroprotection, anti-microthrombosis, cerebral ischemic tolerance and promotes endothelial cell function [5]. Further evidence suggests that eNOS and neuronal nitric oxide synthase (nNOS) play a major role in the progression of SAH, and are possible targets for future therapy.

Nitric Oxide and Vasoconstriction

NO provides protective anti-vasoconstricting properties, where it inhibits large vessel responsiveness to several vasoconstrictors such as 5-HT, PGE2 and thromboxane. In SAH, impaired relaxation may result from (1) Haemoglobin related vasospasm. Hb results in direct dysfunction of smooth muscles and scavenging of NO [6, 7]. Haemoglobin also produces superoxide radicals, which reacts and breaks down NO to form peroxynitrite that facilitating the dysfunction of eNOS, exacerbating both the vasospasm and subsequent secondary complications [6, 8]. Haemoglobin is also associated with the direct reduction of cGMP levels. (2) Reduction in the endothelium dependent-relaxation caused by loss of cGMP. This will result in reduced phosphorylation of eNOS, thus decreased NO. (3) Inflammatory response induced activation of neutrophils and macrophages. This

M. Sabri, J. Ai, and R.L. Macdonald (✉)
Division of Neurosurgery, St. Michael's Hospital, Keenan Research Centre in the Li Ka Shing Knowledge Institute of St. Michael's Hospital and Department of Surgery, University of Toronto, Toronto, ON, Canada
e-mail: macdonaldlo@smh.ca

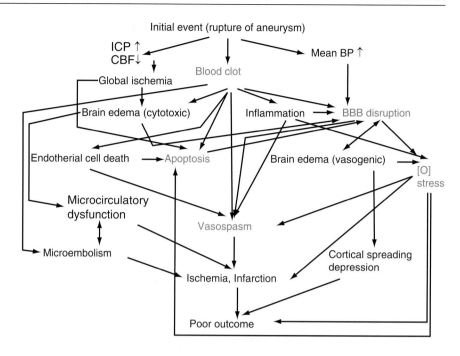

Fig. 1 Schematic representation of the multiple pathogenic complications that are observed after subarachnoid hemorrhage and the interrelationships that exists within them

results in the breakdown of NO, therefore facilitating vasoconstriction. It is evident that the presence of the blood clot in subarachnoid patients or in experimental models is a key activator of cerebral vasospasm, due to the direct link between haemoglobin and the scavenging of NO.

Pathogenesis of Cerebral Vasospasm and the Role of eNOS

NO availability directs the progression of SAH significantly. NO was readily scavenged from canine basilar arteries (BA) when haemoglobin was applied [9]. This was responsible for the subsequent vasoconstriction observed. Byrne et al demonstrated that haemoglobin not only inhibited NO but efficiently scavenged the protective molecules [10]. It is evident, therefore, that the role of NO is crucial in the progression of SAH and in modulating cerebral vasospasm and possibly other secondary complications. Several studies focused on eNOS in order to investigate if the enzyme was modified adversely by presence of blood in the subarachnoid space.

It has been demonstrated that there is an initial up regulation of eNOS after the onset of SAH, possibly linked to the vasospastic insult that introduces shear stress on the endothelium [11–13]. Harrison et al reported an upregulation of eNOS mRNA levels after exposing endothelial cells to shear stress, indicating a possible link between vasospasm and subsequent up-regulation of eNOS [14, 15]. Other insults, such as increased oxidative stress what was introduced by the haemoglobin break down products, bilirubin oxidation products (BOXes) and superoxides, regulates eNOS as well [16]. It has been hypothesized that this initial eNOS up regulation is a protective mechanism against cerebral vasospasm. However, recent data points to the possibility of upregulation of uncoupled eNOS that exacerbates oxidative stress, vasospasm and secondary pathologies rather than alleviating them [17]. Reports by Griendling et al demonstrated a direct link between oxidative stress and smooth muscle cell hypertrophy and endothelial cell apoptosis leading to the eventual endothelial dysfunction and vasospasm [18].

DIND, Microthrombosis, Radicals and Oxidative Stress

DIND is one of the secondary complications seen in 20–30% of all SAH patients that develop vasospasm. It is a commonly observed complication in experimental models as well, possibly indicating the importance of vasospasm and blood products on the incidence of DIND [19]. The occurrence of clinical DIND was substantiated when autopsies of SAH patients were analyzed and found to be positive for neuronal cell injury in the hippocampus [20]. DIND has also been hypothesized to be a major cause of the neurological and cognitive deficits observed in some SAH survivors [21, 22]. DIND has been hypothesized to be a byproduct of ischemic damage, oxidative stress, vasospasm and a combinatorial effect of several adverse conditions introduced by the onset of bleeding such as BBB disruption, increased ICP and heightened inflammatory conditions. Both eNOS and NO contribute to the progression of DIND indirectly, where the deficiency of NO due to faster than normal breakdown or reduced synthesis has been hypothesized to contribute to the severity of vasospasm and subsequent ischemic damage. Excessive NO production due to the compensatory feedback mechanisms to combat vasospasm have also been shown to have toxic effects on vasomotor function and increase inflammatory insults on neighbouring vessels. Excessive NO also reacts with superoxides introduced by blood products producing peroxynitrites which exacerbate oxidative stress and subsequent neuronal injury.

Recently, several studies on microthrombosis demonstrated that such microcirculatory changes maybe major players in the progression of SAH, vasospasm and the development of delayed cerebral ischemia [23]. Even though vasospasm remains to be a good determinant for cerebral infarction in SAH patients, in 33% of patients with cerebral infarcts vasospasm is not predictive of location or incidence on infarction [24]. Additionally, several SAH patients develop cortical band-like infarcts with no radiographic or clinical evidence of vasospasm, postulating the increasingly important role that microvessels plays in SAH [23–26]. Several studies demonstrated that SAH patients have heightened levels of serological coagulation markers which often correlate with the development of DIND, severity of SAH and poor outcome [23]. Autopsies studies have demonstrated that microthrombi were detected in patients with SAH and cerebral infarct [23, 27, 28]. The reduction of NO has been associated with the production of microthrombi. NO confers an antimicrothrombotic effect that prevents plaques from developing and unwanted platelet activation.

SAH produces several radicals such as reactive oxidative species (ROS), BOXes and superoxides in the brain, which creating an oxidative environment. A recent study reported that malondialdehyde, a by-product of lipid peroxidation and marker of oxidative stress, was selectively elevated in the CSF of SAH patients. Its level at 14 days post SAH correlated with poor outcome [29]. Several experimental and clinical studies demonstrated that SAH introduces a biochemical imbalance that is geared towards producing more radicals and the reduction of anti-oxidative processes [30–33]. It has been demonstrated that the overproduction O^2 reacts with NO to produce peroxynitrite [34], which in turn contributes to neuronal cell injury, endothelial cell injury and eventual vasomotor dysfunction. Oxidative stress due to increase ROS is also associated with increased incidence of DNA breaks in the neurons and therefore may be a major factor in the development of delayed neuronal injury and DIND [35, 36].

Therapeutic Application of NO

Current treatment options for SAH patient revolve around the elimination of delayed cerebral vasospasm and aimed on the improvement of CBF levels though the vasodilatation of vessels. The usefulness of hypervolemic–hypertensive-hemodilution (triple H) therapy is in doubt due to the high rate of complications that often outweigh the benefits [37]. Hemorrhagic clot is the culprit behind several complications observed in SAH. However, no simple surgical intervention can eliminate it from the subarachnoid space [38]. This obstacle complicates the treatment options available for SAH patients. Several clinical trials have been conducted utilizing NO substituting products to dilate constricted vessels in the hopes to reverse secondary complications [39–41]. The success of most NO donor clinical trials was often attributed to the NO-cGMP effect on the smooth muscles, inducing vasorelxation and the reversal of vasospasm. Other mechanisms of NO donor-specifc relief of vasospasm have been hypothesized (1) NO may react with haemoglobin to produce Fe-nitrosyl-hemoglobin which aids in the quenching of deoxyHb. (2) the direct NO-induced closure of potassium channels leading to the hyperpolarization of smooth muscle cells and reverse cerebral vasospasm [42]. One disadvantage of general vasodilators is their role in increasing ICP and lowering perfusion pressure, which becomes a risky treatment option for patients that are hemodynamically unstable and more prone to ischemic complications.

Conclusion

NO and its producing NOSes are closely linked to many of the pathophysiological changes following SAH. These include vasospasm, DIND, microthrombosis and oxidative stress that all contribute to the secondary deterioration in patients. Therefore, therapeutic agent with multiple efficacies on these complications, or the combination of several agents such as NO donors, oxide radical scavengers and neuroprotectants would be more desirable for future development of SAH drugs.

Acknowledgement This research is supported by funding from Physician Service Incorporated Ontario, Brain Aneurism Foundation to Dr. R Loch Macdonald.

Conflict of interest statement Dr. R. Loch Macdonald is a consultant for Actelion Pharmaceuticals. He is chief scientific officer of Edge Therapeutics.

References

1. Taylor TN, Davis PH, Torner JC, Holmes J, Meyer JW, Jacobson MF. Lifetime cost of stroke in the United States. Stroke 1996;27:1459–66.
2. Macdonald RL, Pluta RM, Zhang JH. Cerebral vasospasm after subarachnoid hemorrhage: the emerging revolution. Nat Clin Pract Neurol. 2007;3:256–63.
3. Pluta RM, Hansen-Schwartz J, Dreier J, Vajkoczy P, Macdonald RL, Nishizawa S, et al. Cerebral vasospasm following subarachnoid hemorrhage: time for a new world of thought. Neurol Res. 2009;31:151–8.
4. Forstermann U, Munzel, T. Endothelial nitric oxide synthase in vascular disease: from marvel to menace. Circulation 2006;113:1708–14.
5. Hashiguchi A, Yano S, Morioka M, Hamada J, Ushio Y, Takeuchi Y, et al. Up-regulation of endothelial nitric oxide synthase via phosphatidylinositol 3-kinase pathway contributes to ischemic tolerance in the CA1 subfield of gerbil hippocampus. J Cereb Blood Flow Metab. 2004;24:271–79.
6. Ignarro LJ. Biosynthesis and metabolism of endothelium-derived nitric oxide. Annu Rev Pharmacol Toxicol. 1990;30, 535–60.
7. Wennmalm A, Benthin G, Petersson AS. Dependence of the metabolism of nitric oxide (NO) in healthy human whole blood on the oxygenation of its red cell haemoglobin. Br J Pharmacol. 1992;106:507–8.
8. Fujiwara S, Kassell NF, Sasaki T, Nakagomi T, Lehman RM. Selective hemoglobin inhibition of endothelium-dependent vasodilation of rabbit basilar artery. J Neurosurg. 1986;64:445–52.
9. Kanamaru K, Waga S, Kojima T, Fujimoto K, Niwa S. Endothelium-dependent relaxation of canine basilar arteries. Part 2: Inhibition by hemoglobin and cerebrospinal fluid from patients with aneurysmal subarachnoid hemorrhage. Stroke 1987;18:938–43.
10. Byrne JV, Griffith TM, Edwards DH, Harrison TJ, Johnston KR. Investigation of the vasoconstrictor action of subarachnoid haemoglobin in the pig cerebral circulation in vivo. Br J Pharmacol. 1989;97:669–74.
11. Black SM, Fineman JR, Steinhorn RH, Bristow J, Soifer SJ. Increased endothelial NOS in lambs with increased pulmonary blood flow and pulmonary hypertension. Am J Physiol. 1998;275:H1643–51.
12. Mattsson EJ, Kohler TR, Vergel SM, Clowes AW. Increased blood flow induces regression of intimal hyperplasia. Arterioscler Thromb Vasc Biol. 1997;17:2245–49.
13. Mazumder B, Seshadri V, Fox PL. Translational control by the 3'-UTR: the ends specify the means. Trends Biochem Sci. 2003;28:91–8.
14. Harrison DG, Kurz MA, Quillen JE, Sellke FW, Mugge A. Normal and pathophysiologic considerations of endothelial regulation of vascular tone and their relevance to nitrate therapy. Am J Cardiol. 1992;70:11B–7B.
15. Harrison DG. The endothelial cell. Heart Dis Stroke 1992;1:95–9.
16. Ayer RE, Zhang JH. Oxidative stress in subarachnoid haemorrhage: significance in acute brain injury and vasospasm. Acta Neurochir Suppl. 2008;104:33–41.
17. Osuka K, Watanabe Y, Usuda N, Atsuzawa K, Yoshida J, Takayasu M. Modification of endothelial nitric oxide synthase through AMPK after experimental subarachnoid hemorrhage. J Neurotrauma. 2009;26(7):1157–65.
18. Griendling KK, Ushio-Fukai M. Redox control of vascular smooth muscle proliferation. J Lab Clin Med. 1998;132:9–15.
19. Sabri M, Kawashima A, Ai J, Macdonald RL. Neuronal and astrocytic apoptosis after subarachnoid hemorrhage: a possible cause for poor prognosis. Brain Res. 2008;1238:163–71.
20. Nau R, Haase S, Bunkowski S, Bruck W. Neuronal apoptosis in the dentate gyrus in humans with subarachnoid hemorrhage and cerebral hypoxia. Brain Pathol. 2002;12:329–36.
21. Jeon H, Ai J, Sabri M, Tariq A, Shang X, Chen G, et al. Neurological and neurobehavioral assessment of experimental subarachnoid hemorrhage. BMC Neurosci. 2009;10:103.
22. Schievink WI. Intracranial aneurysms. N Engl J Med. 1997;336:28–40.
23. Vergouwen MD, Vermeulen M, Coert BA, Stroes ES, Roos YB. Microthrombosis after aneurysmal subarachnoid hemorrhage: an additional explanation for delayed cerebral ischemia. J Cereb Blood Flow Metab. 2008;28:1761–70.
24. Weidauer S, Vatter H, Beck J, Raabe A, Lanfermann H, Seifert V., et al. Focal laminar cortical infarcts following aneurysmal subarachnoid haemorrhage. Neuroradiology 2008;50:1–8.
25. Naidech AM, Drescher J, Ault ML, Shaibani, A, Batjer, HH, Alberts, MJ. Higher hemoglobin is associated with less cerebral infarction, poor outcome, and death after subarachnoid hemorrhage. Neurosurgery 2006;59:775–9.
26. Naidech AM, Drescher J, Tamul P, Shaibani A, Batjer HH, Alberts MJ. Acute physiological derangement is associated with early radiographic cerebral infarction after subarachnoid haemorrhage. J Neurol Neurosurg Psychiatry. 2006;77:1340–44.
27. Suzuki N, Nakamura T, Imabayashi S, Ishikawa Y, Sasaki T, Asano T. Identification of 5-hydroxy eicosatetraenoic acid in cerebrospinal fluid after subarachnoid hemorrhage. J Neurochem. 1983;41:1186–9.
28. Ohkuma H, Suzuki S, Nonogaki Y, Sohma M. [Disturbance of inhibitory capacity of endothelial cell for platelet adhesion or aggregation following experimental subarachnoid hemorrhage]. No Shinkei Geka. 1990;18:47–52.
29. Kaneda K, Fujita M, Yamashita S, Kaneko T, Kawamura Y, Izumi T, et al. Prognostic value of biochemical markers of brain damage and oxidative stress in post-surgical aneurysmal subarachnoid hemorrhage patients. Brain Res Bull. 2010;81:173–7.
30. Gaetani P, Pasqualin A, Baena R, Borasio E, Marzatico F. Oxidative stress in the human brain after subarachnoid hemorrhage. J Neurosurg. 1998;89:748–54.
31. Kaynar MY, Tanriverdi T, Kemerdere R, Atukeren P, Gumustas K. Cerebrospinal fluid superoxide dismutase and serum malondialdehyde levels in patients with aneurysmal subarachnoid hemorrhage: preliminary results. Neurol Res. 2005;27:562–7.
32. Marzatico F, Gaetani P, Cafe C, Spanu G, Baena R. Antioxidant enzymatic activities after experimental subarachnoid hemorrhage in rats. Acta Neurol Scand. 1993;87:62–6.
33. Marzatico F, Gaetani P, Tartara F, Bertorelli L, Feletti F, Adinolfi D, et al. Antioxidant status and alpha1-antiproteinase activity in subarachnoid hemorrhage patients. Life Sci. 1998;63:821–6.
34. Gilgun-Sherki Y, Rosenbaum Z, Melamed E, Offen D. Antioxidant therapy in acute central nervous system injury: current state. Pharmacol Rev. 2002;54:271–84.
35. Facchinetti F, Dawson VL, Dawson TM. Free radicals as mediators of neuronal injury. Cell Mol Neurobiol. 1998;18:667–82.
36. Lewen A, Matz P, Chan PH. Free radical pathways in CNS injury. J Neurotrauma. 2000;17:871–90.
37. Egge A, Waterloo K, Sjoholm H, Solberg T, Ingebrigtsen T, Romner B. Prophylactic hyperdynamic postoperative fluid therapy

after aneurysmal subarachnoid hemorrhage: a clinical, prospective, randomized, controlled study. Neurosurgery 2001;49: 593–605.
38. Handa Y, Weir BK, Nosko M, Mosewich R, Tsuji T, Grace M. The effect of timing of clot removal on chronic vasospasm in a primate model. J Neurosurg. 1987;67:558–64.
39. Dorsch NW. Therapeutic approaches to vasospasm in subarachnoid hemorrhage. Curr Opin Crit Care. 2002;8:128–33.
40. Pluta RM. Delayed cerebral vasospasm and nitric oxide: review, new hypothesis, and proposed treatment. Pharmacol Ther. 2005;105:23–56.
41. Pluta RM. Dysfunction of nitric oxide synthases as a cause and therapeutic target in delayed cerebral vasospasm after SAH. Neurol Res. 2006;28:730–7.
42. Hanggi D, Steiger HJ. Nitric oxide in subarachnoid haemorrhage and its therapeutics implications. Acta Neurochir (Wien). 2006; 148:605–13.

Endothelin-1₍₁₋₃₁₎ Induces Spreading Depolarization in Rats

D. Jorks, S. Major, A.I. Oliveira-Ferreira, J. Kleeberg, and J.P. Dreier

Abstract *Background*: The vasoconstrictor endothelin-1$_{(1-21)}$ (ET-1) seems to induce cerebral vasospasm after aneurismal subarachnoid hemorrhage (aSAH). Moreover, ET-1 causes spreading depolarization (SD) via vasoconstriction/ischemia. ET-1$_{(1-31)}$ is an alternate metabolic intermediate in the generation of ET-1. Our aim was to investigate whether endothelin-1$_{(1-31)}$ causes SD in a similar fashion to ET-1.

Method: Increasing concentrations of either ET-1, ET-1$_{(1-31)}$ or vehicle were brain topically applied in 29 rats. Each concentration was superfused for one hour while regional cerebral blood flow (rCBF) and direct current electrocorticogram (DC-ECoG) were recorded.

Findings: In response to the highest concentration of 10^{-6}M, all animals of both ET groups developed typical SD. At concentrations below 10^{-6}M only ET-1 induced SD (n = 14 of 19 rats). Thus, the efficacy of ET-1$_{(1-31)}$ to induce SD was significantly lower ($P < 0.001$, two-tailed Fisher's Exact Test).

Conclusions: Our findings suggest that ET-1$_{(1-31)}$ less potently induces SD compared to ET-1 which implicates that it is a less potent vasoconstrictor. Speculatively, it could be interesting to shift the metabolic pathway towards the alternate intermediate ET-1$_{(1-31)}$ after aSAH as an alternative strategy to ET$_A$ receptor inhibition. This could decrease ET-induced vasoconstriction and SD generation while a potentially beneficial basal ET$_A$ receptor activation is maintained.

Keywords Electrocorticography · Endothelin-1 · Ischemia · Spreading depression · Vasospasm · Stroke

Introduction

Delayed ischemic neurological deficit (DIND) is the predominant in-hospital complication after aSAH. The risk of developing DIND correlates with the amount of blood observed in the initial CT [1], and its onset coincides with the peak of subarachnoid hemolysis after aSAH [2]. This led to the hypothesis that breakdown products of erythrocytes induce DIND [3].

Proximal vasospasm develops in 40–70% of cases with aSAH [4]. In addition, there is clinical evidence of chronic vasospasm in intraparenchymal arterioles [5] as well as sudden pial and intraparenchymal arteriolar spasm triggered by SD. The latter process has been termed spreading ischemia and is assumed to occur superimposed on chronic vasospasm [6, 7]. Based on experimental and clinical evidence, it is increasingly recognized that all three types of vasospasm contribute to the development of delayed ischemia.

It has been suggested that ET-1 plays a role in chronic vasospasm after aSAH [8]. Recognized as a neuropeptide with neurotransmitter/neuromodulator functions, ET-1 is also a potent vasoconstrictor. Thus, a concentration of 10^{-6}M directly applied to the middle cerebral artery was sufficient to produce severe arterial spasm and ischemic damage in the vascular territory [9]. Similarly, brain topical application of ET-1 induced ischemic damage through pial and intraparenchymal vasospasm [10, 11]. ET$_A$ receptor antagonists attenuated proximal vasospasm in animal models [12, 13] and a double-blind, randomized clinical trial of the selective ET_A receptor antagonist clazosentan showed a robust (65% at the highest drug dose) reduction in the relative risk of angiographic vasospasm [14]. In contrast to a possible role in proximal vasospasm, experimental evidence suggested that ET-1 is not involved in spreading ischemia since ET_A and ET_B receptor antagonists failed to antagonize this neuronally induced arteriolar spasm whereas L-type calcium antagonists such as nimodipine or nitric oxide donors effectively caused spreading ischemia to revert to spreading hyperemia in response to SD [6, 15, 16].

ET-1 is a 21-amino acid polypeptide (Fig. 1a). Its effects are mediated by ET_A and ET_B receptors (Fig. 1b). ET_A receptors reside on vascular smooth muscle cells and mediate vasoconstriction while ET_B receptors reside on endothelium and mediate vasodilatation through the release of NO and prostacyclin [17]. ET-1 is generated from pro-ET-1 in a two-step enzymatic pathway. Firstly, subtilisin-like convertases and a carboxypeptidase produce the 38-amino acid precursor big-ET-1. Then, cleavage of big-ET-1 by endothelin-converting enzyme (ECE) yields ET-1 [18]. In addition, there is an alternate intermediate ET-1$_{(1-31)}$ (Fig. 1a) that results from cleavage of the Tyr^{31}–Gly^{32} bond of big-ET-1 by mast-cell derived chymase [19]. In contrast to the direct production of ET-1 from big-ET-1, neutral endopeptidase 24.11 (NEP) and, to a lesser extent, ECE are involved in the generation of ET-1 from ET-1$_{(1-31)}$ [20]. To our knowledge, it has not been demonstrated directly that ET-1$_{(1-31)}$ exists in the brain. However, chymase, the key enzyme of ET-1$_{(1-31)}$ production, is expressed in human brain which implicates the presence of ET-1$_{(1-31)}$ [21].

It has been found previously that ET-1 induced vasoconstriction causes SD as part of the process that transforms viable neurons into necrotic ones [11, 22, 23]. Here, we investigated whether brain topical application of the alternate metabolic intermediate ET-1$_{(1-31)}$ would induce SD in a similar fashion to ET-1.

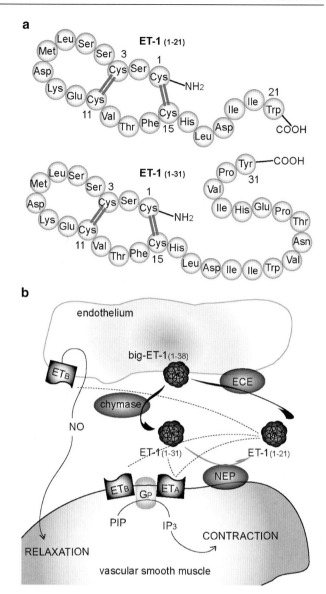

Fig. 1 ET-1 peptides & receptors (**a**) The two disulfide bridges represent an important structural feature of both peptides (*gray double bars*) that lead to the formation of loops. (**b**) In the cerebrovasculature, physiological vasoconstriction of ET-1 is exclusively mediated by smooth muscle ET_A and vasodilatation by endothelial ET_B receptors. It is controversial whether a contractile smooth muscle ET_B receptor subtype is expressed in brain under pathological conditions such as aSAH [13]

Materials and Methods

Animals

Male Wistar rats (n = 29, 220–410 g) were anesthetized with thiopental sodium intraperitoneally (Trapanal, BYK Pharmaceuticals; Konstanz, Germany), tracheotomized and artificially ventilated. The left femoral artery and vein were cannulated and continuously infused with a saline solution. Body temperature was maintained at $37.5 \pm 0.5°C$. Systemic arterial pressure (RFT Biomonitor; Zwönitz, Germany), endexpiratory pCO_2 (Heyer CO_2 Monitor EGM I; Bad Ems, Germany) and arterial blood gases were monitored.

An open cranial window of 4×7 mm was implanted over the somatosensory cortex using a saline-cooled drill as reported previously (Fig. 2a) [22]. The dura mater was removed and the cortical surface was continuously superfused with artificial cerebrospinal fluid (aCSF). RCBF was monitored by two laser-Doppler flow probes (Perimed AB, Järfälla, Sweden). DC-ECoG was measured with a subarachnoid Ag-AgCl electrode connected to a differential amplifier

(Jens Meyer, Munich, Germany) (Fig. 2a). Data were recorded using Spike 2 software (version 5, Cambridge Electronic Design Limited, Cambridge, UK). Animals were killed immediately after the experiment by intravenous administration of KCl.

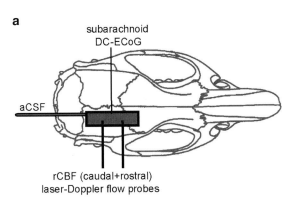

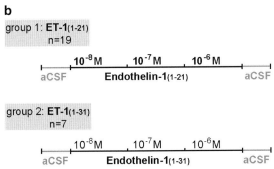

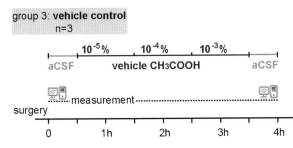

Fig. 2 Experimental setup & paradigms (**a**) An open cranial window of 4 × 7 mm was implanted over the right somatosensory cortex and superfused with aCSF. DC-ECoG and rostral and caudal rCBF were recorded continuously while using the same experimental time schedule (**b**) for each group

Experimental Protocols

In group 1 (n = 19), ET-1 (Sigma-Aldrich inc., Steinheim, Germany) was brain topically administered (stepwise increases from 10^{-8} to 10^{-7} to 10^{-6}M at one hour intervals) (Fig. 2b). In group 2, ET-1$_{(1-31)}$ (Peptide Institute inc., Osaka, Japan) was applied instead of ET-1 (n = 7). Group 3 (n = 3) served as vehicle control for group 2 (aCSF containing acetic acid in stepwise increases from 10^{-5} to 10^{-3}% at one hour intervals).

Data Analysis

Data were analyzed by comparing absolute changes of the DC potential and relative changes of rCBF calculated in relation to baseline (100%) at the onset of the measurement. Data in text and figures are given as median value and first and third quartile. Statistical tests are mentioned in the results section. A *P*-value of <0.05 was considered statistically significant.

Results

The physiological variables remained within the normal range in the three groups (Table 1). In group 1, administration of ET-1 led to SDs in all 19 animals. Three animals developed SDs in response to 10^{-8}M (15.8%), eleven animals in response to 10^{7}M (57.9%) and five in response to 10^{-6}M (26.3%). All animals of group 2 showed SDs after administration of ET-1$_{(1-31)}$. However, in contrast to group 1, ET-1$_{(1-31)}$ only induced SDs at a concentration of 10^{-6}M. Thus, at concentrations below 10^{-6}M, ET-1 led to SDs more frequently than ET-1$_{(1-31)}$ (Fig. 3a). This difference was statistically significant (*P* < 0.001, two-tailed Fisher's Exact Test). No significant differences were observed between ET-1 and ET-1$_{(1-31)}$ induced SDs regarding changes of DC-ECoG and rCBF (Table 2, two-tailed Mann-Whitney U tests, Fig. 3b). In both groups a similar spreading depression of high-frequency ECoG activity was observed but not quantified (Fig. 3a). Vehicle controls (n = 3) did not show SDs.

Table 1 Physiological variables in median and first and third quartile

	Mean arterial pressure (mmHg)	Arterial pCO$_2$ (mmHg)	Arterial pO$_2$ (mmHg)	Arterial pH
Group 1 ET-1$_{(1-21)}$	99.0 (93.5–138.8)	35.5 (32.5–39.2)	118.1 (115.1–125.3)	7.40 (7.39–7.43)
Group 2 ET-1$_{(1-31)}$	122.0 (104.5–133.0)	38.2 (35.3–42.0)	90.6 (88.2–103.5)	7.42 (7.41–7.44)
Group 3 vehicle control	131.5 (121.5–134.0)	41.6 (40.2–42.3)	107.7 (95.4–107.8)	7.41 (7.41–7.44)

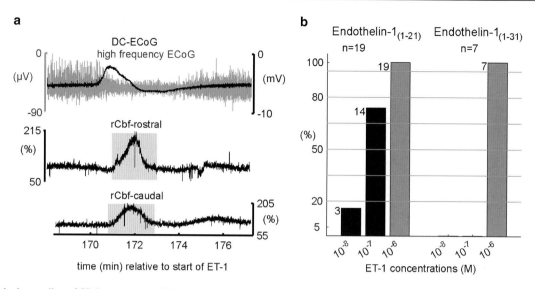

Fig. 3 Original recording of SD in response to ET-1$_{(1-31)}$ & plot showing concentrations of ET-1 and ET-1$_{(1-31)}$ inducing SD (**a**) An ET-1$_{(1-31)}$ induced SD is shown. The first trace gives the high frequency ECoG (*gray*, bandpass filter: 0.5–45 Hz) and the DC-ECoG (*black*, bandpass filter: 0–45 Hz). Note simultaneous depression of high-frequency ECoG activity and negative DC shift typical of SD. The two lower traces demonstrate the typical increase in rCBF (in % of baseline) during SD. Note the small time delay between rostral and caudal rCBF indicating SD propagation. (**b**) Comparison between threshold concentrations of ET-1 (three bars on the left, n = 19) and ET-1$_{(1-31)}$ (bar on the right, n = 7) inducing SD suggest a weaker effect of ET-1$_{(1-31)}$. Three rats generated SD in response to 10^8M of ET-1, 14 rats at 10^7M and all rats at 10^6 M. In contrast, ET-1$_{(1-31)}$ only induced SD at a concentration of 10^{-6}M

Table 2 SD parameters in median and first and third quartile

	Negative DC-shift amplitude (mV)	Negative DC-shift duration (s)	rCBF bevor SD (%)	Hyperemia (%)	Hyperemia duration (s)
Group 1 ET-1$_{(1-21)}$	3.5 (2.8–5.3)	73 (64–95)	89 (78–114)	208 (144–234)	86 (78–98)
Group 2 ET-1$_{(1-31)}$	3.8 (3.0–4.4)	97 (83–139)	91 (86–98)	179 (168–185)	93 (84–108)

Discussion

We here showed that ET-1$_{(1-31)}$ induced SDs in a similar fashion to ET-1. This could be explained by either a direct effect of ET-1$_{(1-31)}$ on ET$_A$ receptors or an indirect effect if ET-1$_{(1-31)}$ is first metabolized to ET-1. The efficacy of ET-1$_{(1-31)}$ was less than that of ET-1. This is consistent with the weaker vasocontractile potency of ET-1$_{(1-31)}$ compared to ET-1 in different vascular beds [24, 25].

SD

Experimental and clinical evidence suggests that SD represents a state that brain cortical tissue undergoes before it dies [26]. Consistently, clusters of SDs occurred time-locked to the development of delayed ischemic stroke in aSAH patients [7, 27] and in patients with malignant hemispheric stroke [28]. SD is ignited by an imbalance between dendritic inward currents such as slowly inactivating sodium and N-methyl-D-aspartate receptor controlled currents and outward currents driven by membrane Ca- and Na, K-ATPases. Near-complete sustained neuronal depolarization and breakdown of ion homeostasis represent the hallmarks characterizing SD. SD presumably mediates the death of neurons through the initiation and maintenance of intracellular calcium overload [26]. However, in principle SD is reversible until the so called commitment point. Whether or not the tissue recovers from SD depends on additional recruitment of Ca- and Na, K-ATPase activities [26]. Therefore, recovery from SD is energy dependent [29]. In focal ischemia long-lasting, pharmacoresistant and harmful SD starts in the center of the low perfusion area and changes to a progressively shorter-lasting, pharmacosensitive, and benign SD as it spreads through the metabolically compromised penumbra and surrounding healthy tissue [30–33]. SDs recur in clusters during focal ischemia. Experimental evidence suggests that each SD causes the infarct to grow [11, 30, 33].

ET-1 Induced SD

Experimental evidence has increasingly supported that ET-1 induces SD via the induction of ischemia although the measured changes of rCBF using laser-Doppler flowmetry are only in the upper range for an ischemic penumbra [22]. Thus, it was found that (a) the receptor profile of ET-1-induced SD is consistent with arterial constriction, as ET_A receptors only mediated ET-1-induced SD [23]; (b) it was shown with K^+-sensitive microelectrodes that a slow rise of the extracellular K^+ concentration typical of ischemia preceded SDs under ET-1; (c) ET-1 failed to elicit SD in brain slices which lack a blood circulation [22]; and (d) an area with selective neuronal necrosis was previously found in the ET-1 exposed cortex whenever ET-1 elicited SD, but not when ET-1 failed to trigger SD [11].

ET-1 in Vasospasm After aSAH

Synthesis of ET-1 is stimulated at the level of gene transcription by a number of factors released from blood clot after aSAH including hemoglobin, thrombin and prostaglandin $F_{2\alpha}$ [34–36]. Yet, measured cerebrospinal concentrations of ET-1 are lower after aSAH than concentrations necessary for induction of ischemia under normal conditions. However, sensitivity of vascular smooth muscle to ET-1 markedly increases after aSAH [13, 37] and ET-1 concentrations in the relevant abluminal compartment for vasoconstriction are possibly higher than those in cerebrospinal fluid [38]. In fact, cerebrospinal ET-1 may not reflect increased abluminal ET-1 release of endothelium stimulated by subarachnoid clot but release by astrocytes in response to oxidative substrate depletion [39]. Thus, elevation of cerebrospinal ET-1 occurred time-locked to the neuronal damage after aSAH rather than to the development of angiographic vasospasm [40].

$ET-1_{(1-31)}$

$ET-1_{(1-31)}$ was first described by Nakano et al. in 1997 [19]. Early after discovery, it received attention as an endogenous selective ET_A receptor agonist since it mainly showed potent ET_A mediated effects such as vasoconstriction [25], intracellular calcium increase and smooth muscle proliferation in isolated arteries [41, 42]. It even displaced ET-1 binding to ET_A but not to ET_B receptors in isolated human arteries [43]. Vasoconstriction by $ET-1_{(1-31)}$ in humans in vivo was first described in the skin, where big-$ET-1_{(1-38)}$ and $ET-1_{(1-31)}$ were 30-fold less potent than ET-1 [24].

However, it was later found that $ET-1_{(1-31)}$ may have an additional indirect effect on both ET_A and ET_B receptors when cleaved to ET-1. Conversion to ET-1 is presumably responsible for the biological activity of $ET-1_{(1-31)}$ in cultured bronchial smooth muscle cells [44] and the central cardiovascular effects of $ET-1_{(1-31)}$ in rats [45]. In contrast, conversion to ET-1 was not likely to be involved in effects of $ET-1_{(1-31)}$ in isolated human coronary and internal mammary arteries since vasoconstriction and the increase of the intracellular Ca^{2+} concentration were not significantly inhibited by ECE/NEP inhibitors [25, 41]. If $ET-1_{(1-31)}$ acts directly on ET_A receptors in cerebral vessels this alternate metabolic pathway of big-ET-1 suggests that ECE inhibitors less effectively inhibit vasospasm than ET_A receptor blockers as demonstrated for cardiovascular effects [46].

$ET-1_{(1-31)}$ could play a pathophysiological role in both the early and delayed period after aSAH if chymase, converting big-ET-1 to $ET-1_{(1-31)}$, is expressed in the tissue in a considerable amount. E.g., chymase is released by mast cells that infiltrate inflammatory sites. In addition $ET-1_{(1-31)}$ was found to be the predominant ET in neutrophils attracted by inflammatory mediators. Inflammatory sites develop after aSAH in response to subarachnoid blood products and ischemia [47]. Similarly to ET-1, $ET-1_{(1-31)}$ may have adverse effects acutely being a vasoconstrictor while it is possible that it shows subacutely beneficial effects, e.g., in inflammatory processes or angiogenesis following ischemia [48]. Therefore, it would be interesting to further characterize potentially beneficial effects of ET-1 and $ET-1_{(1-31)}$. Then, it should be determined whether adverse and beneficial effects correlate in a similar fashion in ET-1 and $ET-1_{(1-31)}$ or whether $ET-1_{(1-31)}$ has relatively stronger beneficial effects. If this were the case, it could be interesting to divert the metabolic pathways after aSAH using ECE and NEP inhibitors to antagonize adverse effects of ET-1 while keeping a basal level of ET_A receptor activation with $ET-1_{(1-31)}$. In this respect, it is interesting that the adverse effect of $ET-1_{(1-31)}$ to induce SD was weaker than that of ET-1 in our study.

Acknowledgement Supported by grants of the Deutsche Forschungsgemeinschaft (DFG DR 323/2–2), the Bundesministerium für Bildung und Forschung (Center for Stroke Research Berlin, 01 EO 0801) and the Kompetenznetz Schlaganfall to Dr. Dreier.

Conflict of interest statement We declare that we have no conflict of interest.

References

1. Kistler JP, Crowell RM, Davis KR, Heros R, Ojemann RG, Zervas T, et al. The relation of cerebral vasospasm to the extent and location of subarachnoid blood visualized by CT scan: a prospective study. Neurology 1983;33:424–36.
2. Pluta RM, Afshar JK, Boock RJ, Oldfield EH. Temporal changes in perivascular concentrations of oxyhemoglobin, deoxyhemoglobin, and methemoglobin after subarachnoid hemorrhage. J Neurosurg. 1998;88:557–61.

3. Macdonald RL, Pluta RM, Zhang JH. Cerebral vasospasm after subarachnoid hemorrhage: the emerging revolution. Nat Clin Pract Neurol. 2007;3:256–63.
4. Schuknecht B, Fandino J, Yuksel C, Yonekawa Y, Valavanis A. Endovascular treatment of cerebral vasospasm: assessment of treatment effect by cerebral angiography and transcranial colour Doppler sonography. Neuroradiology 1999;41:453–62.
5. Ohkuma H, Manabe H, Tanaka M, Suzuki S. Impact of cerebral microcirculatory changes on cerebral blood flow during cerebral vasospasm after aneurysmal subarachnoid hemorrhage. Stroke 2000;31:1621–27.
6. Dreier JP, Korner K, Ebert N, Gorner A, Rubin I, Back T, et al. Nitric oxide scavenging by hemoglobin or nitric oxide synthase inhibition by N-nitro-L-arginine induces cortical spreading ischemia when K+ is increased in the subarachnoid space. J Cereb Blood Flow Metab. 1998;18:978–90.
7. Dreier JP, Major S, Manning A, Woitzik J, Drenckhahn C, Steinbrink J, et al. Cortical spreading ischaemia is a novel process involved in ischaemic damage in patients with aneurysmal subarachnoid haemorrhage. Brain 2009;132:1866–81.
8. Zimmermann MMD, Seifert VMDP. Endothelin and subarachnoid hemorrhage: an overview. Neurosurgery 1998;43:863–75.
9. Macrae IM, Robinson MJ, Graham DI, Reid JL, McCulloch J. Endothelin-1-induced reductions in cerebral blood-flow – dose dependency, time course, and neuropathological consequences. J Cereb Blood Flow Metab. 1993;13:276–84.
10. Fuxe K, Bjelke B, Andbjer B, Grahn H, Rimondini R, Agnati LF. Endothelin-1 induced lesions of the frontoparietal cortex of the rat. A possible model of focal cortical ischemia. Neuroreport 1997;8:2623–29.
11. Dreier JP, Kleeberg J, Alam M, Major S, Kohl-Bareis M, Petzold GC, et al. Endothelin-1-induced spreading depression in rats is associated with a microarea of selective neuronal necrosis. Exp Biol Med (Maywood). 2007;232:204–13.
12. Chow M, Dumont AS, Kassell NF. Endothelin receptor antagonists and cerebral vasospasm: an update. Neurosurgery 2002;51:1333–41; discussion 1342.
13. Vatter H, Konczalla J, Weidauer S, Preibisch C, Zimmermann M, Raabe A, et al. Effect of delayed cerebral vasospasm on cerebrovascular endothelin A receptor expression and function. J Neurosurg. 2007;107:121–27.
14. Macdonald RL, Kassell NF, Mayer S, Ruefenacht D, Schmiedek P, Weidauer S, et al. Clazosentan to overcome neurological ischemia and infarction occurring after subarachnoid hemorrhage (CONSCIOUS-1): randomized, double-blind, placebo-controlled phase 2 dose-finding trial. Stroke 2008;39:3015–21.
15. Dreier JP, Petzold G, Tille K, Lindauer U, Arnold G, Heinemann U, et al. Ischaemia triggered by spreading neuronal activation is inhibited by vasodilators in rats. J Physiol. 2001;531:515–26.
16. Petzold GC, Einhaupl KM, Dirnagl U, Dreier JP. Ischemia triggered by spreading neuronal activation is induced by endothelin-1 and hemoglobin in the subarachnoid space. Ann Neurol. 2003;54:591–98.
17. Cosenzi A. Enrasentan, an antagonist of endothelin receptors. Cardiovasc Drug Rev. 2003;21:1–16.
18. D'Orleans-Juste P, Plante M, Honore JC, Carrier E, Labonte J. Synthesis and degradation of endothelin-1. Can J Physiol Pharmacol. 2003;81:503–10.
19. Nakano A, Kishi F, Minami K, Wakabayashi H, Nakaya Y, Kido H. Selective conversion of big endothelins to tracheal smooth muscle-constricting 31-amino acid-length endothelins by chymase from human mast cells. J Immunol. 1997;159:1987–92.
20. Fecteau MH, Honore JC, Plante M, Labonte J, Rae GA, D'Orleans-Juste P. Endothelin-1 (1–31) is an intermediate in the production of endothelin-1 after big endothelin-1 administration in vivo. Hypertension 2005;46:87–92.
21. Baltatu O, Nishimura H, Hoffmann S, Stoltenburg G, Haulica ID, Lippoldt A, et al. High levels of human chymase expression in the pineal and pituitary glands. Brain Res. 1997;752:269–78.
22. Dreier JP, Kleeberg J, Petzold G, Priller J, Windmuller O, Orzechowski HD, et al. Endothelin-1 potently induces Leao's cortical spreading depression in vivo in the rat: a model for an endothelial trigger of migrainous aura? Brain 2002;125:102–12.
23. Kleeberg J, Petzold GC, Major S, Dirnagl U, Dreier JP. ET-1 induces cortical spreading depression via activation of the ETA receptor/phospholipase C pathway in vivo. Am J Physiol Heart Circ Physiol. 2004;286:H1339–46.
24. Leslie SJ, Rahman MQ, Denvir MA, Newby DE, Webb DJ. Endothelins and their inhibition in the human skin microcirculation: ET[1–31], a new vasoconstrictor peptide. Br J Clin Pharmacol. 2004;57:720–25.
25. Maguire JJ, Kuc RE, Davenport AP. Vasoconstrictor activity of novel endothelin peptide, ET-1(1–31), in human mammary and coronary arteries in vitro. Br J Pharmacol. 2001;134:1360–66.
26. Somjen GG. Ions in the brain. Normal function, seizures and stroke. New York: Oxford University Press; 2004.
27. Dreier JP, Woitzik J, Fabricius M, Bhatia R, Major S, Drenckhahn C, et al. Delayed ischaemic neurological deficits after subarachnoid haemorrhage are associated with clusters of spreading depolarizations. Brain 2006;129:3224–37.
28. Dohmen C, Sakowitz OW, Fabricius M, Bosche B, Reithmeier T, Ernestus RI, et al. Spreading depolarizations occur in human ischemic stroke with high incidence. Ann Neurol. 2008;63:720–28.
29. Mies G, Paschen W. Regional changes of blood flow, glucose, and ATP content determined on brain sections during a single passage of spreading depression in rat brain cortex. Exp Neurol. 1984;84:249–58.
30. Busch E, Gyngell ML, Eis M, Hoehn-Berlage M, Hossmann KA. Potassium-induced cortical spreading depressions during focal cerebral ischemia in rats: contribution to lesion growth assessed by diffusion-weighted NMR and biochemical imaging. J Cereb Blood Flow Metab. 1996;16:1090–99.
31. Koroleva VI, Bures J. Circulation of cortical spreading depression around electrically stimulated areas and epileptic foci in the neocortex of rats. Brain Res. 1979;173:209–15.
32. Nedergaard M, Hansen AJ. Characterization of cortical depolarizations evoked in focal cerebral ischemia. J Cereb Blood Flow Metab. 1993;13:568–74.
33. Takano K, Latour LL, Formato JE, Carano RA, Helmer KG, Hasegawa Y, et al. The role of spreading depression in focal ischemia evaluated by diffusion mapping. Ann Neurol. 1996;39:308–18.
34. Kasuya H, Weir BK, White DM, Stefansson K. Mechanism of oxyhemoglobin-induced release of endothelin-1 from cultured vascular endothelial cells and smooth-muscle cells. J Neurosurg. 1993;79:892–98.
35. Ohlstein EH, Storer BL. Oxyhemoglobin stimulation of endothelin production in cultured endothelial cells. J Neurosurg. 1992;77:274–78.
36. Schini VB, Hendrickson H, Heublein DM, Burnett JC, Jr., Vanhoutte PM. Thrombin enhances the release of endothelin from cultured porcine aortic endothelial cells. Eur J Pharmacol. 1989;165:333–34.
37. Xie A, Aihara Y, Bouryi VA, Nikitina E, Jahromi BS, Zhang ZD, et al. Novel mechanism of endothelin-1-induced vasospasm after subarachnoid hemorrhage. J Cereb Blood Flow Metab. 2007;27:1692–701.
38. Kastner S, Oertel MF, Scharbrodt W, Krause M, Boker DK, Deinsberger W. Endothelin-1 in plasma, cisternal CSF and microdialysate following aneurysmal SAH. Acta Neurochir (Wien). 2005;147:1271–79; discussion 1279.

39. Pluta RM, Boock RJ, Afshar JK, Clouse K, Bacic M, Ehrenreich H, et al. Source and cause of endothelin-1 release into cerebrospinal fluid after subarachnoid hemorrhage. J Neurosurg. 1997;87:287–93.
40. Mascia L, Fedorko L, Stewart DJ, Mohamed F, terBrugge K, Ranieri VM, et al. Temporal relationship between endothelin-1 concentrations and cerebral vasospasm in patients with aneurysmal subarachnoid hemorrhage. Stroke 2001;32:1185–90.
41. Yoshizumi M, Inui D, Okishima N, Houchi H, Tsuchiya K, Wakabayashi H, et al. Endothelin-1-(1–31), a novel vasoactive peptide, increases [Ca2+]i in human coronary artery smooth muscle cells. Eur J Pharmacol. 1998;348:305–9.
42. Yoshizumi M, Kim S, Kagami S, Hamaguchi A, Tsuchiya K, Houchi H, et al. Effect of endothelin-1 (1–31) on extracellular signal-regulated kinase and proliferation of human coronary artery smooth muscle cells. Br J Pharmacol. 1998;125:1019–27.
43. Rossi GP, Andreis PG, Colonna S, Albertin G, Aragona F, Belloni AS, et al. Endothelin-1[1–31]: a novel autocrine-paracrine regulator of human adrenal cortex secretion and growth. J Clin Endocrinol Metab. 2002;87:322–28.
44. Hayasaki-Kajiwara Y, Naya N, Shimamura T, Iwasaki T, Nakajima M. Endothelin generating pathway through endothelin1–31 in human cultured bronchial smooth muscle cells. Br J Pharmacol. 1999;127:1415–21.
45. Lu Y, Wang LG, Liao Z, Tang CS, Wang WZ, Yuan WJ. Cardiovascular effects of centrally applied endothelin-1 1–31 and its relationship to endothelin-1 1–21 in rats. Auton Neurosci. 2007;133:146–52.
46. Wada A, Tsutamoto T, Ohnishi M, Sawaki M, Fukai D, Maeda Y, et al. Effects of a specific endothelin-converting enzyme inhibitor on cardiac, renal, and neurohumoral functions in congestive heart failure: comparison of effects with those of endothelin A receptor antagonism. Circulation 1999;99:570–77.
47. Strbian D, Kovanen PT, Karjalainen-Lindsberg ML, Tatlisumak T, Lindsberg PJ. An emerging role of mast cells in cerebral ischemia and hemorrhage. Ann Med. 2009;1:1–13
48. Cui P, Tani K, Kitamura H, Okumura Y, Yano M, Inui D, et al. A novel bioactive 31-amino acid endothelin-1 is a potent chemotactic peptide for human neutrophils and monocytes. J Leukoc Biol. 2001;70:306–12.

The Gamut of Blood Flow Responses Coupled to Spreading Depolarization in Rat and Human Brain: from Hyperemia to Prolonged Ischemia

N. Offenhauser, O. Windmüller, A.J. Strong, S. Fuhr, and J.P. Dreier

Abstract Cortical spreading depolarizations (SD) have been shown to occur frequently in patients with aneurysmal subarachnoid hemorrhage (SAH) and are associated with delayed ischemic brain damage. In animal models the link between SD and cell damage is the microvascular spasm coupled to the passage of SDs, resulting in spreading ischemia. Here we compared the hemodynamic changes induced by SD between human and rat cerebral cortex. Specifically, we addressed the question, whether the full spectrum of regional cerebral blood flow (rCBF) responses to SD is found in the human brain in a similar fashion to animal models. SDs were identified by slow potential changes in electrocorticographic recordings and the rCBF response profiles and magnitudes were analyzed. We found a large variability of rCBF changes concomitant to SDs in rat and in human recordings. The spectrum ranged from normal hyperemic responses to prolonged cortical spreading ischemia with intermediate forms characterized by biphasic (hypoemic–hyperemic) responses. The bandwidths of rCBF responses were comparable and the relative response magnitudes of hypo- and hyperperfusion phases did not differ significantly between rats and humans. The correspondence of the rCBF response spectrum to SD between human and animal brain underscores the importance of animal models to learn more about the mechanisms underlying the early and delayed pathological sequelae of SAH.

Keywords Cerebral blood flow · Depolarization · Electrophysiology · Inverse coupling · Spreading depression · Spreading ischemia · Subarachnoid hemorrhage · Vasospasm

Introduction

Blood in the subarachnoid space is the initial step in a detrimental cascade potentially leading to tissue damage in patients with aneurysmal subarachnoid haemorrhage (SAH) [1]. Identification of decisive factors in the pathogenesis of delayed ischemia after SAH is a prerequisite to improve quality of diagnosis, monitoring and treatment. Up to now the complex and interrelated cascade from hemoglobin and ion changes in the subarachnoid space to vasospasm, regional cerebral blood flow (rCBF) reduction and neuronal injury remain poorly understood [2]. Translational research is a basic principle for developing pathophysiological, diagnostic and therapeutic concepts in the treatment of ischemic brain damage [3]. Cortical spreading depolarization (SD) and cortical spreading ischemia (CSI) have been extensively studied in a multitude of animal models and paradigms. SD is a wave of neuronal/astroglial depolarization propagating at a rate of approximately 3 mm min^{-1} in the cerebral cortex. Restoration of ion homeostasis after SD is energetically expensive and requires adequate supply of energy substrates with the blood flow. SDs in the healthy brain are associated with a marked increase in rCBF, serving the increased demand of energy metabolism during SD [4], thus preventing neuronal damage [5]. In animal models of acute brain injury like ischemia, trauma and SAH, SDs arise spontaneously

N. Offenhauser
Center for Stroke Research Berlin, Charité-University Medicine Berlin, Berlin, Germany
Department of Experimental Neurology, Charité University Medicine Berlin, Berlin, Germany

O. Windmüller and S. Fuhr
Department of Experimental Neurology, Charité University Medicine Berlin, Berlin, Germany

A.J. Strong
Department of Clinical Neuroscience, King's College London, London, UK

J.P. Dreier (✉)
Center for Stroke Research Berlin, Charité-University Medicine Berlin, Berlin, Germany
Department of Experimental Neurology, Charité University Medicine Berlin, Berlin, Germany
Department of Neurology, Charité University Medicine Berlin, Berlin, Germany
e-mail: jens.dreier@charite.de

and repetitively and contribute to neuronal damage and lesion progression as they occur in an already energy compromised tissue [6–10]. SDs induced in experimental SAH models cause microvascular spasm and ischemia which propagate together with the depolarization wave [11]. This spreading hypoperfusion has been termed CSI and is sufficient to induce cortical necrosis [8]. SDs recently have been shown to occur with high incidence in patients with SAH and are closely interrelated with ischemic cell damage and lesion progression [12, 13]. In the latter study the inversion of the rCBF response from physiological hyperemia to hypoperfusion and prolonged ischemia has been demonstrated. This suggests a close similarity between the SD induced rCBF changes in experimental SAH models and in patients with SAH. The aim of the current work was to directly compare the magnitude of cortical depolarization induced blood flow changes and to specify similarities and differences between the experimentally observed spectrum of rCBF responses and the spectrum of rCBF responses recorded from the diseased human brain. To this end, we analyzed rCBF changes induced by SD in patients with SAH and in a rat model known to develop cerebral microvascular spasm in response to SD [11].

Materials and Methods

Animal Recordings

The analysis was based on experiments on anesthetized (thiopental), artificially ventilated, male Wistar rats (n = 10). All experiments were approved by the German authorities and are in line with the European convention for the protection of vertebrate animals used for experimental and other scientific purposes. A closed cranial window was implanted over the frontoparietal cortex and superfused with aCSF as described [11, 14]. At this site, rCBF was assessed by laser Doppler flowmetry (LDF; Perimed, Järfalla Sweden) and the cortical DC potential (DC-ECoG) was measured by an adjacent Ag/AgCl electrode (filter: 0–45 Hz). To induce SD associated with CSI the artificial cerebrospinal fluid (aCSF) contained hemoglobin (2.5 mM) in combination with an elevated K+ level (35 mM), (for a detailed description see [14]). A regime known to result in SD to which CSI is coupled instead of spreading hyperemia [8].

Human Recordings

ECoG and rCBF recordings from patients with major SAH were analyzed (8 patients, 14 electrode positions). SAH diagnosis was based on assessment of CT scans. After the clinical decision had been made to offer surgical treatment, clinical and research consents were obtained according to the Declaration of Helsinki. A single, linear, 6 contact electrocorticography recording strip (Wyler, 5 mm diamter, Ad-Tech Medical, Racine, Wisconsin, USA) was placed on the cortex. Filter settings for the ECoG recordings were 0.01–45 Hz. The electrode strip was equipped additionally with optodes for concurrent rCBF measurements by LDF (Perimed) and enabled combined rCBF/ECoG measurements from closely adjacent brain regions (for details see [12]).

Data Analysis

Data were analyzed for the rCBF response profiles coupled to SD. SDs were identified by propagating large amplitude slow potential changes (SPCs) in the ECoG and the heterogeneity of rCBF response profiles and the magnitudes of the relative rCBF changes (hyperemia and hypoperfusion) were analyzed. For better comparison between the SD induced potential changes of rats and humans, animal data (DC-ECoG recordings) were additionally filtered off-line with filter settings comparable to the human recordings (lower frequency limit: 0.01 Hz; higher frequency limit: 45 Hz). Clinical ECoG recordings are typically made with AC-coupled amplifiers. Their inbuilt lower frequency limit (here 0.01 Hz) does not allow recordings of true negative DC potential shifts, which are the standard for experimental studies on SDs. Nevertheless, they are suitable for identification of SDs in human ECoGs by the occurrence of typical multiphasic SPCs with an initial negative component [13, 15]. The major drawback compared to DC recordings is the distortion of the waveform, which excludes simple analysis of SD durations [16].

SD induced rCBF and potential changes which were not accompanied by physiological (initial hyperemic) responses, were further analyzed and compared (eight recording sites from seven patients and recordings from ten animals). The absolute change of the DC potential during the SD wave (animal recordings) and the peak to peak amplitude of the propagating SPC (human and rat recordings) were calculated [13]. The relative change of the rCBF was calculated in relation to baseline before the occurrence of SD and is shown as percent of rCBF decrease (hypoperfusion) and percent of rCBF increase (hyperemia). The duration of the rCBF decrease was assessed additionally. All data are given as mean values ± standard deviations.

Results

In animal and human cerebral cortex a broad spectrum of rCBF changes associated with the propagating SD wave was identified. Original recordings of characteristic

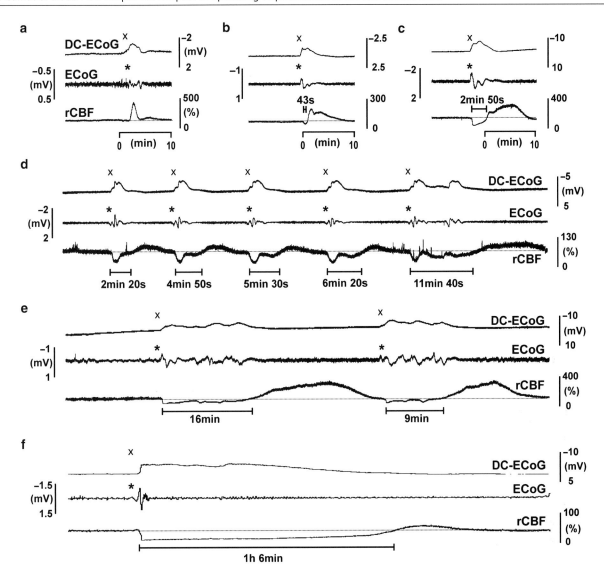

Fig. 1 The spectrum of hemodynamic responses to SD in rat cerebral cortex. The upper two traces in a–f show original traces of subdural ECoG recordings. The lower traces show the corresponding rCBF changes measured by LDF. The upper traces are true DC-ECoG (0–45 Hz) recordings, enabling clear identification of spreading depolarizations by the negative DC potential shift (x) of high amplitude. The middle traces show the same recordings after high pass filtering (0.01–45 Hz) with frequency limits comparable to the human ECoG recordings (see Fig. 2). Despite the distortion of the SPC by applying a high pass filter, SDs can be identified by the occurrence of multiphasic slow potential changes. Onset of SDs are marked by *asterisks*. (a) Characteristic hyperemia in response to SD under physiological conditions (physiological aCSF). (b–f) Spectrum of SD induced rCBF responses observed in the presence of hemoglobin and elevated K^+ in the aCSF. (b) A small and brief initial hypoperfusion precedes the hyperemia. (c) Biphasic rCBF response with initial hypoperfusion for 2 min 50 s, reaching ischemic levels and followed by a slowly developing hyperemia. (d) Series of SDs associated with hypoperfusions of variable duration and only small degrees of hyperemia. (e) Longer lasting hypoperfusions associated with prolonged DC potential shifts and slow rCBF recovery and delayed hyperemia. (f) SD induced pronounced and long lasting hypoperfusion for more than 1 h and associated with only minor hyperemia. *Dotted lines* in the rCBF traces illustrate baseline rCBF values before the onset of SDs. Note that the negative DC potential shifts last as long as the rCBF decreases

response profiles are shown in Fig. 1 (rat) and 2 (human). Overall the rCBF responses to SD in rat and humans ranged from typical physiological hemodynamic responses (Figs. 1a, 2a) to prolonged CSIs (Figs. 1f, 2e). Most frequently CSIs in rat and humans were biphasic (initial hypoperfusion followed by delayed hyperemia) and the two phases were of variable duration and degree (Figs. 1b–f, 2b–e).

In four patients single recording sites showed normal physiological responses to SD (like observed under control conditions in the animal model). All rCBF changes in the presence of elevated K^+ and hemoglobin in the animal model showed a biphasic pattern. In contrast, three of the human recording sites showed no significant hyperemia above baseline after the initial hypoperfusion phase, and one recording site showed no recovery to baseline.

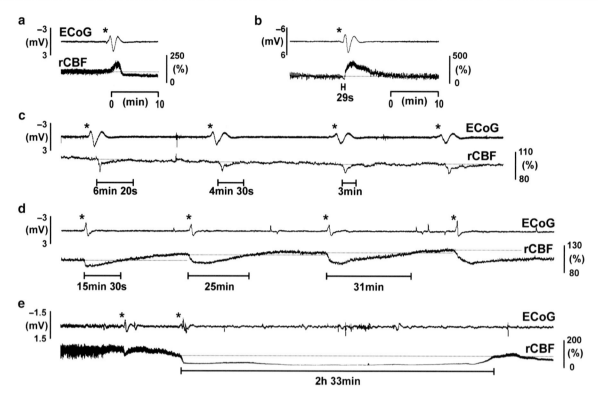

Fig. 2 The spectrum of hemodynamic responses to SD in human cerebral cortex of patients with SAH. The upper traces in a–e show original traces of subdural ECoG recordings (filter settings: 0.01–45 Hz). Onset of SDs can be identified by multiphasic slow potential changes and are marked by *asterisks*. Lower traces show the corresponding rCBF changes measured by LDF. (**a**) Example of a physiological hyperemic response to SD, characterized by the typical initial hyperemic rCBF response, followed by mild relative oligemia. (**b–e**) SD induced rCBF responses with initial hypoperfusion indicating impaired (inverse) neurovascular coupling. (**b**) A small and brief initial hypoperfusion precedes the hyperemic response to SD. (**c**) Repetitive SDs associated with hypoperfusions of variable duration and without relevant hyperemia. (**d**) Series of four SDs associated with long lasting hypoperfusions of increasing duration, followed by minor hyperemia. (**e**) SD induced pronounced and long lasting hypoperfusion lasting for more than 2.5 h followed by minor hyperperfusion. *Dotted lines* in the rCBF traces illustrate baseline rCBF values before the onset of individual SDs

The mean SD induced rCBF reduction was 58.3 ± 24.9% in rats and 47.6 ± 29.5% in humans (Fig. 3a). The mean duration of this initial rCBF decrease was slightly longer in humans (42 min ± 62 min) than in rats (20 min ± 35 min), but this difference was not statistically significant (Fig. 3d). The hyperperfusion after the initial hypoperfusion led to a similar rCBF increase of 53.7 ± 35.6% in rats and 51.6 ± 95.7% in humans (Fig. 3c).

The amplitudes of the SPC (0.01–45 Hz) did not differ significantly in rats and humans (rat: 2.4 ± 1.4 mV; human: 2.7 ± 2.3 mV), but mean SPC amplitudes of rat and human SDs were significantly smaller than the mean amplitude of the rat DC potential change (5.8 ± 2.0, $p < 0.05$, ANOVA followed by Tukey Test, Fig. 3b).

Discussion

We investigated the spectrum of rCBF changes coupled to the propagation of neuronal/astroglial depolarization waves in the cerebral cortex of patients with SAH and in an animal model of CSI. We demonstrated that rCBF changes during SD exhibit a comparable broad spectrum in humans and rats. The mean magnitudes of SD associated rCBF changes did not differ significantly, despite an apparent intraindividual and interindividual heterogeneity of responses. We found no significant difference in the magnitude of SPC changes associated with SD between rats and humans, in line with previous studies [16]. The comparability between the spectra and the similarity of the CBF change magnitudes during CSI supports the idea, that in rats and humans the same underlying pathophysiological cascade causes the inversion of the rCBF response to SD. A number of experimental studies established a linear relationship between the duration of the characteristic negative DC-potential shift accompanying SDs and the duration of the associated rCBF reduction [14, 17, 18]. This finding was recently confirmed for the human brain [12] and further supports the similarity between human CSI and experimental models. Several pathophysiological conditions have been investigated in animal studies, which were found to be associated with an inversion of the rCBF response to SD. E.g. it was possible to replace the nitric

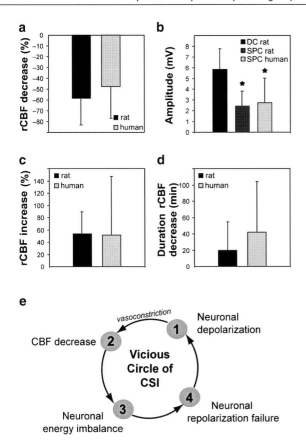

Fig. 3 Magnitudes of non-physiological rCBF responses and slow potential changes induced by SD in rats and humans. (**a**) Graph illustrating the magnitude of the initial hypoperfusion in relation to the baseline level before SD. (**b**) Comparison of the SD amplitudes of different ECoG recordings. The mean amplitude of SD induced DC potential shifts in rat DC-ECoG recordings was significantly greater compared to the corresponding filtered SPC from rat or human (ANOVA followed by Tukey Test; $p < 0.001$). SPC amplitudes between rats and humans did not show a significant difference. (**c**) Graph showing the magnitude of the rCBF increase (hyperperfusion) after the initial hypoperfusion in relation to baseline level before SD. (**d**) Duration of the initial hypoperfusion. The means ± standard deviations are plotted. Significant differences between groups are indicated by asterisks. (**e**) The vicious circle underlying CSI. The propagating SD wave is characterized by neuronal/astroglial depolarization and induces vasoconstriction (inverted coupling between neuronal energy metabolism and rCBF). This reduces the supply of oxygen and glucose at sites of vasoconstriction and limits neuronal energy supply. The energy depletion leads to a failure of neuronal repolarization so that the vasoconstriction persists

oxide (NO) scavenger oxyhemoglobin with a NO synthase inhibitor in the protocol inducing CSI [11]. CSI was also observed in hypotension and in models of focal ischemia in the penumbra [9, 18]. The common feature of these paradigms is a reduction of energy supply. Restoration of ion homeostasis after the neuronal/astroglial depolarization is highly dependent on activation of ATP-dependent ion pumps, causing an increase in ATP use, oxygen and glucose consumption [4, 19–21]. Under normal conditions energy supply is sufficient for the brain to cope with the increased demand and is additionally supported by the increased rCBF. Ischemia, hypoxia or CSI curtail energy availability and, beyond a critical threshold, will prevent recovery from depolarization. In this way, rCBF level and rCBF response on one side and the grade of energy consumption on the other side, determine energy availability for ion pumping and thus dictate the ability of neurons to repolarize. In SAH the pathophysiological features of CSI induced by SDs were hypothesized to reach a self-perpetuating level, finally entering a vicious circle [14].

It has been demonstrated, that the propagating SPC and DC potential shifts precede the onset of the rCBF decrease [12]. This implies that vasoconstriction and the resulting rCBF decrease are a consequence of the SD. Despite the decreased rCBF, the energy demand increases with SD and creates a critical mismatch between demand and supply. This will lead to prolonged depolarization which in turn leads to prolonged ischemia (Fig. 3e). According to this hypothesis, the different response types observed in the animal, as well as in the human recordings, might represent CSIs at different stages of the vicious circle. This might explain the bandwidth of responses to CSI. It will be of fundamental importance for our understanding of the pathophysiology of CSIs, and their prevention, to elucidate the factors which determine whether a certain brain region stays in the vicious circle, or is able to escape and recover. In the case of a persistent energy deficiency, repeated CSIs will increasingly prolong depolarization and ischemia in that region. The duration of the negative DC shift is therefore suggested to indicate transformation of normal SDs to harmful events, as they are indicative of critically impaired blood flow responses and a marker of the rising mismatch between energy supply and demand. This idea is the basis for the suggested clinical use of DC potential recordings as real time indicator of energy depletion and progressive ischemic brain damage in patients with SAH [13], or otherwise acutely injured brain [22–24]. By application of specific inverse filtering techniques it is possible to recover DC potential changes from high pass filtered AC coupled ECoG recordings [16]. However, most recently it has also become possible to perform true DC recordings in the human brain [13].

Taken together we demonstrated a wide spectrum of rCBF responses to SD in the cerebral cortex of patients with SAH and in an animal model of SAH. The observed spectra showed great similarities and ranged from normal hyperemia to prolonged spreading ischemia. This similarity points to the existence of a common mechanism driving the normal rCBF response into an inverted response type. Our findings underscore the importance of animal models and translational research approaches to understand the pathophysiology of brain damage after SAH.

Acknowledgement Supported by grants of the Deutsche Forschungsgemeinschaft (DFG DR 323/3-1, DFG DR 323/5-1), the Bundesministerium für Bildung und Forschung (Center for Stroke Research Berlin, 01 EO 0801) and the Kompetenznetz Schlaganfall to Dr. Dreier.

Conflict of interest statement We declare that we have no conflict of interest.

References

1. Cahill J, Zhang JH. Pre-vasospasm: early brain injury. Acta Neurochir Suppl (Wien). 2008;104:7–10.
2. Kawashima A, Macdonald RL. Electrophysiology of cerebral vasospasm. Acta Neurochir Suppl (Wien). 2008;104:87–93.
3. Fisher M, Henninger N. Translational research in stroke: taking advances in the pathophysiology and treatment of stroke from the experimental setting to clinical trials. Curr Neurol Neurosci Rep. 2007;7:35–41.
4. Piilgaard H, Lauritzen M. Persistent increase in oxygen consumption and impaired neurovascular coupling after spreading depression in rat neocortex. J Cereb Blood Flow Metab. 2009;29:1517–27.
5. Nedergaard M, Hansen AJ. Spreading depression is not associated with neuronal injury in the normal brain. Brain Res. 1988;449:395–98.
6. Back T, Ginsberg MD, Dietrich WD, Watson BD. Induction of spreading depression in the ischemic hemisphere following experimental middle cerebral artery occlusion: effect on infarct morphology. J Cereb Blood Flow Metab. 1996;16:202–13.
7. Busch E, Gyngell ML, Eis M, Hoehn-Berlage M, Hossmann KA. Potassium-induced cortical spreading depressions during focal cerebral ischemia in rats: contribution to lesion growth assessed by diffusion-weighted NMR and biochemical imaging. J Cereb Blood Flow Metab. 1996;16:1090–99.
8. Dreier JP, Ebert N, Priller J, Megow D, Lindauer U, Klee R, et al. Products of hemolysis in the subarachnoid space inducing spreading ischemia in the cortex and focal necrosis in rats: a model for delayed ischemic neurological deficits after subarachnoid hemorrhage? J Neurosurg. 2000;93:658–66.
9. Shin HK, Dunn AK, Jones PB, Boas DA, Moskowitz MA, Ayata C. Vasoconstrictive neurovascular coupling during focal ischemic depolarizations. J Cereb Blood Flow Metab. 2006;26:1018–30.
10. Strong AJ, Anderson PJ, Watts HR, Virley DJ, Lloyd A, Irving EA, et al. Peri-infarct depolarizations lead to loss of perfusion in ischaemic gyrencephalic cerebral cortex. Brain 2007;130:995–1008.
11. Dreier JP, Korner K, Ebert N, Gorner A, Rubin I, Back T, et al. Nitric oxide scavenging by hemoglobin or nitric oxide synthase inhibition by N-nitro-L-arginine induces cortical spreading ischemia when K^+ is increased in the subarachnoid space. J Cereb Blood Flow Metab. 1998;18:978–90.
12. Dreier JP, Major S, Manning A, Woitzik J, Drenckhahn C, Steinbrink J, et al. Cortical spreading ischaemia is a novel process involved in ischaemic damage in patients with aneurysmal subarachnoid haemorrhage. Brain 2009;132:1866–81.
13. Dreier JP, Woitzik J, Fabricius M, Bhatia R, Major S, Drenckhahn C, et al. Delayed ischaemic neurological deficits after subarachnoid haemorrhage are associated with clusters of spreading depolarizations. Brain 2006;129:3224–37.
14. Dreier JP, Windmuller O, Petzold G, Lindauer U, Einhaupl KM, Dirnagl U. Ischemia triggered by red blood cell products in the subarachnoid space is inhibited by nimodipine administration or moderate volume expansion/hemodilution in rats. Neurosurgery 2002;51:1457–65.
15. Fabricius M, Fuhr S, Bhatia R, Boutelle M, Hashemi P, Strong AJ, et al. Cortical spreading depression and peri-infarct depolarization in acutely injured human cerebral cortex. Brain 2006;129:778–90.
16. Hartings JA, Watanabe T, Dreier JP, Major S, Vendelbo L, Fabricius M. Recovery of slow potentials in AC-coupled electrocorticography: application to spreading depolarizations in rat and human cerebral cortex. J Neurophysiol. 2009;102:2563–75.
17. Dreier JP, Windmuller O, Petzold G, Lindauer U, Einhaupl KM, Dirnagl U. Ischemia caused by inverse coupling between neuronal activation and cerebral blood flow in rats. Int Congr Ser. 2002;1235:487–92.
18. Sukhotinsky I, Dilekoz E, Moskowitz MA, Ayata C. Hypoxia and hypotension transform the blood flow response to cortical spreading depression from hyperemia into hypoperfusion in the rat. J Cereb Blood Flow Metab. 2008;28:1369–76.
19. Hashemi P, Bhatia R, Nakamura H, Dreier JP, Graf R, Strong AJ, et al. Persisting depletion of brain glucose following cortical spreading depression, despite apparent hyperaemia: evidence for risk of an adverse effect of Leao's spreading depression. J Cereb Blood Flow Metab. 2009;29:166–75.
20. Mies G, Paschen W. Regional changes of blood flow, glucose, and ATP content determined on brain sections during a single passage of spreading depression in rat brain cortex. Exp Neurol. 1984;84:249–58.
21. Sonn J, Mayevsky A. Effects of brain oxygenation on metabolic, hemodynamic, ionic and electrical responses to spreading depression in the rat. Brain Res. 2000;882:212–16.
22. Dohmen C, Sakowitz OW, Fabricius M, Bosche B, Reithmeier T, Ernestus RI, et al. Spreading depolarizations occur in human ischemic stroke with high incidence. Ann Neurol. 2008;63:720–28.
23. Fabricius M, Fuhr S, Willumsen L, Dreier JP, Bhatia R, Boutelle MG, et al. Association of seizures with cortical spreading depression and peri-infarct depolarisations in the acutely injured human brain. Clin Neurophysiol. 2008;119:1973–84.
24. Hartings JA, Strong AJ, Fabricius M, Manning A, Bhatia R, Dreier JP, et al. Spreading depolarizations and late secondary insults after traumatic brain injury. J Neurotrauma. 2009;26:1857–66.

Cerebral Microdialysis in Acutely Brain-Injured Patients with Spreading Depolarizations

K.L. Krajewski, B. Orakcioglu, D. Haux, D.N. Hertle, E. Santos, K.L. Kiening, A.W. Unterberg, and O.W. Sakowitz

Abstract Multimodal cerebral monitoring was utilized to examine the relationship between pathological changes in microdialysis parameters and the occurrence of spreading depolarizations (SD) in brain-injured patients. SD are a relatively newly discovered phenomenon in man found to be linked to secondary insults and infarct growth and they can be detected via electrocorticography (ECoG). A total of 24 brain-injured patients (mean age: 52 ± 11 years) requiring craniotomy took part in this prospective observational study. Each patient was monitored with a linear strip electrode for ECoG data and a cerebral microdialysis probe. SD were detected in 13 of the 24 patients. Pathological concentrations of glucose and lactate in brain parenchyma were significantly correlated with various time points prior to and/or immediately following the SD. Severe systemic hyperglycemia and systemic hypoglycemia were also found to be correlated with the occurrence of SD. The present study shows a clear relationship between SD and pathological changes in cerebral metabolism; further studies are needed to elucidate these complex interactions with the ultimate goal of developing therapeutic strategies for improving outcome in brain-injured patients.

Keywords Electrocorticography · Microdialysis · Neuromonitoring · Spreading depolarizations

K.L. Krajewski, B. Orakcioglu, D. Haux, D.N. Hertle, E. Santos, K.L. Kiening, and A.W. Unterberg
From the Department of Neurosurgery, University of Heidelberg, Heidelberg, Germany

O.W. Sakowitz (✉)
Department of Neurosurgery, University Hospital Heidelberg, Im Neuenheimer Feld 400, 69120 Heidelberg, Germany
e-mail: oliver.sakowitz@med.uni-heidelberg.de

Introduction

Until recently, standard neurointensive care monitoring did not extend beyond cardiopulmonary surveillance, neurological assessments, and occasional imaging studies. The concept of multimodal cerebral monitoring techniques was introduced several years ago and has evolved into an integral part of neurointensive research and care [1]. The common goal of these invasive measures is to detect secondary ischemic brain injuries, though much of it is still experimental and the pathophysiology is often not fully understood.

Microdialysis (MD) is a tool that allows one to analyze extracellular concentrations of substances such as products of glucose metabolism, neurotransmitters and other amino acids in living tissues. Analyzing these concentrations in brain tissues allows one to directly assess secondary ischemic injuries. Pathophysiologically, glutamate is released from the cell and accumulates in the extracellular space during periods of ischemia [2, 3]. Similarly, an increase in lactate, and more specifically the lactate/pyruvate (L/P) ratio, are also general markers of suboptimal cerebral metabolism and/or ischemia; in fact, the L/P ratio was found to be the most sensitive and specific marker of ischemia in several studies [4, 5]. Further, extracellular concentrations of lactate and glutamate have been used to diagnose vasospasm after subarachnoid hemorrhage (SAH), as confirmed by transcranial doppler (TCD), angiography and delayed ischemic neurological deficits (DIND) [6, 7]. Extracellular concentrations of glucose, on the other hand, are more difficult to interpret; low cerebral glucose levels have a weaker correlation with poor outcome as compared to glutamate and L/P. It has already been long-established that *systemic* hyperglycemia should be avoided in the brain-injured patient and studies on systemic hyperglycemia and vasospasm have found a positive correlation between the two [8].

Electrocortigraphy (ECoG) is an invasive form of electroencephalography that has found use mainly in the diagnosis and research of epilepsy and epilepsy surgery. Sum potentials are directly recorded by arrays of electrodes placed directly on the brain. In 2002, Strong et al. [9] were the first to determine that spreading depolarizations can be found in the vicinity of brain hemorrhage in man and that these were similar to cortical spreading depressions that had been exclusively found in animals so far. They hypothesized that this phenomenon may contribute to the secondary insult seen in brain-injured patients and that this phenomenon is related to peri-infarct depolarizations, which have been shown to enhance ischemic zone enlargement following ischemic stroke and SAH [10, 11]. The "Cooperative Study on Brain Injury Depolarisations" (COSBID) was recently established as an international group of basic science and clinical researchers who are investigating exactly these questions [12]. The present project was carried out on the basis of the COSBID study protocol in order to investigate the relationship of cerebral metabolism as assessed by microdialysis in regards to the occurrence of SD.

Methods

Patients

A total of 24 patients with a mean age of 52 ± 11 years were included in the study. The target group of patients were those who required craniotomy or invasive intracranial monitoring as the result of traumatic brain injury, subarachnoid hemorrhage, spontaneous intracerebral hemorrhage or ischemic infarction. Exclusion criteria were age < 6 years, Glasgow Coma Score < 4 and/or bilateral dilated and unresponsive pupils or other signs of imminent death as well as a history of trauma/bleed < 5 days prior to admission.

Ethics approval was obtained from the Ethics Committee for the University of Heidelberg Medical School. Written informed consent was obtained from the patient's legal representative or next-of-kin, whoever was available at the time of emergency craniotomy.

Operative Procedures

The strip electrode and other probes were placed in the parenchyma ipsilateral to the insult after craniotomy was completed and appropriate hemostasis was obtained. All patients received an invasive intracranial pressure probe, a cerebral microdialysis probe (CMA70/71, CMA, Solna, Sweden) and either a regional cerebral blood flow (rCBF) probe via thermodiffusion (QFlow500, Hemedex Inc., Cambridge, MA) or an oxygen partial pressure probe (Licox™, Integra, Plainsboro, NJ). These probes were placed in parenchyma corresponding to the ECoG lead closest to the hemorrhage.

Postoperative Care

All patients returned to the intensive care unit for sedation and mechanical ventilation as long as indicated by their primary disease, and/or other organ system disorders. The patients were maintained in a normotensive, normovolemic, normoglycemic, and normothermic state as much as possible. In patients with SAH, one aimed to keep cerebral perfusion pressures in the upper range of normal. Treatment of increased intracranial pressure was initiated, when necessary, according to the guidelines for severe head injury. Treatment of vasospasm was initiated as necessary with hypertensive, hypervolemic and hemodilutional therapy, as diagnosed by the clinical appreciation of neurostatus deterioration in combination with parameters of invasive monitoring (i.e. rCBF, MD), angiographic studies (if needed) and/or TCD studies (defined by flow velocities > 200 cm/s) and with the exclusion of other possible causes such as hydrocephalus, hemorrhage, sepsis, etc. In addition, a postoperative CT scan was carried out in every patient in order to check the location of the probes. Neurological, GCS and pupil exams were carried out hourly.

Monitoring

"Standard" neurointensive care monitoring parameters included end-hourly readings of core body temperature, pulse, systolic and diastolic blood pressure, mean arterial pressure, arterial oxygen saturation, and arterial blood gas analysis every 4 h including blood chemistry (systemic blood sugar, electrolytes) as well as regular complete blood counts. Minute-by-minute data were transmitted from the intensive care unit monitoring system via TCP/ICP, the Infinity Gateway Software Suite (Dräger Medical Deutschland GmbH, Lübeck, Germany) and the respective client plugin of the ICU Pilot™ (CMA Microdialysis AB, Solna, Sweden) software. Others were transferred manually from the patients' charts.

MD catheters were perfused with sterile Ringer's solution at constant flow rates of 0.3 µl/min (CMA106/107 model pumps, Solna, Sweden). Glucose, lactate, pyruvate and glutamate were assayed using a bedside automatic, photometric, enzyme-kinetic analyzer (CMA600, Solna, Sweden). These values were obtained hourly and the vials were placed in frozen storage for off-line analysis at a later time. Values were not corrected for recovery, which is known to be approximately 0.70 (for the CMA70-10 mm probe perfused at 0.3 μl/min relative recovery was shown to be 0.65–0.72). Decreases in glucose, an increase in lactate and the lactate/pyruvate ratio and increases in glutamate were interpreted as a deterioration of cerebral metabolism.

A representative band of cortex approximately 5 cm wide centrifugally related to the lesion was monitored with a subdural linear strip electrode (six or eight platinum contacts; Wyler, 5/10 mm; Ad-Tech Medical Instrument Corp., Racine, WI; interelectrode distance: 1 cm). Recordings were acquired in 4–7 active channels with electrodes connected in bipolar montage to one Octal™ or two Dual Bioamp™ amplifiers (0.01–200 Hz) (ADInstruments, New South Wales, Australia). Recording and review was accomplished with the Powerlab 16/SP analog/digital converter coupled with the Chart-5 software (ADInstruments, New South Wales, Australia). SD were recognized by their characteristic slow potential change that spreads between adjacent channels and that is accompanied by transient depression of ECoG activity. Most of these SDs appeared repetitively in clusters.

In addition to the electrocorticographical data, the chart program interface was used by nursing and medical staff to record the start and finish of the following events: patient transport, nursing maneuvers (such as sponge-bathing, wound care, etc.), suctioning, physical therapy, patient repositioning (decubital ulcer prevention), blood gas analysis, sedation, machine calibration, etc. These events were noted as a "time-stamp" labeled "nursing maneuvers" and could not be further differentiated for analyses.

Data Reduction and Statistics

The EcoG data was reviewed for SD for each patient. A summary of the number as well as the temporal occurrence ("early", within 72 h; "subacute", day 3–7 post-trauma; "late", after day 7) was completed for each patient. SPSS software was used for statistical analyses (SPSS v. 13.0, Chicago, USA). Correlations were calculated by Spearman's rho. The partial correlations routine of the same software package allowed to correct for covariates "initial GCS score", "anisocoria" and "age".

Table 1 Percentage of spreading depolarizations with pathological measurements in intracranial pressure (ICP), cerebral perfusion pressure (CPP), extracellular concentrations in glucose, lactate and lactate–pyruvate ratios

Parameter	Threshold	Pathological (%)
ICP	>20 mmHg	<1
CPP	<60 mmHg	<1
Glucose	<1 mM; >3 mM	41
Lactate	>4 mM	60
Lactate/Pyruvate	>20	83

The hemodynamic and metabolic data were then reviewed for pathological values at the start of the first SPC for each SD (at "time zero") and summarized as a percentage. Next, the 60 min prior to SD start and the 120 min following the SD start were analyzed for the percentage of pathological hemodynamic and metabolic values (as averaged over 10-min periods). A frequency distribution of pathological values within this time frame was completed for each parameter. The Friedman test was employed to determine whether this course was statistically significant; if deemed significant, time-pairs were then individually tested with the Wilcoxon Signed Ranks test. P-values < 0.05 were regarded as significant.

Results

In 13 of the 24 (54%) patients in the study, one or more spreading depolarizations manifested with a range of 4–94, and a mean of 31 ± 24. The mean time in hours to the first spreading depolarization was 85.5 ± 43.2 h and the mean time between spreading depolarizations was 5.2 ± 6.1 h with a weighted average of 2.6 h. In all pathologies except in one patient with spontaneous intracerebral hemorrhage spreading depolarizations were observed (8/17 SAH, 2/3 TBI, 3/3 stroke, 0/1 intracerebral hemorrhage).

The first analysis of the microdialysis parameters at the time of the first slow potential change for a given SD revealed the percentages of pathological values as displayed in Table 1. Only 6% of SD occurred at a time when the patient was being handled by medical personnel, which lowers the chance that the SD had much artifact interference (e.g. probes/electrodes were being manipulated/checked and possibly causing waves that could imitate a SD).

In Fig. 1 the frequency distribution of pathological glucose, glutamate and lactate values for the 80 min prior to and 100 min after the SD (averaged over 10-min periods) is depicted. Cerebral hypoglycemia (e.c. glucose <1 mM) and hyperglycemia (e.c. glucose > 3 mM) alone did not display any significant differences (data not shown); thus the glucose pathologies were combined, which can be summarized as "deteriorated cerebral glucose". There is a normalization in extracellular concentrations of glucose in the 10 minutes prior to SD. The number of pathological values 20 min after SD is significantly reduced with respect to those 20 min prior to SD. A peak of pathological glutamate values (again as calculated with respect to glutamate peaks 20% > baseline) at "time zero" was not found statistically significant. The percentage of pathological lactate values manifests a general tendency towards poor cerebral metabolic states leading up to SD, similarly to glucose. Instead of a "peak" of pathological values at "time zero", there appears to be a

Fig. 1 Percentages of pathological monitoring values relative to the onset of spreading depolarizations (SD) in minutes of time and as indicated by the dashed lines

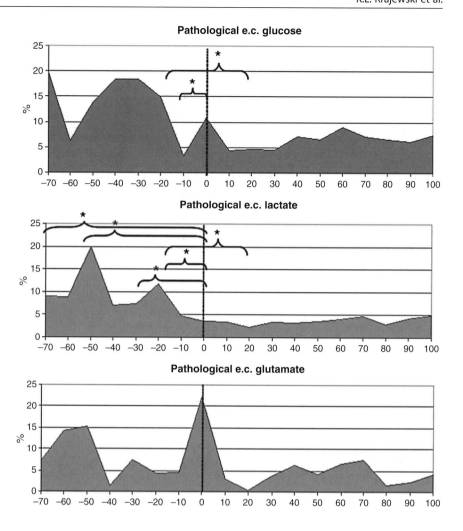

Table 2 Partial correlations between monitoring abnormalities and the numerical appearance of SD

	SD total	SD ≤ 72 h	SD Day 3–7
Severe systemic hyperglycemia	0.464 *	n.s.	n.s.
Systemic hypoglycemia	n.s.	n.s.	0.485 *

Only significant correlations after correcting for age, presence of anisocoria and GCS score on the initial presentation are given
Values listed are r values * p < 0.05

general improvement of pathological lactate levels at "time zero" as compared to the time leading up to SD that continues at least 20 min afterwards.

All monitoring events were quantified according to number, hours and percent monitoring time and then tested against the total number of SD, the number of SD within 72 h ("early"), the number of SD between days 3 and 7 ("subacute"), and the number of SDs after day 7 ("late"), after correcting for age, presence of anisocoria and GCS score on the initial presentation. Only glucose events were found significantly correlated with the number of SD. The results of this partial correlation can be found in Table 2.

Discussion

Microdialysis Technique

The surveillance of cerebral metabolism in neurointensive care patients is a challenging task and despite significant progress, there are several technical shortcomings which require modification. Commercially available equipment is restricted to only one supplier and temporal resolution (sampling rate of typically 1 to maximally 3 measurements/hour) is rather poor. With these hourly measurements one assumes information on long-term changes is obtained. Only one other group has reported its findings of microdialysis measurements in patients with ECoG-proven occurrence of SD to date [13]. In a small sample of 11 patients with brain contusions and spontaneous intracerebral hemorrhage, a custom-built "rapid-online microdialysis" system was used and lactate and glucose measurements were referenced to the occurrence of SD. In that study, with minute-by-minute sampling, good time-locking with SD-events could be observed. Several patterns of MD response to SD, namely *transient* increases, decreases, and even oscillations could be identified. Overall, similarly to our own results, there was a good correlation between a progressive reduction in dialysate glucose and the aggregate number of SD. However, the results were too heterogenous to draw final conclusions on whether SD appear with impaired glucose metabolism or vice versa.

It should again be mentioned that MD, as every regional measurement, can be affected by artifacts arising from regular activities around the bedside. Though the number of nursing maneuvers varied widely, an association with SD in only 6% suggests that nursing maneuvers as did not play a large role in their pathogenesis.

Glucose and Lactate

The combined glucose chart yielded significant differences between several minutes before SD and at SD start. The plateau of pathological values leading up to an SD could demonstrate the poor metabolic state of the brain leading up to SD. Upon closer scrutiny, it became evident that the majority of the pathological glucose values prior to the SD were too low rather than too high; thus, e.c. glucose concentrations tended to *increase* around the SD. In contrast, Hopwood and colleagues found a reduction in cerebral glucose in the 10 minutes after SD in an experimental model, with anecdotal episodes of temporary normalization and then further reductions [14], possibly due to increased utilization or reduced vascular supply. Our findings suggest that SD are involved in long-term metabolic changes (at least 20 min post-SD), and not just momentary fluctuations.

Similarly we observed a *marked improvement* of e.c. lactate concentrations post-SD that continues for over an hour afterwards. Without further differentiation of the SD-phenomena we were unable to confirm Hopwood and colleagues' findings that lactate increases in the 30 min post-SD and stabilizes at this higher, pathological level for the following 3 h [14]. The "improvement" in lactate may, in fact, be a sign that the tissue at risk between the penumbra and the unaffected parenchyma recovered- or that the penumbra was extended rendering the tissue metabolically inert. In contrast to experimental studies, it is impossible to clinically determine the exact location of the penumbra; thus, many results may have been skewed solely based on uncertain probe placement.

Total SD were positively correlated with severe systemic hyperglycemia, whereas late SD (days 3–7) were positively correlated with systemic hypoglycemia. These findings support the hypothesis of an inverse relationship between SD and plasma glucose [13, 14].

Glutamate

We have put forward evidence that SD generation in patients may depend on N-methyl-D-aspartate-receptor-based mechanisms [15]. Though the glutamate chart demonstrated an impressive increase of SD-associated peaks at time zero, this course was not statistically significant. One would expect an increase of glutamate after SD, similarly to lactate, based on the assumption of similar ischemia-related metabolic changes. The efficacy of glutamate inhibitors on ischemia in animal models has not yet been confirmed in clinical trials; thus, further studies are needed to confirm the neuroprotective effects of such inhibitors and to explore this evidently complex relationship between glutamate and SD.

Outlook

Two important observations by Fabricius and colleagues that may help clarifying the picture are that there are different *types* of SD (slow potential changes that accompany CSD, "classical" CSD vs. PID) as well as the *direction* of SD can differ (they found that 43% of SD originated from the injury site and spread outward, while 57% did the opposite) [16]. Although the average weighted time between SD exceeded 2 h in the present study, many other groups have reported "clusters" of SD, which could have caused overlap in some cases, skewing the present analyses. There are several aspects of SD that need to be further explored in order to elucidate the true nature of their effects. There is ongoing research related to the occurrence of SD. As previously mentioned, a more refined spatio-temporal analysis as well as a more differentiated subtype analysis are the next step in elucidating this phenomenon.

Conclusion

Our findings corroborated the presence of spreading depolarizations in brain-injured patients. We were able to confirm significant associated changes in cerebral glucose and lactate concentrations. In addition, we were able to show an association between SD and elevated as well as reduced blood glucose concentrations. Taken together, these findings both warrant further investigations on this phenomenon and provide a good direction for future studies.

Conflict of interest statement We declare that we have no conflict of interest.

References

1. Bardt TF, Unterberg AW, Kiening KL, Schneider GH, Lanksch WR. Multimodal cerebral monitoring in comatose head-injured patients. Acta Neurochir 1998;140:357–65.
2. Kett-White R, Hutchinson PJ, Al-Rawi PG, Gupta AK, Pickard JD, Kirkpatrick PJ. Adverse cerebral events detected after subarachnoid hemorrhage using brain oxygen and microdialysis probes. Neurosurgery 2002;50:1213–21.
3. Sarrafzadeh AS, Haux D, Lüdemann L, Amthauer H, Plotkin M, Küchler I, et al. Cerebral ischemia in aneurysmal subarachnoid hemorrhage: a correlative microdialysis-PET study. Stroke 2004;35:638–43.
4. Persson L, Hillered L. Chemical monitoring of neurosurgical intensive care patients using intracerebral microdialysis. J Neurosurg 1992;76:72–80.
5. Hutchinson PJ, al-Rawi PG, O'Connell MT, Gupta AK, Maskell LB, Hutchinson DB, et al. Head injury monitoring using cerebral microdialysis and Paratrend multiparameter sensors. Zentralbl Neurochir 2000;61:88–94.
6. Skjøth-Rasmussen J, Schulz M, Kristensen SR, Bjerre P. Delayed neurological deficits detected by an ischemic pattern in the extracellular cerebral metabolites in patients with aneurysmal subarachnoid hemorrhage. J Neurosurg 2004;100:8–15.
7. Unterberg AW, Sakowitz OW, Sarrafzadeh AS, Benndorf G, Lanksch WR. Role of bedside microdialysis in the diagnosis of cerebral vasospasm following aneurysmal subarachnoid hemorrhage J Neurosurg 2001;94:740–9.
8. Frontera JA, Fernandez A, Claassen J, Schmidt M, Schumacher HC, Wartenberg K, et al. Hyperglycemia after SAH: predictors, associated complications, and impact on outcome. Stroke 2006;37:199–203.
9. Strong AJ, Fabricius M, Boutelle MG, Hibbins SJ, Hopwood SE, Jones R, et al. Spreading and synchronous depressions of cortical activity in acutely injured human brain. Stroke 2002;33:2738–43.
10. Mies G, Iijima T, Hossmann KA. Correlation between peri-infarct DC shifts and ischaemic neuronal damage in rat. Neuroreport 1993;4:709–11.
11. Dreier JP, Ebert N, Priller J, Megow D, Lindauer U, Klee R, et al. Products of hemolysis in the subarachnoid space inducing spreading ischemia in the cortex and focal necrosis in rats: a model for delayed ischemic neurological deficits after subarachnoid hemorrhage? J Neurosurg 2000;93:658–66.
12. Strong AJ, Hartings JA, Dreier JP. Cortical spreading depression: an adverse but treatable factor in intensive care? Curr Opin Crit Care 2007;13:126–33.
13. Parkin M, Hopwood S, Jones DA, Hashemi P, Landolt H, Fabricius M, et al. Dynamic changes in brain glucose and lactate in pericontusional areas of the human cerebral cortex, monitored with rapid sampling on-line microdialysis: relationship with depolarisation-like events. J Cereb Blood Flow Metab 2005;25:402–13.
14. Hopwood SE, Parkin MC, Bezzina EL, Boutelle MG, Strong AJ. Transient changes in cortical glucose and lactate levels associated with peri-infarct depolarisations, studied with rapid-sampling microdialysis. J Cereb Blood Flow Metab 2005;25:391–401.
15. Sakowitz OW, Kiening KL, Krajewski KL, Sarrafzadeh AS, Fabricius M, Strong AJ, et al. Preliminary evidence that ketamine inhibits spreading depolarizations in acute human brain injury Stroke 2009;40:e519–22.
16. Fabricius M, Fuhr S, Bhatia R, Boutelle M, Hashemi P, Strong AJ, et al. Cortical spreading depression and peri-infarct depolarization in acutely injured human cerebral cortex. Brain 2006;129:778–90.

Section V: Pathophysiology of Cerebral Vasospasm

Mitogen-Activated Protein Kinases in Cerebral Vasospasm After Subarachnoid Hemorrhage: A Review

Hidenori Suzuki, Yu Hasegawa, Kenji Kanamaru, and John H. Zhang

Abstract *Background*: Mitogen-activated protein kinases (MAPKs) have been implicated in the pathogenesis of cerebral vasospasm after subarachnoid hemorrhage. The goal of this review is to bring together recent diverse data concerning the roles of MAPKs in cerebral vasospasm and to consider the future research.

Method: A review of publications in the National Library of Medicine and National Institutes of Health database was conducted in August 2009 using specific keyword search terms pertaining to subarachnoid hemorrhage and MAPKs.

Findings: There are nine in vitro studies and 17 in vivo studies published. Most of previous studies used MAPK inhibitors or their upstream molecule inhibitors, and showed that MAPK inhibitions prevented vasospasm. The MAPK cascade appears to interact with other signaling molecules, and MAPK may be an important final common pathway for the signaling transduction during cerebral vasospasm. However, the mechanism by which MAPK causes sustained vascular smooth muscle contraction remains unclear. In addition, the role of endogenous MAPK inhibitors, MAPK phosphatases, has not been investigated in cerebral vasospasm.

Conclusions: The experimental data support the causative role of MAPK in cerebral vasospasm and warrant further research.

Keywords Cerebral vasospasm · Mitogen-activated protein kinase · Signaling transduction · Subarachnoid hemorrhage

Introduction

Arterial smooth muscle contraction is initiated by Ca^{2+}-dependent mechanisms activating actin–myosin coupling and cross-bridge cycling, but additional proteins have been proposed to participate in the sustained contractile phase to explain the dissociation between maintained force and rapidly decreasing intracellular Ca^{2+} concentration and phosphorylation of myosin light chain. In smooth muscle cells, the thin filament-binding protein caldesmon and calponin have been localized in close proximity to actin, myosin, and tropomyosin. Caldesmon and calponin block myosin binding to actin and inhibit actin-dependent myosin ATPase activity (so-called latch-state), and these inhibitory effects are reversed on the phosphorylation of caldesmon and calponin [1]. Caldesmon and calponin are substrates for mitogen-activated protein kinases (MAPKs), and therefore MAPKs are considered likely modulators of prolonged smooth muscle contraction [2, 3].

Phosphorylation of the small heat shock protein 27 (HSP27), downstream of p38 MAPK, is another MAPK-mediated mechanism proposed to modulate the sustained phase of smooth muscle contraction [4, 5]. Elevated phosphorylation of HSP27 has been observed after stimulation with a variety of contractile agonists such as thrombin [6] and endothelin-1 (ET-1) [7]. Phosphorylated HSP27 promotes actin remodeling by enhancing actin polymerization, which is an important event in the mechanism of force maintenance during smooth muscle contraction [8], while phosphorylated HSP27 inhibits HSP20 phosphorylation by protein kinases A and G, preventing both cyclic adenosine monophosphate and cyclic guanosine monophosphate-dependent vasorelaxation [9]. Thus, it is possible that the p38 MAPK/HSP27 pathway plays a role in the sustained vascular smooth muscle contraction [10].

In addition to sustained vasocontraction and impaired vasorelaxation, MAPK is involved in tissue proliferation, apoptosis and inflammation development, all of which are

H. Suzuki and Y. Hasegawa
Department of Physiology, Loma Linda University School of Medicine, Risley Hall, Room 223, Loma Linda, CA 92354, USA

K. Kanamaru
Department of Neurosurgery, Suzuka Kaisei Hospital, Suzuka, Japan

J.H. Zhang (✉)
Department of Physiology, Loma Linda University School of Medicine, Risley Hall, Room 223, Loma Linda, CA 92354, USA
Department of Neurosurgery, Loma Linda University School of Medicine, Risley Hall, Room 223, Loma Linda, CA 92354, USA
e-mail: johnzhang3910@yahoo.com

key features of cerebral vasospasm [11]. These mechanisms may be involved in a complex pathological process of cerebral vasospasm characterized by persistent contraction of arterial smooth muscle and morphological changes in the arterial wall.

A review of the National Library of Medicine and National Institutes of Health database until August, 2009 yielded 26 publications (in vitro, 9; in vivo, 17) pertaining to the role of MAPK in cerebral vasospasm after subarachnoid hemorrhage (SAH). We review these publications and consider the future research.

Overview of In Vitro Studies (Table 1)

Most studies have focused on extracellular signal-regulated kinase (ERK)1/2. Hemolysate, oxyhemoglobin (oxyHb), bloody cerebrospinal fluid (CSF) and endothelin (ET)-1 enhanced total ERK1/2 levels and ERK1/2 activity within 3–5 min that was maintained up to 2–4 h in rabbit basilar arteries (BAs) [13, 14]. MAPK/ERK kinase (MEK) inhibitor PD98059 and U0126 significantly inhibited hemolysate-, oxyHb-, bloody CSF- and ET-1-induced contraction and ERK1/2 upregulation and activation in rabbit BAs [13–15].

Genistein, an inhibitor of tyrosine kinases, and PD098059 were also effective in the reduction of oxyHb-induced contraction of isolated BAs from a canine double-hemorrhagic model or a healthy control, and OxyHb-induced ERK2 and c-Src upregulation in cultured canine cerebral smooth muscle cells from BA and middle cerebral artery (MCA) of untreated dogs [12]. ET-1 enhanced total ERK1/2 levels and produced contraction in rabbit BA by activation of ET_A but not ET_B receptors [14]. On the other hand, Henriksson et al. [18] reported that the ET-1-induced vasoconstriction of rat MCAs was increased after incubation with SB386023 (an inhibitor of Raf, the MAPK kinase kinase of ERK1/2), while unaffected by U0126. Jamali and Edvinsson [19] also reported that RO-31-7549 (a protein kinase C [PKC] inhibitor), SB386023 and SP600125 (a c-Jun N-Terminal kinase [JNK] inhibitor) attenuated the contraction induced by S6c (an ET_B receptor agonist) in the rat BAs, but that they had no effect on ET_A receptor-mediated contraction. These studies suggested that the PKC, ERK1/2, and JNK (especially ERK1/2) are important for the upregulation of contractile ET_B receptors in cerebral arteries after organ culture [18, 19]. PKC is known to activate the MEK/ERK pathway at several levels [21]. The ET_A receptor is a contractile receptor situated on the smooth-muscle cells of the vessels, whereas the ET_B receptor is mainly found on the

Table 1 Summary of in vitro studies regarding a role for MAPK in cerebral vasospasm

Reference	Tissue	Agonist	MAPK	Antagonist	Effect
Vollrath et al. (1998) [12]	Dog BA	OxyHb	ERK1/2	PD98059	Contraction↓
				Genistein	Contraction↓
	Dog BA (DHM)	OxyHb	ERK1/2	PD98059	Contraction↓
				Genistein	Contraction↓
Zubkov et al. (1999) [13]	Rabbit BA	Hemolysate	ERK1/2	PD98059	Contraction↓
Zubkov et al. (2000) [14]	Rabbit BA	Endothelin-1	ERK1/2	PD98059	Contraction↓
				U0126	Contraction↓
Zubkov et al. (2001) [15]	Rabbit BA	Hemolysate	ERK1/2	U0126	Contraction↓
		OxyHb	ERK1/2	U0126	Contraction↓
		Bloody CSF	ERK1/2	U0126	Contraction↓
Sasaki et al. (2004) [16]	Human UA	Hemolysate	p38	FR167653	Contraction→
Maeda et al. (2004) [17]	Bovine MCA	Oxidative stress & Bradykinin	p38	SB203580	Contraction↓ (Relaxation→)
Henriksson et al. (2004) [18]	Rat MCA	Endothelin-1	ERK1/2	SB386023	Contraction↑
			ERK1/2	U0126	Contraction→
			p38	SB239063	Contraction↑
Jamali et al. (2006) [19]	Rat BA	S6c	ERK1/2	SB386023	Contraction↓
			JNK	SP600125	Contraction↓
		Endothelin-1 & S6c desensitization	ERK1/2	SB386023	Contraction→
			JNK	SP600125	Contraction→
Beg et al. (2006) [20]	Rat BA & MCA (SHM)	Endothelin-1	ERK1/2	SB386023-b	Contraction↓

BA basilar artery, *CSF* cerebrospinal fluid, *DHM* double hemorrhage model, *ERK* extracellular signal-regulated kinase, *JNK* c-Jun N-Terminal kinase, *MAPK* mitogen-activated protein kinase, *MCA* middle cerebral artery, *OxyHb* oxyhemoglobin, *SHM* single hemorrhage model, *UA* umbilical artery

PD98059, U0126 an inhibitor of the MAPK/ERK kinase (MEK)1/2 (the MAPK kinase of ERK1/2), *SB386023, SB386023-b* an inhibitor of Raf (the MAPK kinase kinase of ERK1/2), *Genistein* an inhibitor of tyrosine kinases, *FR167653, SB203580, SB239063* a p38 MAPK inhibitor, *SP600125* a JNK inhibitor, *S6c* an endothelin type B receptor agonist

endothelium, mediating dilation. In addition, there is a small population of contractile ET$_B$ receptors expressed on the smooth-muscle cells in some arteries and veins [22].

SB203580, a p38 MAPK inhibitor, and genistein prevented the oxidative stress-induced endothelial dysfunction of the bovine MCA [17]. Oxidative stress was reported to cause apoptosis via an apoptosis signal-regulating kinase 1-p38 MAPK pathway [23]. In human arterial smooth muscle cells from umbilical artery, hemolysate induced interleukin (IL)-1α, IL-1β and IL-8, and activated p38 after 48 h. These effects were inhibited by FR167653, a selective inhibitor of p38. However, FR167653 did not reduce the hemolysate-induced contraction of the artery in an isometric tension study, suggesting that p38MAPK may not be involved directly in signal transduction to sustained contraction of smooth muscle cells [16]. In contrast, Henriksson et al. [18] reported that the ET-1-induced vasoconstriction of rat MCAs was increased after incubation with SB239063 (a specific inhibitor of p38).

Overview of In Vivo Studies (Table 2)

ERK1/2 is the best studied of MAPKs. The activation of ERK1/2 is reported to peak early in the course of vasospasm and remain elevated up to day 7 after SAH. In a dog double hemorrhage model, phosphorylated ERK1/2 peaked on day 2 (before the second injection) or day 3, and this enhancement of phosphorylated ERK1/2 sustained above the baseline up to day 7 [24, 28]. Strong staining of phosphorylated ERK1/2 was observed in all layers of the BA, especially in the adventitial layer and in the endothelial cells [31]. There was no change in ERK1 and ERK2 expression during vasospasm. PD98059 but not U0126 significantly reduced phosphorylated ERK1/2 and prevented angiographic vasospasm of the BA in a dog double hemorrhage model [26–28], while both PD98059 and U0126 reduced vasospasm of the penetrating arteries and improved clinical scores [26]. In a rabbit double hemorrhage model, in contrast, expression of phosphorylated ERK1/2 and proliferating cell nuclear

Table 2 Summary of in vivo studies regarding a role for MAPK in cerebral vasospasm

Reference	Model	MAPK	Antagonist	Effect
Fujikawa et al. (1999) [24]	Dog DHM	Shc, Raf1, ERK1/2 activation	Genistein	Vasospasm↓
				Shc activation↓
Tibbs et al. (2000) [25]	Dog DHM	ERK1/2 activation	–	–
Zubkov et al. (2000) [26]	Dog DHM	ERK1/2, basilar artery	PD98059	Vasospasm↓
		ERK1/2, perforating artery	PD98059	Vasospasm↓
		ERK1/2, basilar artery	U0126	Vasospasm→
		ERK1/2, perforating artery	U0126	Vasospasm↓
Yin et al. (2001) [27]	Dog DHM	ERK1/2	PD98059	Vasospasm↓
			U0126	Vasospasm→
Aoki et al. (2002) [28]	Dog DHM	ERK1/2 activation	PD98059	Vasospasm↓
Satoh et al. (2002) [29]	Rat SHM	ERK1/2 activation	Antisense	Vasospasm↓
	Rat DHM	ERK1/2 activation	Antisense	Vasospasm↓
Tsurutani et al. (2003) [30]	Rabbit DHM	ERK1/2 activation	Antithrombin-III	Vasospasm↓
Yamaguchi et al. (2004) [31]	Dog DHM	Ras, ERK1/2 activation	FTI-277	Vasospasm↓
			FTase inhibitor I	Vasospasm↓
Kusaka et al. (2003) [32]	Dog DHM	Src, ERK1/2 activation	PP2	Vasospasm↓
			Damnacanthal	Vasospasm↓
Kusaka et al. (2004) [33]	Rat EPM	ERK1/2, p38, JNK activation	PP1	–
Sasaki et al. (2004) [16]	Dog DHM	p38 activation	FR167653	Vasospasm↓
Yatsushige et al. (2005) [34]	Dog DHM	JNK, c-Jun activation	SP600125	Vasospasm↓
Beg et al. (2006) [20]	Rat SHM	ERK1/2	SB386023-b	CBF↑
Vikman et al. (2007) [35]	Rat SHM	ERK1/2, p38, JNK activation	–	–
		ATF-2, Elk-1, c-Jun upregulation		
Vikman et al. (2007) [36]	Rat SHM	ERK1/2, p38, Elk-1,	–	–
		ATF-2 activation		
Ansar et al. (2008) [37]	Rat SHM	ERK1/2, p38, JNK activation	RO-31–7549	ERK1/2↓
			SB386023-b	ERK1/2↓
Chen et al. (2009) [38]	Rabbit DHM	ERK1/2 activation	PD98059	Vasospasm↓

ATF activating transcription factor, *CBF* cerebral blood flow, *DHM* double hemorrhage model, *EPM* endovascular perforation model, *ERK* extracellular signal-regulated kinase, *JNK* c-Jun N-Terminal kinase, *MAPK* mitogen-activated protein kinase, *SHM* single hemorrhage model *Genistein* an inhibitor of tyrosine kinases, *PD98059, U0126* an inhibitor of the MAPK/ERK kinase (MEK)1/2 (the MAPK kinase of ERK1/2), *FTI-277* FTase inhibitor I, an inhibitor of Ras farnesyltransferase (FTase), *PP1, PP2* damnacanthal, an Src-family kinase inhibitor, *FR167653* a selective inhibitor of p38, *SP600125* a JNK inhibitor, *SB386023-b* a Raf inhibitor, *RO-31–7549* a protein kinase C inhibitor

antigen (PCNA) began to increase significantly on day 3 and reached peak on day 7 [38]. Total ERK1/2 expression showed no significant change. PD98059 significantly reduced angiographic and morphological vasospasm associated with reduced phosphorylated ERK1/2 and PCNA expression [38]. Tsurutani et al. [30] reported that ERK1/2 was activated in the vascular smooth muscle cell layer of spastic BA on day 4, and that an intracisternal injection of antithrombin-III (inhibition of thrombin activity) suppressed cerebral vasospasm and ERK1/2 activation in a rabbit double hemorrhage model. ERK1/2 was also activated in the spastic BA on day 2 in a single-hemorrhage rat SAH model and on day 7 in a double-hemorrhage rat SAH model [29]. ERK1/2 immunoreactivity was mainly localized in the cytoplasm and partially in the nucleus of the smooth muscle cells. Total ERK1/2 (ERK1/2 expression) was not altered between normal tissues before SAH and spastic tissues within 2 days after SAH. Antisense ERK1/2 oligodeoxynucleotide therapy inhibited vasospasm in both rat SAH models. In a rat single-hemorrhage model (a blood injection into the prechiasmatic cistern), G-protein-coupled receptors (ET_B and 5-hydroxytryptamine 1B [$5-HT_{1B}$] receptors) were upregulated in the smooth muscle layers of MCA and BA 48 h post-SAH and this upregulation was prevented by the ERK1/2 inhibitor SB386023-b [20]. The level of ET_A receptor was unchanged after SAH. The contractile responses to ET-1 were markedly increased in MCA and BA after SAH, which was ET_B receptor dependent. SB386023-b also reduced the ET-1-induced contraction of MCA and BA and prevented the reduction in regional and global cerebral blood flow seen after SAH [20].

Several upstream regulators of MAPK have been suggested to contribute to MAPK activation and the development of cerebral vasospasm [39]. Among them, Shc, Src, Raf-1 and Ras were activated in the canine spastic BAs [24, 31, 32]. While Shc is upstream of Src [39], Raf-1, an effector of Ras, activates MAPK. In addition, PKC may phosphorylate Raf-1, either bypassing or activating Ras, to activate MAPK [11]. In a canine double hemorrhage model of SAH, genistein reduced, in a concentration-dependent manner, tyrosine phosphorylation, generation of protein kinase M (a catalytic fragment of PKCα) and cerebral vasospasm, suggesting the link among PKC, tyrosine kinase and MAPK [24]. In a canine double hemorrhage model, an Src inhibitor, PP2 or damnacanthal, and the inhibitors of Ras farnesyltransferase abolished ERK1/2 activation, attenuated angiographic vasospasm and improved clinical scores [31, 32]. In an endovascular perforation model of SAH in rats, PP1, an Src-family kinase inhibitor, decreased SAH-induced phosphorylation of ERK1/2, p38 and JNK in the cerebral arteries 24 h post-SAH [33]. In a rat single-hemorrhage model (a blood injection into the prechiasmatic cistern), PKCδ was activated at 1 h and at 48 h, whereas PKCα was activated in large circle of Willis cerebral arteries at 48 h after SAH [37]. The phosphorylated ERK1/2 level was increased at 1, 6, and 48 h after SAH, whereas JNK and p38 showed enhanced phosphorylation only at 48 h after SAH. Treatment with either the PKC (RO-31-7549) or the Raf (SB386023-b) inhibitor prevented the kinase activation other than JNK and p38 [37]. These findings suggest that ERK1/2 and PKCδ are key pathways for the initiation of cerebral vasospasm after SAH, while PKCα, JNK, and p38 may have a role in the late phase of events (the maintenance of vasospasm) in cerebral arteries after SAH.

MAPK may cause vasospasm by inducing inflammatory reaction. In a canine double-hemorrhage model, IL-1α, IL-1β, IL-8, and phosphorylated p38 was induced in the BA on day 7 (total p38 was similar) [16]. FR167653, a selective inhibitor of p38, inhibited the p38 activation and cytokine induction, and prevented vasospasm. The JNK signaling pathway (the ratio of phosphorylated JNK to total JNK and the ratio of phosphorylated c-Jun to total c-Jun) was also activated in the BA on day 7 after SAH, and SP600125 a JNK inhibitor reduced vasospasm with a concomitant reduction of infiltrated leukocytes (T cells, neutrophils, and macrophages) in the adventitia layer or the subarachnoid space and IL-6 production in CSF [34]. Strong positive staining of phosphorylated c-Jun was observed in all layers of BA wall. In a rat single-hemorrhage model (a blood injection into the prechiasmatic cistern), phosphorylated ERK1/2, phosphorylated JNK, phosphorylated p38, their downstream transcription factors (activating transcription factor [ATF]-2, Elk-1, c-Jun), and inflammatory genes (IL-6, inducible nitric oxide synthase, tumor necrosis factor [TNF]-α, IL-1β) were upregulated in the smooth muscle layers of MCA and BA 24 h post-SAH [35, 36]. The pattern of activation consisted of a rapid phase within the first few hours and a late phase that occurred from 24 to 48 h [36].

Possible Pathway for MAPK to Induce Vasospasm

MAPKs are present in vascular smooth muscle cells, and the MAPK cascade appears to interact with other signaling molecules. Activation of G protein-coupled receptors by spasmogens such as ET-1, adenosine triphosphate or bilirubin oxidation product (BOX) leads to activation of phospholipase C (PLC), generating inositol-1, 4, 5-trisphosphate and diacylglycerol (DAG), which are involved in intracellular Ca^{2+} mobilization and PKC activation, respectively. Ca^{2+} and PKC activate protein tyrosine kinase, which in turn activates Src or Ras proteins, eventually leading to the activation of MAPK [13, 40]. Growth factors such as platelet-derived growth factor or epidermal growth factor released during vasospasm activate growth factor receptors (receptor tyrosine kinase) and lead to Src and Ras activation, assisted with adapter proteins Grb2 or Shc and exchange factor son of sevenless [41]. Ras stimulates Raf-1, leading to the activation of MAPK. PKC can activate Raf-1 directly. OxyHb and BOX generate free radicals and lipid peroxide and may activate the phosphatidylcholine and phosphatidylethanolamine pool to sustain a prolonged elevation of DAG, leading to PKC activation and then MAPK activation [11]. Free radicals also promote Ras activation, causing MAPK activation [42]. Cytokines, such as IL-1β or TNF-α, also have been shown to activate MAPK in smooth muscle cells [43] with or without generating DAG, a well-known activator of PKC, by stimulating a phosphatidylcholine-specific PLC [44]. Thus, MAPK may be an important "final common pathway" for the signaling transduction during cerebral vasospasm (Fig. 1).

However, the mechanism by which MAPK causes sustained vascular smooth muscle contraction remains unclear. Potential mediators for MAPK to induce sustained vascular smooth muscle contraction are caldesmon, calponin and HSP27 [10, 45]. Caldesmon and calponin have been reported to be involved in the pathogenesis of cerebral vasospasm, but the link between MAPK and caldesmon or calponin has not been investigated in cerebral vasospasm. Macomson et al. [46] reported that impaired endothelium-independent and endothelium-dependent relaxation occurred in the MCAs 48 h after SAH in a rat model of endovascular perforation. These changes were associated with decreased expression of both total and phosphorylated HSP20 and increases in the amount of phosphorylated HSP27. HSP20 may represent a final point at which the cyclic nucleotide-dependent signaling pathways converge to induce relaxation. Phosphorylated HSP27 inhibits HSP20 activation, preventing vasorelaxation. These mechanisms may account for the impaired relaxation observed in the cerebral vasculature after SAH, but the link between MAPK and HSP27/HSP20 also has not been investigated in cerebral vasospasm. In this regard, thus, further studies are needed.

Conclusion

Since MAPK pathways are activated through phosphorylation, dephosphorylation of MAPKs mediated by phosphatases represents a highly efficient mode of kinase deactivation. In mammalian cells, the dual-specificity protein phosphatases are the primary phosphatases responsible for dephosphorylation/deactivation of MAPKs, and therefore these phosphatases are often referred to as MAPK phosphatases (MKPs) [47]. To date, at least ten MKPs have been identified in mammalian cells, with MKP-1 being the archetype [48, 49]. However, MKP has not been investigated in cerebral vasospasm after SAH. Therapeutic induction of MKP may prove to be a novel approach for the prevention and treatment of cerebral vasospasm.

Acknowledgments This study was partially supported by grants (NS053407) from the National Institutes of Health to J.H.Z.

Conflict of interest statement We declare that we have no conflict of interest.

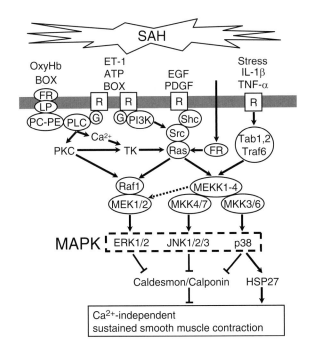

Fig. 1 Possible pathway for mitogen-activated protein kinases (MAPKs) to induce vasospasm *ATP* adenosine triphosphate, *BOX* bilirubin oxidation product, *DAG* diacylglycerol, *EGF* epidermal growth factor, *ERK* extracellular signal-regulated kinase, *ET-1* endothelin-1, *FR* free radicals, *G* G protein, *HSP* heat shock protein, *IL-1β* interleukin-1β, *JNK* c-Jun N-Terminal kinase, *LP* lipid peroxide, *MAPK* mitogen-activated protein kinase, *MEK* MAPK/ERK kinase, *MEKK* MEK kinase, *MKK* MAPK kinase, *OxyHb* oxyhemoglobin, *PC* phosphatidylcholine, *PDGF* platelet-derived growth factor, *PE* phosphatidylethanolamine, *PI3K* phosphatidylinositol-3 kinase, *PKC* protein kinase C, *PLC* phospholipase C, *R* receptor, *SAH* subarachnoid hemorrhage, *TK* protein tyrosine kinase, *TNF-α* tumor necrosis factor-α

References

1. Zhang Y, Moreland S, Moreland RS. Regulation of vascular smooth muscle contraction: myosin light chain phosphorylation dependent and independent pathways. Can J Physiol Pharmacol. 1994;72:1386–91.
2. Menice CB, Hulvershorn J, Adam LP, Wang CA, Morgan KG. Calponin and mitogen-activated protein kinase signaling in differentiated vascular smooth muscle. J Biol Chem. 1997;272:25157–61.

3. Hedges JC, Oxhorn BC, Carty M, Adam LP, Yamboliev IA, Gerthoffer WT. Phosphorylation of caldesmon by ERK MAP kinase in smooth muscle. Am J Physiol Cell Physiol. 2000;278: C718–26.
4. Beall A, Epstein A, Woodrum D, Brophy CM. Cyclosporine-induced renal artery smooth muscle contraction is associated with increases in the phosphorylation of specific contractile regulatory proteins. Biochim Biophys Acta. 1999;1449:41–9.
5. Bitar KN, Kaminski MS, Hailat N, Cease KB, Strahler JR. Hsp27 is a mediator of sustained smooth muscle contraction in response to bombesin. Biochem Biophys Res Commun. 1991;181:1192–200.
6. Brophy CM, Woodrum D, Dickinson M, Beall A. Thrombin activates MAPKAP2 kinase in vascular smooth muscle. J Vasc Surg. 1998;27:963–969.
7. Wang P, Bitar KN. Rho A regulates sustained smooth muscle contraction through cytoskeletal reorganization of HSP27. Am J Physiol Gastrointest Liver Physiol. 1998;275:G1454–62.
8. Gerthoffer W, Gunst SJ. Invited review: focal adhesion and small heat shock proteins in the regulation of actin remodeling and contractility in smooth muscle. J Appl Physiol. 2001;91:963–72.
9. McLemore EC, Tessier DJ, Thresher J, Komalavilas P, Brophy CM. Role of the small heat shock proteins in regulating vascular smooth muscle tone. J Am Coll Surg. 2005;201:30–6.
10. Yamboliev IA, Hedges JC, Mutnick JL-M, Adam LP, Gerthoffer WT. Evidence for modulation of smooth muscle force by the p38 MAP kinase/HSP27 pathway. Am J Physiol Heart Circ Physiol. 2000;278:1899–1907.
11. Laher I, Zhang JH. Protein kinase C and cerebral vasospasm. J Cereb Blood Flow Metab. 2001;21:887–906.
12. Vollrath B, Cook D, Megyesi J, Findlay JM, Ohkuma H. Novel mechanism by which hemoglobin induces constriction of cerebral arteries. Eur J Pharmacol. 1998;361:311–19
13. Zubkov AY, Ogihara K, Tumu P, Patlolla A, Lewis AI, Parent AD, Zhang J. Mitogen-activated protein kinase mediation of hemolysate-induced contraction in rabbit basilar artery. J Neurosurg. 1999;90:1091–97.
14. Zubkov AY, Rollins KS, Parent AD, Zhang J. Mechanism of endothelin-1-induced contraction in rabbit basilar artery. Stroke 2000;31:526–33.
15. Zubkov AY, Rollins KS, McGehee B, Parent AD, Zhang J. Relaxant effect of U0126 in hemolysate-, oxyhemoglobin-, and bloody cerebrospinal fluid-induced contraction in rabbit basilar artery. Stroke 2001;32:154–61.
16. Sasaki T, Kasuya H, Onda H, Sasahara A, Goto S, Hori T, Inoue I. Role of p38 mitogen-activated protein kinase on cerebral vasospasm after subarachnoid hemorrhage. Stroke 2004;35:1466–70.
17. Maeda Y, Hirano K, Nishimura J, Sasaki T, Kanaide H. Endothelial dysfunction and altered bradykinin response due to oxidative stress induced by serum deprivation in the bovine cerebral artery. Eur J Pharmacol. 2004;491:53–60.
18. Henriksson M, Xu C-B, Edvinsson L. Importance of ERK1/2 in upregulation of endothelin type B receptors in cerebral arteries. Br J Pharmacol. 2004;142:1155–61.
19. Jamali R, Edvinsson L. Involvement of protein kinases on the upregulation of endothelin receptors in rat basilar and mesenteric arteries. Exp Biol Med. 2006;231:403–11
20. Beg SAS, Hansen-Schwartz JA, Vikman PJ, Xu C-B, Edvinsson LIH. ERK1/2 inhibition attenuates cerebral blood flow reduction and abolishes ET_B and $5-HT_{1B}$ receptor upregulation after subarachnoid hemorrhage in rat. J Cereb Blood Flow Metab. 2006; 26:846–56.
21. Schonwasser DC, Marais RM, Marshall CJ, Parker PJ. Activation of the mitogen-activated protein kinase/extracellular signal-regulated kinase pathway by conventional, novel, and atypical protein kinase C isotypes. Mol Cell Biol. 1998;18:790–98.
22. Uddman E, Moller S, Adner M, Edvinsson L. Cytokines induce increased endothelin ET(B) receptor-mediated contraction. Eur J Pharmacol. 1999;376:223–32.
23. Ichijo H, Nishida E, Irie K, ten Dijke P, Saitoh M, Moriguchi T, Takagi M, Matsumoto K, Miyazono K, Gotoh Y. Induction of apoptosis by ASK1, a mammalian MAPKKK that activates SAPK/JNK and p38 signaling pathways. Science 1997; 275:90–4.
24. Fujikawa H, Tani E, Yamaura I, Ozaki I, Miyaji K, Sato M, Takahashi K, Imajoh-Ohmi S. Activation of protein kinases in canine basilar artery in vasospasm. J Cereb Blood Flow Metab. 1999;19:44–52.
25. Tibbs R, Zubkov A, Aoki K, Meguro T, Badr A, Parent A, Zhang J. Effects of mitogen-activated protein kinase inhibitors on cerebral vasospasm in a double-hemorrhage model in dogs. J Neurosurg. 2000;93:1041–47.
26. Zubkov AY, Tibbs RE, Aoki K, Zhang JH. Prevention of vasospasm in penetrating arteries with MAPK inhibitors in dog double-hemorrhage model. Surg Neurol. 2000;54:221–28
27. Yin W, Tibbs R, Aoki K, Badr A, Zhang J. Metabolic alterations in cerebrospinal fluid from double hemorrhage model of dogs. Neurol Res. 2001;23:87–92
28. Aoki K, Zubkov AY, Tibbs RE, Zhang JH. Role of MAPK in chronic cerebral vasospasm. Life Sci. 2002;70:1901–08.
29. Satoh M, Parent AD, Zhang JH. Inhibitory effect with antisense mitogen-activated protein kinase oligodeoxynucleotide against cerebral vasospasm in rats. Stroke 2002;33:775–781.
30. Tsurutani H, Ohkuma H, Suzuki S. Effects of thrombin inhibitor on thrombin-related signal transduction and cerebral vasospasm in the rabbit subarachnoid hemorrhage model. Stroke 2003;34: 1497–1500
31. Yamaguchi M, Zhou C, Nanda A, Zhang JH. Ras protein contributes to cerebral vasospasm in a canine double-hemorrhage model. Stroke 2004;35:1750–55.
32. Kusaka G, Kimura H, Kusaka I, Perkins E, Nanda A, Zhang JH. Contribution of Src tyrosine kinase to cerebral vasospasm after subarachnoid hemorrhage. J Neurosurg. 2003;99:383–90.
33. Kusaka G, Ishikawa M, Nanda A, Granger DN, Zhang JH. Signaling pathways for early brain injury after subarachnoid hemorrhage. J Cereb Blood Flow Metab. 2004;24:916–25.
34. Yatsushige H, Yamaguchi M, Zhou C, Calvert JW, Zhang JH. Role of c-Jun N-Terminal kinase in cerebral vasospasm after experimental subarachnoid hemorrhage. Stroke 2005;36:1538–43.
35. Vikman P, Ansar S, Henriksson M, Stenman E, Edvinsson L. Cerebral ischemia induces transcription of inflammatory and extracellular-matrix-related genes in rat cerebral arteries. Exp Brain Res. 2007;183:499–510.
36. Vikman P, Ansar S, Edvinsson L. Transcriptional regulation of inflammatory and extracellular matrix-regulating genes in cerebral arteries following experimental subarachnoid hemorrhage in rats. J Neurosurg. 2007;107:1015–22.
37. Ansar S, Edvinsson L. Subtype activation and interaction of protein kinase C and mitogen-activated protein kinase controlling receptor expression in cerebral arteries and microvessels after subarachnoid hemorrhage. Stroke 2008;39:185–90.
38. Chen D, Chen J-J, Yin Q, Guan c-H, Liu Y-H. Role of ERK1/2 and vascular cell proliferation in cerebral vasospasm after experimental subarachnoid hemorrhage. Acta Neurochir. 2009;151:1127–34. doi:10.1007/s00701-009-0385-3.
39. Zhang JH. Role of MAPK in cerebral vasospasm. Drug News Perspect. 2001;14:261–67.
40. Zhang JH. Role of protein kinase C in cerebral vasospasm: past and future. Neurol Res. 2000;22:369–78.
41. Berk BC, Corson MA. Angiotensin signal transduction in vascular smooth muscle: role of tyrosine kinase. Circ Res. 1997;80:607–16.

42. Lander HM, Ogiste JS, Teng KK, Novogrodsky A. p21ras as a common signal target of reactive free radicals and cellular redox stress. J Biol Chem. 1995;270:21195–98.
43. Yan CM, Luo SF, Wang CC, Chiu CT, Chien CS, Lin CC, Hsiao LD. Tumour necrosis factor-alpha- and interleukin-1beta-stimulated cell proliferation through activation of mitogen-activated protein kinase in canine tracheal smooth muscle cell. Br J Pharmacol. 2000;130:891–99.
44. Schütze S, Berkovic D, Tomsing O, Unger C, Krönke M. Tumor necrosis factor induces rapid production of 1'2'diacylglycerol by a phosphatidylcholine-specific phospholipase C. J Exp Med. 1991;174:975–88.
45. Zubkov AY, Nanda A, Zhang JH. Signal transduction pathways in cerebral vasospasm. Pathophysiology 2003;9:47–61.
46. Macomson SD, Brophy CM, Miller AW, Harris VA, Shaver EG. Heat shock protein expression in cerebral vessels after subarachnoid hemorrhage. Neurosurgery 2002;51:204–11.
47. Wang X, Liu Y. Regulation of innate immune response by MAP kinase phosphatase-1. Cell Signal. 200719:1372–82.
48. Boutros T, Chevet E, Metrakos P. Mitogen-activated protein (MAP) kinase/MAP kinase phosphatase regulation: roles in cell growth, death, and cancer. Pharmacol Rev. 2008;60:261–310.
49. Keyse SM. Dual-specificity MAP kinase phosphatases (MKPs) and cancer. Cancer Metastasis Rev. 2008;27:253–61.

Association of Apolipoprotein E Polymorphisms with Cerebral Vasospasm After Spontaneous Subarachnoid Hemorrhage

Hai-tao Wu, Xiao-dong Zhang, Hai Su, Yong Jiang, Shuai Zhou, and Xiao-chuan Sun

Abstract Cerebral vasospasm (CVS) is the main complication of spontaneous subarachnoid hemorrhage (SAH), severely affecting clinical outcome of patients with SAH. Apolipoprotein E gene (APOE) is associated with prognosis of spontaneous subarachnoid hemorrhage (SAH), and APOEε4 allele is reported to be apt to CVS after SAH. The current study aimed to investigate the association of APOE polymorphisms with CVS after SAH. One hundred and eighty-five patients with spontaneous SAH were recruited in the study. APOE genotypes were determined by polymerase chain reaction-restriction fragment length polymorphism (PCR-RFLP). CVS was judged by Transcranial Doppler sonography (TCD) combined with patients' condition. χ^2-test and logistic regression analysis were done by SPSS (version 11.5). The distributions of APOE genotypes and alleles matched Hardy–Weinberg Law. In 185 patients, 21 of 32 (65.7%) patients with APOEε4 allele showed CVS, which was significantly different from those without APOE ε4 allele (56 of 153 patients, 36.6%, $P = 0.022$). However, neither the presence of ε2 nor ε3 was significantly different from those absent of it ($P > 0.05$). Logistic regression analysis demonstrated that ApoEε4 allele was a risk factor (OR = 2.842.95%CI1.072–6.124.$P = 0.019$) to predispose to CVS after adjusting for age, sex, hypertension or not, hyperlipemia or not, Fisher grade, and Hunt–Hess grade after SAH. Our finding suggests that the patients with APOEε4 allele predispose to CVS after spontaneous SAH.

Keywords Apolipoprotein E · Cerebral vasospasm · Polymorphisms · Spontaneous subarachnoid hemorrhage

Introduction

Apolipoprotein E (ape-protein, APOE-gene) is one of the most important apoproteins in human body, which is encoded by APOE. This polymorphic gene locates on chromosome 19q13.2, having four exons. The three human APOE alleles, APOEε2, APOEε3 and APOEε4, encode three isoforms apoE2, apoE3 and apoE4 respectively. Brain is the second largest organ for the synthesis of apoE, seconded only to liver. ApoE in brain is related to physiological and pathological changes of central nervous system (CNS). More and more studies show that, APOEε4 allele predispose to poor outcome of Alzheimer's diseases (AD) and traumatic brain injury (TBI) [2, 7]. Meanwhile, accumulating evidence indicates that APOEε4 is associated with poor outcome after spontaneous subarachnoid hemorrhage (SAH) [3]. One hundred and eighty-five Chinese Mainland patients with SAH were recruited to the current study, the correlation between APOE genotype and cerebral vasospasm (CVS) was analyzed, aimed to uncover the association of APOE polymorphisms and CVS after SAH.

H.-t. Wu, X.-d. Zhang, S. Zhou, and X.-c. Sun (✉)
Department of Neurosurgery, the First Affiliated Hospital of Chongqing Medical University, Chongqing, 400016, Prople's Republic of China
e-mail: sunxch1445@gmail.com

H. Su
Department of Neurosurgery, the Second People's Hospital of Chongqing, Chongqing 402160, People's Republic of China

Y. Jiang
Department of Neurosurgery, the Affiliated Hospital of Luzhou Medical College, Sichuan 646000, People's Republic of China

Materials and Methods

Patient Population

A total of 185 patients with SAH admitted to Department of Neurosurgery, the First Affiliated Hospitals of Chongqing Medical University (Chongqing, China) from Dec. 2007 to May 2009 were selected and studied prospectively. The following inclusion and exclusion criteria were used to determine eligibility for the study. Inclusion criteria (1) patients with spontaneous SAH, (2) SAH was certified by computer tomography (CT) or bloody cerebrospinal fluid (CSF), (3) clinical data were recorded completely. Exclusion criteria (1) having a suspicious history of traumatic brain injury (TBI), (2) brain hernia occurs or patients died within 3 days after SAH. This study was approved by the ethics committee of the Dept. of Medical Research. An informed consent was obtained from the patient himself/herself directly or their family members if the status of patients' consciousness restricted such procedure.

Judgement of CVS

All 185 patients undertook condition, especially CVS assessment, and accepted Transcranial Doppler sonography (TCD) examination. Refered to Ionita's research [6], clinical CVS was defined as the onset of new focal neurological deficit attributed to delayed ischemic injury, and TCD CVS was defined as anterior circulation peak mean velocity (PMV) > 160 cm/s, basilar artery (BA) PMV > 90 cm/s, and Lindegaard ratio (LR) > 6. Therefore, sufferers displayed symptomatic CVS or PMV ≥ 140 cm/s were deemed to present CVS, then asymptomatic patients with PMV < 140 cm/s could be ruled out.

APOE Genotyping

Venous blood was collected from patients on admission, and then frozen and stored for extraction of DNA by standard techniques. APOEε2, ε3, ε4 genotyping was completed using the method of polymerase chain reaction–restriction fragment length polymorphism (PCR–RFLP). Genomic DNA was amplified by PCR, using reaction conditions modified from those previously described [17]. A 250-bp fragment was amplified containing the coding regions. The PCR amplification was undertaken in a reaction volume of 50 μL (35 cycles of consisting 94°C for 30 s, 62°C for 30 s, and 72°C for 40 s). Primers were as follows: P1:5′-TAAGCTTGGCACGG- CTGTCCAAGGA-3′ (upstream) and P2: 5′-ACAGAATTCGCCCCGGCCTGGTA –CAC-3′(downstream). The PCR products were digested by *Hha*I and the fragments were separated by electrophoresis on 4% ethidium bromide-containing agarose gels for genotype determination. DNA fragments were visualized by ultraviolet illumination.

Statistical Analysis

Allele frequencies in SAH patients were estimated by counting the number of alleles and calculating the sample proportions. The SPSS software (version 11.5) was used. Univariate analysis was performed using the χ^2-test and the Fisher Exact test when necessary. In the multivariate analysis, logistic regression analysis was performed to control other related factors including age, sex, hyperlipemia or not, hypertension or not, Fisher grade, Hunt–Hess grade as well as APOE status and to test interactions between APOE genotypes and clinical status after SAH. Adjusted odds ratios (OR) and 95% confidence intervals (CI) were calculated from logistic regression model coefficients.

Results

The enrolled 185 consecutive patients (84 males and 101 females, with mean age of 54.89 years) with SAH in this study, whose general information (age, sex, hyperlipemia or not, hypertension or not), Fisher grade, Hunt–Hess grade and genotypes were available. Seventy-seven sufferers presented CVS post hospitalization. χ^2-test showed no statistical difference in clinical characteristics between the 77 patients and the other 108 cases without CVS (Table 1).

The distributions of APOE allele frequencies and genotypes of 185 patients were given in Table 2, Among 185 patients, 153 patients were APOEε4 (−) and 32 were APOEε4(+). Genotypic distribution was consistent with Hardy–Weinberg equilibrium ($P > 0.05$).

Table 1 Comparison of characteristics in 185 patients and patient condition

Items		CVS(−)	CVS(+)	P value
Age	<60	57	37	0.526
	≥60	51	40	
Sex	Male	49	35	0.991
	Female	59	42	
Hypertension	Yes	37	25	0.799
	No	71	52	
Hyperlipemia	Yes	35	29	0.549
	No	73	48	
Hunt–Hess grade	1–2	95	61	0.107
	3–5	13	16	
Fisher grade	1–2	75	40	0.016
	3–4	33	37	

Table 2 Distribution of APOE genotype

Genotype						Allele frequency		
ε2/2	ε2/3	ε2/4	ε3/3	ε3/4	ε4/4	ε2	ε3	ε4
0	26	7	127	23	2	8.9%	81.9%	9.2%

Table 3 Association of APOE ε2, ε3, ε4 status and CVS

Items	ε2 allele Carriers	Non-carriers	ε3 allele Carriers	Non-carriers	ε3 allele Carriers	Non-carriers
No-CVS	20	88	105	3	11	97
CVS	13	64	71	6	21	56
P	0.753		0.249		0.022	

Of 185 patients, 21 of 32 patients with APOEε4 (65.7%) showed CVS which was significantly different from those without APOEε4 (56 of 153 patients, 36.7%, $P = 0.022$). However, neither the presence of ε2 nor of ε3 was significantly different from those absent of it ($P > 0.05$) (Table 3). After the adjustment by binary logistic regression for general information (age, sex, hyperlipemia or not, hypertension or not), Fisher grade, and Hunt–Hess grade, only APOE ε4 was found to be a risk factor to predispose to CVS ($P = 0.010$, 95% CI 1.2057.116, OR = 2.713). And the further multiple logistic regression showed that APOEε4 was still a risk factor to predispose to CVS ($P = 0.019$, 95% CI 1.0726.124, OR = 2.842).

Discussion

SAH is a potentially disastrous disease. Though controversy has been existing [8], increasing evidence indicates the APOEε4 genotype as having a negative effect on neuropsychological outcomes following SAH [12]. In 2006, a Meta-analysis was used to 610 SAH sufferers [14], arriving at the conclusion that APOE may differentially affect outcome after SAH. Meanwhile, the author indicated that, large studies are needed to confirm or refute these findings. It has been known that, CVS is the common complication of SAH, and is one of the important reasons leading to death and disability of SAH victims. Moreover, CVS plays an important part in affecting the survival rate and the quality of life after SAH. To the best of our knowledge, few studies so far have been performed to investigate the association of APOE genotype with SAH induced CVS. A research [11] indicated that, the presence of an ε4 allele increases the risk of delayed ischemic neurologic deficit. Similar to most CVS related studies, the above research was carried out at least 6 months after the SAH. The current study aimed to explore relationship between APOE genotype and CVS in acute stage of SAH (≤ 14 days after SAH).

This study found that APOE polymorphism was related to the presence of CVS at acute phase of SAH. APOEε4 carriers showed significantly higher incidence of CVS than that of non-ε4 carriers ($P = 0.022$). Furthermore, uni- and multivariate logistic regression analysis also led to the conclusion that APOEε4 was likely to be a risk factor of CVS. As to each phenotype, incidence of CVS in genotype ε2/4 (4/7) was significantly higher than that in genotype ε2/3 (9/26), and ε3/4 (15/23) was higher than ε3/3 (47/127) as well. Unfortunately, the proportion of genotype ε4/4 is extremely low, which were only two cases in the current study. However, one of the two cases presented severe CVS, which further indicated the negative effect of ε4 allele. There was no statistical difference in Hunt–Hess grade between ε4 carriers and non-ε4 carriers (9/32 vs. 20/153, $P = 0.057$). Although the proportion of Fisher grade 34 in ε4 carriers (15/32) was higher than that in non-ε4 carriers (55/153), but this difference was out of significance ($P = 0.246$)

Since the pathological nature of CVS is very complex, the mechanisms by which APOEε4 carriers predisposing to CVS is not fully understood, and several supposed mechanisms are as follow (1) inflammation. It has been known that, inflammation plays an important part in post-haemorrhagic vasospasm [4, 16]. Meanwhile, Lynch [13] found that animals expressing the E4 allele had significantly greater systemic and brain elevations of the pro-inflammatory cytokines as compared with their APOEε2 and ε3 counterparts. Therefore, we suppose that ε4 carriers may be more likely to present CVS than non-ε4 carriers because of post-haemorrhagic inflammation. (2) Beta-amyloid induced vasoactivity. Paris [15] indicated that, soluble beta-amyloid (Abeta) exhibited vasoactive properties, being able to promote vasoconstriction, and apoE4 isoform synergistically enhanced the rate of vasoconstriction induced by Abeta. At the same time, Kay [9] found that, the decrease of Abeta concentration in CSF correlated significantly with that of apoE. supporting the concept that interactions between apoE and Abeta influence outcome after SAH. (3) Endothelin (ET) B receptor. ET-1 plays an important role in the pathogenesis of cerebral vasospasm. Hansen [5] observed a significantly increased expression of ET (B) receptor in the spasmodic cerebral vessels in a rats SAH model. Meanwhile, apoE4 isoform was in accord with ET-1 induced CVS [13]. (4) ApoE4 participated in regulating CVS by means of interacting with intracellular Ca(2+) [1]. The above mentioned factors and some unknown factors may act synergistically, and lead to CVS after SAH eventually.

Conclusion

With the increasing understanding of molecular mechanisms of CVS, neurologists have been able to predict the onset and development of the SAH induced severe complication, and to take proper measures to reduce the incidence of CVS, and to decrease neurological damage thus incurred. Nowadays, more and more scholars give high expectations to APOE genetic therapy to nerve injury after SAH. It has been confirmed that, transfecting of APOEε3 had a protective effect on nerve cells both in vivo and in vitro [10]. The results of this study not only help to predict the occurrence of CVS post SAH through APOE genotyping, but imply a new path of genetic therapy on CVS.

Conflict of interest statement We declare that we have no conflict of interest.

References

1. Alexander SA, Kerr ME, Balzer J, Horowitz M, Kassam A, Kim Y, et al. Cerebrospinal fluid apolipoprotein E, calcium and cerebral vasospasm after subarachnoid hemorrhage. Biol Res Nurs. 2008;10:102–12.
2. Fan J, Donkin J, Wellington C Greasing the wheels of Abeta clearance in Alzheimer's disease: the role of lipids and apolipoprotein E. Biofactors 2009;35:239–48.
3. Gallek MJ, Conley YP, Sherwood PR, Horowitz MB, Kassam A, Alexander SA. APOE genotype and functional outcome following aneurysmal subarachnoid hemorrhage. Biol Res Nurs. 2009;10: 205–212.
4. Hakan T, Berkman MZ, Ersoy T, Karatas I, San T, Arabk S Anti-inflammatory effect of meloxicam on experimental vasospasm in the rat femoral artery. J Clin Neurosci. 2008;15:55–59.
5. Hansen-Schwartz J, Hoel NL, Zbou M, Xu CB, Svendgaard NA, Edvinsson L. Subarachnoid hemorrhage enhances endothelin receptor expression and function in rat cerebral arteries. Neurosurgery 2003;52:1188–95.
6. Ionita CC, Graffagnino C, Alexander MJ, Zaidat OO. The value of CT angiography and traunscranial doppler sonography in triaging suspected cerebral vasospasm in SAH prior to endovascular therapy. Neurocrit Care. 2008;9:8–12.
7. Jiang Y, Sun X, Xia Y, Tang W, Cao Y, et al. Effect of APOE polymorphisms on early responses to traumatic brain injury. Neurosci Lett. 2006;408:155–8.
8. Juvela S, Siironen J, Lappalainen J. Apolipoprotein E genotype and outcome after aneurysmal subarachnoid hemorrhage. J Neurosurg. 2009;110:989–95.
9. Kay A, Petzold A, Kerr M, Keir G, Thompson E, Nicoll J. Temporal alterations in cerebrospinal fluid amyloid beta-protein and apolipoprotein E after subarachnoid hemorrhage. Stroke 2003;34:240–43.
10. Lahiri DK. Apolipoprotein E as a target for developing new therapeutics for Alzheimer's disease based on studies from protein, RNA, and regulatory region of the gene. Mol Neurosci. 2004;23:225–33.
11. Lanterna LA, Rigoldi M, Tredici G, Biroli F, Cesana C, Gaini SM, et al. APOE influences vasospasm and cognition of noncomatose patients with subarachnoid hemorrhage. Neurology 2005;64:1238–44.
12. Louko AM, Vilkki J, Niskakangas T ApoE genotype and cognition after subarachnoid hemorrhage: a longitudinal study. Acta Neurol Scand. 2006;114:315–19.
13. Lynch JR, Tang W, Wang H, Vitek MP, Bennett ER, Sullivan PM, et al. APOE genotype and an ApoE-mimetic peptide modify the systemic and central nervous system inflammatory response. J Biol Chem. 2003;278:48529–33.
14. Martínez-González NA, Sudlow CL. Effects of apolipoprotein E genotype on outcome after ischaemic stroke, intracerebral haemorrhage and subarachnoid haemorrhage. J Neurol Neurosrug Psychiatry. 2006;77:1329–35.
15. Paris D, Town T, Parker TA, Humphrey J, Mullan M. Isoform-specific vasoconstriction induced by apolipoprotein E and modulation of this effect Alzheimer's beta-amyloid peptide. Neurosci Lett. 1998;256:73–6.
16. Prunell GF. Svendgaard NA, Alkass K, Mathiesen T. Inflammation in the brain after experimental subarachnoid hemorrhage. Neurosurgery 2005;56:l082–92.
17. Wenham PR, Price WH, Blundell G. Apolipoprotein E genotyping by one-stage PCR. Lancet 1991;337:1158–59.

Impact of Subarachnoid Hemorrhage on Local and Global Calcium Signaling in Cerebral Artery Myocytes

Masayo Koide[1], Matthew A. Nystoriak[1], Joseph E. Brayden, and George C. Wellman

Abstract *Background*: Ca^{2+} signaling mechanisms are crucial for proper regulation of vascular smooth muscle contractility and vessel diameter. In cerebral artery myocytes, a rise in global cytosolic Ca^{2+} concentration ($[Ca^{2+}]_i$) causes contraction while an increase in local Ca^{2+} release events from the sarcoplasmic reticulum (Ca^{2+} sparks) leads to increased activity of large-conductance Ca^{2+}-activated (BK) K^+ channels, hyperpolarization and relaxation. Here, we examined the impact of SAH on Ca^{2+} spark activity and $[Ca^{2+}]_i$ in cerebral artery myocytes following SAH.
Methods: A rabbit double injection SAH model was used in this study. Five days after the initial intracisternal injection of whole blood, small diameter cerebral arteries were dissected from the brain for study. For simultaneous measurement of arterial wall $[Ca^{2+}]_i$ and diameter, vessels were cannulated and loaded with the ratiometric Ca^{2+} indicator fura-2. For measurement of Ca^{2+} sparks, individual myocytes were enzymatically isolated from cerebral arteries and loaded with the Ca^{2+} indicator fluo-4. Sparks were visualized using laser scanning confocal microscopy. *Results*: Arterial wall $[Ca^{2+}]_i$ was significantly elevated and greater levels of myogenic tone developed in arteries isolated from SAH animals compared with arteries isolated from healthy animals. The L-type voltage-dependent Ca^{2+} channel (VDCC) blocker nifedipine attenuated increases in $[Ca^{2+}]_i$ and tone in both groups suggesting increased VDCC activity following SAH. Membrane potential measurement using intracellular microelectrodes revealed significant depolarization of vascular smooth muscle following SAH. Further, myocytes from SAH animals exhibited significantly reduced Ca^{2+} spark frequency (50%). *Conclusions:* Our findings suggest decreased Ca^{2+} spark frequency leads to reduced BK channel activity in cerebral artery myocytes following SAH. This results in membrane potential depolarization, increased VDCC activity, elevated $[Ca^{2+}]_i$ and decreased vessel diameter. We propose this mechanism of enhanced cerebral artery myocyte contractility may contribute to decreased cerebral blood flow and development of neurological deficits in SAH patients.

Keywords Ca^{2+} channels · K^+ channels · Ca^{2+} sparks · Vascular smooth muscle · Vasospasm

Introduction

Intracellular Ca^{2+} is a ubiquitous second messenger, playing critical roles in a wide array of physiological processes including muscle contraction [1]. In the cerebral vasculature, average intracellular Ca^{2+} concentration or global cytosolic Ca^{2+} ($[Ca^{2+}]_i$) dictates smooth muscle contraction (and arterial diameter) via regulation of myosin light chain kinase activity [2]. Thus, an elevation in global cytosolic Ca^{2+} leads to enhanced vasoconstriction and potentially a decrease in cerebral blood flow [3]. Paradoxically, localized intracellular Ca^{2+} release events, termed Ca^{2+} sparks, promote a decrease in $[Ca^{2+}]_i$ and relaxation of cerebral artery myocytes [4, 5]. Ca^{2+} sparks are generated by the coordinated opening of ryanodine receptors (RyRs) located on the sarcoplasmic reticulum of smooth muscle cells and activate plasmamemmal large conductance Ca^{2+}-activated K^+ (BK) channels leading to membrane potential hyperpolarization, decreased activity of voltage-dependent Ca^{2+} channels (VDCCs), decreased $[Ca^{2+}]_i$, and vasodilation. Currently, the impact of subarachnoid hemorrhage on local and/or global Ca^{2+} signals in myocytes from small diameter cerebral arteries is unclear [6].

M. Koide, M.A. Nystoriak, J.E. Brayden, and G.C. Wellman (✉)
Department of Pharmacology, University of Vermont College of Medicine, Burlington, VT 05405-0068, USA
e-mail: george.wellman@uvm.edu

[1] M. Koide and M. Nystoriak contributed equally to this work.

Methods

SAH Model

A rabbit double-injection model of SAH was used in this study. Briefly, anesthetized New Zealand white rabbits (males, 3.0–3.5 kg) received an intracisternal injection of autologous arterial blood (2.5 ml) using a previously described surgical procedure [7, 8]. Forty-eight hours after the initial injection, the procedure was repeated with animals receiving a second injection of 2.5 ml of arterial blood. Five days after the initial surgery, rabbits were euthanized and posterior cerebral and cerebellar arteries (100–200 µm diameters) were dissected for in vitro studies. All protocols were conducted in accordance with the guidelines for the care and use of laboratory animals (NIH publication 85–23, 1985) and followed protocols approved by the Institutional Animal Use and Care Committee of the University of Vermont, USA.

Simultaneous Measurement of Global Cytosolic Ca^{2+} and Arterial Diameter

Intact cerebral arteries were cannulated on glass micropipettes mounted in a Living Systems Inc. (Burlington, VT) arteriograph chamber. Arteries were loaded, in the dark, with the ratiometric Ca^{2+} indicator fura-2-AM (5 µM) in a MOPS solution containing pluronic acid (0.05%) for 45 min at room temperature. The MOPS loading solution had the following composition (in mM): 145 NaCl, 5 KCl, 1 $MgSO_4$, 2.5 $CaCl_2$, 1 KH_2PO_4, 0.02 EDTA, 3 3-(N-morpholino) propanesulfonic acid (MOPS), 2 pyruvate, 5 glucose, 1% bovine serum albumin (pH 7.4). Arteries were then continuously superfused with aerated artificial cerebral spinal fluid (aCSF) at 37°C for the remainder of the experiment. The composition of the aCSF was (in mM): 125 NaCl, 3 KCl, 18 $NaHCO_3$, 1.25 NaH_2PO_4, 1 $MgCl_2$, 2 $CaCl_2$, 5 glucose aerated with 5% CO_2, 20% O_2, 75% N_2 (pH 7.35). Ratio images of the arterial wall were obtained from background corrected images of the 510 nm emission from arteries alternately excited at 340 and 380 nm using software developed by IonOptix Inc. (Milton, MA). Arterial wall $[Ca^{2+}]$ is calculated using the following equation [9]: $[Ca^{2+}] = K_d \times \beta \times (R - R_{min})/(R_{max} - R)$. An apparent K_d of 282 nM of fura-2 for Ca^{2+} was used [3]. Arterial constriction was expressed as a percent decrease from the maximal (fully dilated) diameter obtained at the end of each experiment in Ca^{2+}-free aCSF containing the vasodilators nifedipine (1 µM) and forskolin (1 µM). In some studies, intracellular microelectrodes were used to measure smooth muscle membrane potential in intact pressurized arteries, as described previously [10].

Measurement of Ca^{2+} Sparks in Isolated Cerebral Artery Myocytes

Individual smooth muscle cells were enzymatically isolated from posterior cerebral and cerebellar artery segments [11]. Isolated myocytes were then loaded with fluo-4-AM (10 µM) for 60 min (21°C) in a HEPES-buffered physiological saline solution (PSS) containing pluronic acid (0.05%). The HEPES-PSS had the following composition (in mM): 135 NaCl, 5.4 KCl, 1.8 $CaCl_2$, 1 $MgCl_2$, 10 HEPES, 10 glucose (pH 7.4 with NaOH). Myocyte images were acquired with a Noran Oz laser scanning confocal microscope [12]. Fluo-4 was excited using the 488 nm line of a krypton/argon laser and the light emitted by this dye (520 nm) was separated from the excitation light and collected. Images were acquired at a frequency of ≈60 Hz for a period of 20 s. Ca^{2+} sparks are detected and analyzed using custom software (written by Dr. Adrian Bonev, University of Vermont, using IDL 5.0.2; Research Systems Inc., Boulder, CO). Baseline fluorescence (F_o) was determined by averaging ten images without Ca^{2+} spark activity. Fractional fluorescence increases (F/F_o) are determined in areas (2.1 µm × 2.1 µm) where Ca^{2+} sparks were observed. Ca^{2+} sparks are defined as local fractional fluorescence increases greater than 1.3. All measurements were recorded at room temperature.

Results

Elevated Global Cytosolic Ca^{2+} and Enhanced Myogenic Tone in Small Diameter Cerebral Arteries Following SAH

The relationship between intravascular pressure, arterial Ca^{2+} and myogenic tone was examined in small diameter (150–200 µm) cerebral arteries isolated from healthy control and SAH model rabbits. Arterial wall Ca^{2+} and constriction increased as intravascular pressure was elevated within the range (60–100 mmHg) typically experienced by these arteries in vivo. Arteries from SAH animals exhibited significant elevations in both arterial wall Ca^{2+} and constriction compared to similar arteries from control animals (Fig. 1a). For example, at 100 mmHg, arterial wall Ca^{2+} was 26% higher in arteries isolated from SAH animals (231 ± 17 nM, n = 4) compared with arteries isolated from healthy (184 ± 12 nM, n = 4). The level of constriction (myogenic tone) at 100 mmHg was 1.5-fold higher in arteries isolated from SAH animals (39 ± 3% decrease in diameter, n = 4) compared with arteries isolated from

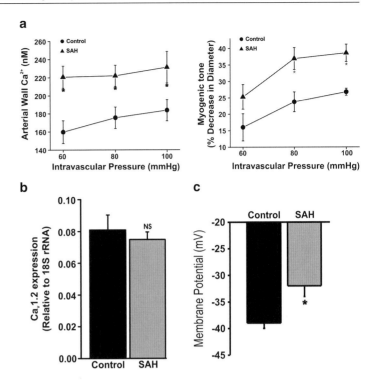

Fig. 1 Elevated global cytosolic Ca^{2+} following SAH: (**a**) Summary data from simultaneous measurement of arterial wall Ca^{2+} (using fura-2) and diameter. Arterial wall Ca^{2+} and tone were significantly increased at intravascular pressures between 60 and 100 mmHg in arteries isolated from SAH animals compared with controls. (**b**) Summary data using quantitative real-time PCR. Total RNA was collected from posterior cerebral arteries. $Ca_V1.2$ expression was not altered following SAH. NS: not statistically significant. (**c**) Summary data from membrane potential measurement using intracellular microelectrodes. Vascular smooth muscle membrane potential in arteries from SAH animals was significantly depolarized following SAH. * $P < 0.05$

healthy animals (27 ± 2% decrease in diameter, n = 4). In the presence of the L-type VDCC blocker nifedipine (1 μM), arterial Ca^{2+} was greatly reduced in arteries from both SAH (141 ± 15 nM) and control (118 ± 7 nM) rabbits. Nifedipine (1 μM) also reduced pressure-induced constrictions by 92 ± 1% and 93 ± 1% in arteries from SAH and control animals, respectively. These data suggest that increased VDCC activity underlies enhanced pressure-induced constriction observed in small diameter cerebral arteries from SAH animals.

Increased VDCC activity could reflect either increased L-type VDCC expression or enhanced VDCC activation due to smooth muscle membrane potential depolarization following SAH. Quantitative real-time PCR was used to assess L-type VDCC expression encoded by the gene $Ca_V1.2$ [13]. Using this approach, no significant difference in $Ca_V1.2$ mRNA levels was detected in cerebral artery homogenates from control and SAH animals (Fig. 1b). Next, we used intracellular microelectrodes to directly measure vascular smooth muscle membrane potential from intact pressurized cerebral arteries. At 80 mmHg, smooth muscle membrane potential was significantly depolarized by approximately 8 mV in arteries isolated from SAH animals compared with arteries from control animals (Fig. 1c). These findings suggest that membrane potential depolarization of vascular smooth muscle leads to increased VDCC activity, elevated global cytosolic Ca^{2+} and enhanced constriction of small diameter cerebral arteries following SAH.

Ca^{2+} Spark Frequency is Decreased in Cerebral Artery Myocytes from SAH Animals

A decrease in Ca^{2+} spark frequency and associated BK activity promotes membrane potential depolarization, elevated global cytosolic Ca^{2+}, and vasoconstriction [4, 5]. To explore whether decreased Ca^{2+} spark frequency may contribute to enhanced cerebral artery constriction, Ca^{2+} sparks were measured in isolated cerebral artery myocytes using laser scanning confocal microscopy and the Ca^{2+} indicator dye fluo-4. As illustrated in Fig. 2, Ca^{2+} sparks were observed in cerebral artery myocytes obtained from both control and SAH animals. However, Ca^{2+} spark frequency was markedly decreased (by approximately 50%) in myocytes isolated from SAH animals. Consistent with the observed decrease in Ca^{2+} spark frequency, the frequency of transient BK currents detected using patch clamp electrophysiology was also reduced by approximately 50% in freshly isolated cerebral artery myocytes from SAH animals (Koide and Wellman, unpublished observations). These data suggest that a decrease in the frequency of Ca^{2+} sparks and their associated BK channel currents may contribute to

Fig. 2 Decreased Ca^{2+} spark frequency in cerebral myocytes from SAH animals: Imaging of Ca^{2+} sparks in cerebral artery myocytes loaded with the fluorescent Ca^{2+} indicator fluo-4. Fluorescent images were detected using laser scanning confocal microscopy with Ca^{2+} sparks defined as a fractional fluorescent increase of greater than 30% within 2.1 μm by 2.1 μm analysis areas. Large size images represent an average of 30 images in *gray scale* without Ca^{2+} spark activity. *White crosses* depict where individual Ca^{2+} sparks occurred during the 20 s recordings. *Scale bars* represent 10 μm. Smaller images illustrate the time course of Ca^{2+} sparks in control and SAH myocytes. Images were obtained every 19 ms

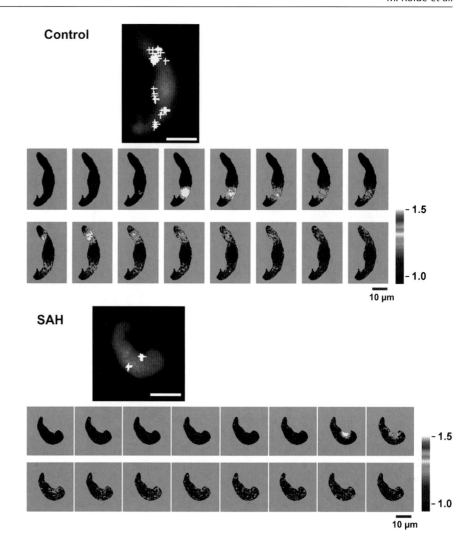

enhanced constriction of small diameter cerebral arteries following SAH.

Discussion

Aneurysmal SAH is associated with high rates of morbidity and mortality [14]. It has been a long-held belief that delayed and sustained large diameter (conduit) cerebral artery vasospasm ("angiographic vasospasm") is a major contributor to SAH-induced death and disability. However, there is a growing appreciation that a host of other factors are also likely involved in the pathological consequences associated with cerebral aneurysm rupture [15, 16]. Here, we provide evidence that SAH enhances the dynamic constriction of small diameter pial arteries in response to physiological increases in intravascular pressure, an effect that could have a pronounced influence to decrease cerebral blood flow. Our findings indicate that this augmented constriction is associated with enhanced smooth muscle contraction due to membrane potential depolarization, enhanced voltage-dependent Ca^{2+} channel activity and elevated global cytosolic calcium. Further, our recent findings suggest a decrease in the frequency of Ca^{2+} sparks and associated BK channel activity may contribute to enhanced cerebral artery constriction and elevated global cytosolic Ca^{2+} (Fig. 3).

The cerebral circulation maintains a constant level of blood flow to the brain despite physiological fluctuations in cerebral perfusion pressure [17]. To achieve stable cerebral blood flow in the face of changes in blood pressure, cerebral arteries must constrict in response to increased intravascular pressure and dilate when intravascular pressure is reduced. In pial arteries from healthy animals, physiological increases in intravascular pressure lead to smooth muscle membrane potential depolarization, an increase in the activity of L-type Ca$_V$1.2 channels (encoded by the gene CACNA1C), and increased global cytosolic Ca^{2+} [3, 13]. The open-state probability of Ca$_V$1.2 is steeply voltage-dependent [18]; thus, small changes in membrane potential can have a

Fig. 3 Summary cartoon: In control cerebral artery myocytes, local Ca^{2+} release events from the sarcoplasmic reticulum (Ca^{2+} sparks) activate large conductance Ca^{2+}-activated (BK) K^+ channels, causing membrane potential hyperpolarization, decreased voltage-dependent Ca^{2+} channel (VDCC) activity and decreased global cytosolic Ca^{2+}. Following SAH, the frequency of Ca^{2+} sparks and therefore BK channel activity is decreased, promoting membrane potential depolarization, increased VDCC activity and increased global cytosolic Ca^{2+} levels

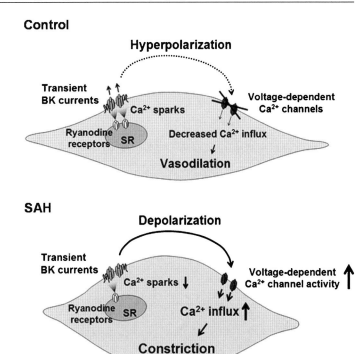

profound impact on smooth muscle Ca^{2+}. Our present results suggest membrane potential depolarization and enhanced L-type VDCC activity in small diameter arteries is likely to contribute to SAH-induced impairment in the autoregulation of cerebral blood flow reported by others [19, 20]. Our evidence also suggests enhanced activity of L-type VDCCs play a large part in the SAH-induced elevation in global cytosolic Ca^{2+}. However, in the presence of the L-type VDCC blocker nifedipine, global Ca^{2+} remained elevated (by approximately 20%) in arteries from SAH animals. This nifedipine-resistant increase in global Ca^{2+} in cerebral arteries from SAH animals may reflect the emergence of R-type VDCC channels [8], or the possible upregulation of additional Ca^{2+} entry pathways.

Our present findings suggest decreased Ca^{2+} spark and associated BK channel activity contribute to SAH-induced membrane potential depolarization and enhanced VDCC activity in cerebral artery myocytes. Harder and colleagues [21] were the first to report that the membrane potential of cerebral artery myocytes is depolarized following SAH and a number of subsequent studies have provided further evidence for decreased voltage-dependent K^+ (K_V) channel activity in pial arteries following SAH [6, 22–26]. Interestingly, BK channel activity and expression have been reported to be unchanged in basilar artery myocytes obtained from a canine SAH model [27]. Our current work demonstrates that decreased BK channel activity following SAH results from a decrease in local Ca^{2+} signaling from the SR to the plasma membrane (i.e. decreased Ca^{2+} spark activity), rather than a direct effect on BK channel properties or expression.

Conclusion

In this study, we examined global and local Ca^{2+} signaling in cerebral artery myocytes following SAH. As for global Ca^{2+}, we observed a significant increase in averaged cytosolic Ca^{2+} and constriction in cerebral arteries from SAH animals at physiological intravascular pressures. Regarding local Ca^{2+} signaling, we report a decrease in the frequency of Ca^{2+} sparks and associated transient outward BK currents, which likely contribute to membrane potential depolarization, increased VDCC activity and enhanced cerebral constriction artery following SAH. These data suggest that increased global Ca^{2+} and impaired local Ca^{2+} signaling may contribute to decreased cerebral blood flow and the development of neurological deficits frequently observed following aneurysmal SAH.

Acknowledgements This work was supported by the Totman Medical Research Trust Fund, the Peter Martin Brain Aneurysm Endowment, the NIH (NIHLBI, R01 HL078983 and NCRR, P20 RR16435) and the American Heart Association (0725837T, 0815736D). The authors wish to thank to Ms. Sheila Russell for her assistance with this study. The authors would also like to acknowledge the University of Vermont Neuroscience COBRE molecular biology and imaging core facilities.

Conflict of interest statement We declare that we have no conflict of interest.

References

1. Clapham DE. Calcium signaling. Cell 1995;80:259–68.
2. Hai CM, Murphy RA. Ca^{2+}, crossbridge phosphorylation, and contraction. Annu Rev Physiol. 1989;51:285–98.
3. Knot HJ, Nelson MT. Regulation of arterial diameter and wall $[Ca^{2+}]$ in cerebral arteries of rat by membrane potential and intravascular pressure. J Physiol. 1998;508(Pt 1):199–209.
4. Nelson MT, Cheng H, Rubart M, Santana LF, Bonev AD, Knot HJ, et al. Relaxation of arterial smooth muscle by calcium sparks. Science 1995;270:633–37.
5. Wellman GC, Nelson MT Signaling between SR and plasmalemma in smooth muscle: sparks and the activation of Ca^{2+}-senstive ion channels. Cell Calcium. 2003;34:211–29.
6. Wellman GC Ion channels and calcium signaling in cerebral arteries following subarachnoid hemorrhage. Neurol Res. 2006;28:690–702.
7. Ishiguro M, Puryear CB, Bisson E, Saundry CM, Nathan DJ, Russell SR, et al. Enhanced myogenic tone in cerebral arteries from a rabbit model of subarachnoid hemorrhage. Am J Physiol Heart Circ Physiol. 2002;283:H2217–225.
8. Ishiguro M, Wellman TL, Honda A, Russell SR, Tranmer BI, Wellman GC. Emergence of a R-type Ca^{2+} channel (CaV 2.3) contributes to cerebral artery constriction after subarachnoid hemorrhage. Circ Res. 2005;96:419–26.
9. Grynkiewicz G, Poenie M, Tsien RY. A new generation of Ca^{2+} indicators with greatly improved fluorescence properties. J Biol Chem. 1985;260:3440–50.
10. Wellman GC, Bonev AD, Nelson MT, Brayden JE. Gender differences in coronary artery diameter involve estrogen, nitric oxide, and Ca^{2+}-dependent K^+ channels. Circ Res. 1996;79:1024–30.
11. Wellman GC, Nathan DJ, Saundry CM, Perez G, Bonev AD, Penar PL, Tranmer BI, Nelson MT. Ca^{2+} sparks and their function in human cerebral arteries. Stroke 2002;33:802–08.
12. Perez GJ, Bonev AD, Patlak JB, Nelson MT. Functional coupling of ryanodine receptors to KCa channels in smooth muscle cells from rat cerebral arteries. J Gen Physiol. 1999;113:229–38.
13. Nystoriak MA, Murakami K, Penar PL, Wellman GC. Ca(v)1.2 splice variant with exon 9* is critical for regulation of cerebral artery diameter. Am J Physiol Heart Circ Physiol. 2009;297: H1820–28.
14. Bederson JB, Connolly ES, Jr., Batjer HH, Dacey RG, Dion JE, Diringer MN, et al. Guidelines for the management of aneurysmal subarachnoid hemorrhage: a statement for healthcare professionals from a special writing group of the Stroke Council, American Heart Association. Stroke 2009;40:994–1025.
15. Hansen-Schwartz J, Vajkoczy P, Macdonald RL, Pluta RM, Zhang JH. Cerebral vasospasm: looking beyond vasoconstriction. Trends Pharmacol Sci. 2007;28:252–56.
16. Pluta RM, Hansen-Schwartz J, Dreier J, Vajkoczy P, Macdonald RL, Nishizawa S, et al. Cerebral vasospasm following subarachnoid hemorrhage: time for a new world of thought. Neurol Res. 2009;31:151–8.
17. Lee KR, Hoff JT. Intracranial pressure. In: Youmans JR, editor. Neurological Surgery. Philadelphia, PA: W. B. Saunders Co.; 1996. p. 491–518.
18. Nelson MT, Patlak JB, Worley JF, Standen NB. Calcium channels, potassium channels, and voltage dependence of arterial smooth muscle tone. Am J Physiol. 1990;259:C3–18.
19. Ohkuma H, Ogane K, Tanaka M, Suzuki S. Assessment of cerebral microcirculatory changes during cerebral vasospasm by analyzing cerebral circulation time on DSA images. Acta Neurochir Suppl. 2001;77:127–30.
20. Takeuchi H, Handa Y, Kobayashi H, Kawano H, Hayashi M. Impairment of cerebral autoregulation during the development of chronic cerebral vasospasm after subarachnoid hemorrhage in primates. Neurosurgery 1991;28:41–8.
21. Harder DR, Dernbach P, Waters A. Possible cellular mechanism for cerebral vasospasm after experimental subarachnoid hemorrhage in the dog. J Clin Invest. 1987;80:875–80.
22. Ishiguro M, Morielli AD, Zvarova K, Tranmer BI, Penar PL, Wellman GC Oxyhemoglobin-induced suppression of voltage-dependent K^+ channels in cerebral arteries by enhanced tyrosine kinase activity. Circ Res. 2006;99:1252–60.
23. Jahromi BS, Aihara Y, Ai J, Zhang ZD, Nikitina E, Macdonald RL. Voltage-gated K^+ channel dysfunction in myocytes from a dog model of subarachnoid hemorrhage. J Cereb Blood Flow Metab. 2008;28:797–811.
24. Koide M, Penar PL, Tranmer BI, Wellman GC. Heparin-binding EGF-like growth factor mediates oxyhemoglobin-induced suppression of voltage-dependent potassium channels in rabbit cerebral artery myocytes. Am J Physiol Heart Circ Physiol. 2007;293: H1750–59.
25. Quan L, Sobey CG. Selective effects of subarachnoid hemorrhage on cerebral vascular responses to 4-aminopyridine in rats. Stroke 2000;31:2460–65.
26. Sobey CG, Faraci FM. Subarachnoid haemorrhage: what happens to the cerebral arteries? Clin Exp Pharmacol Physiol. 1998;25: 867–76.
27. Jahromi BS, Aihara Y, Ai J, Zhang ZD, Weyer G, Nikitina E, et al. Preserved BK channel function in vasospastic myocytes from a dog model of subarachnoid hemorrhage. J Vasc Res. 2008;45:402–15.

Enhanced Angiogenesis and Astrocyte Activation by Ecdysterone Treatment in a Focal Cerebral Ischemia Rat Model[1]

Chunxia Luo, Bin Yi, Wenhui Fan, Kangning Chen, Li Gui, Zhi Chen, Lusi Li, Hua Feng, and Luxiang Chi

Abstract *Background and Purpose*: We reported previously that ecdysterone (EDS) improves neurologic function after experimental stroke. However, the underlying mechanism remained unclear. The present study was conducted to test whether ecdysterone improves neurologic function by enhancing astrocyte activation and angiogenesis after focal cerebral ischemia in rats.

Methods: Focal cerebral ischemia model was conducted by middle cerebral artery occlusion (MCAO). EDS was intraperitoneally injected at 20 mg kg^1 daily for 7 days after MCAO. Neurologic recovery was assessed using the neurologic severity scores. Microvessel density and GFAP expression were detected with immunostaining and analyzed quantitatively with image system.

Results: Treatment with EDS significantly improved functional recovery, along with increases in density of cerebral microvessels and astrocyte activation. Microvessel density was significantly higher in EDS treated group than in ischemia control group at all time points, and reached a peak on day 14. EDS treated group had substantial increment in GFAP immunoreactive cells, darker staining color, more and longer nerve processes, higher GFAP expression and area of immunoreactive cells at each time point.

Conclusion: Our data suggest that EDS treatment enhanced angiogenesis and astrocyte activation which could contribute to functional recovery.

Keywords Angiogenesis · Astrocyte activation · Ecdysterone · Focal cerebral ischemia

Introduction

Ecdysterone (EDS) is a kind of natural active steroid in insect ecdysis, and is also a bioactive component of radix achyranthis, a traditional herbal medicine substance in China [1]. Our previous study has found that [2] EDS has protective effect against secondary neurological injury caused by focal cerebral ischemia, while the underlying mechanism has not been identified. Angiogenesis and astrocyte activation are important repair responses to ischemia injury. We aimed to identify the molecule mechanism for EDS-mediated nerve protection, especially of EDS on astrocyte activation and angiogenesis, in a middle cerebral artery occlusion rat model.

Materials and Methods

Materials

SD rats were provided from the Animal Center of Third Military Medical University, with each weighting 250 ± 30 g. Rabbit anti-rat GFAP polyclonal antibody, rabbit anti-human factor-VIII polyclonal antibody and S-P immunohistochemical staining reagents were provided by Beijing Zhongshan Golden Bridge Biotechnology Co., Ltd. Ecdysterone (99.99% purity) was provided by Kunming Institute of Botany, Chinese Academy of Sciences.

C. Luo, Z. Chen, and H. Feng (✉)
Department of Neurosurgery, Southwest Hospital, Third Military Medical University, Gaotanyan 30, Chongqing 400038, People's Republic of China
e-mail: fenghua8888@yahoo.com.cn

B. Yi
Department of Anesthesiology, Southwest Hospital, Third Military Medical University, Gaotanyan 30, Chongqing 400038, People's Republic of China

W. Fan, K. Chen, L. Gui, L.Li, and L. Chi (✉)
Department of Neurology, Southwest Hospital, Third Military Medical University, Gaotanyan 30, Chongqing 400038, People's Republic of China
e-mail: chi68754271@126.com

[1] Chunxia Luo and Bin Yi contributed equally to this study.

Grouping and Drug Administration

Rats were randomly divided to sham-operated group, ischemia control group and EDS treated group. Middle cerebral artery occlusion (MCAO) was used to study focal cerebral ischemia. Rats in T group (EDS treated group) were intraperitoneally injected EDS 20 mg kg^{-1}·daily for 7 days starting at 24 h after MCAO., while rats in I group (Ischemia control group) were intraperitoneally injected vehicle, with the dose, time and frequency same to group T.

Neurological Scores

Neurological Scores were measured using the neurologic severity scores (NSSs) at 1, 7, 14, and 21 days after MCAO, as previously described [2].

Immunohistostaining and Image Analysis

Five sections of each rat were randomly selected, and their GFAP expression in peripheral tissues of cerebral infarct was examined using S-P method in accordance with the manufacturer's instructions. Rabbit anti-rat GFAP polyclonal antibody was used as primary antibody. The sections were stained with 1:100 DAB regnant, cleared and dehydrated in dimethyl benzene, and mounted in neutral resin. The cell whose cytoplasm is stained into brown is considered positive. Staining results were processed with Leica-MD20 Image Analysis System. PBS was used as negative control in replace of antibody, and known positive section was used as positive control.

Microvessel Density Detection

Microvessel density (MVD) of peripheral tissue of cerebral ischemia was detected by immunohistochemical staining with factor-VIII polyclonal antibody. Positive products of factor –VIII polyclonal antibody are brownish yellow grains located in vascular endothelial cell membrane and cytoplasm. Clearly stained and dense microvessel area was selected with 100× visual field under light microscope, and then counted under 400× visual field. Three non-overlapping visual fields of each section were selected for microvessel counting, and the mean of the three fields was calculated and considered as MVD.

Statistical Analysis

All data were expressed as mean ± SD. Statistical differences among groups were compared by one- way ANOVA followed by Tukey multiple comparison post hoc analysis. Probability value of $P < 0.05$ was considered statistically significant.

Results

EDS Treatment Improved Neurological Recovery

NSS results indicated that there was a significant difference between ischemia control group and EDS treated group t at 14 and 21 days compared with the ischemia control group ($P < 0.05$, see Fig 1).

EDS Treatment Increased the Microvessel Density

For ischemia control group, MVD increased, reached a peak 7 days and slightly decreased 21 days after MCAO. For EDS treated group, angiogenesis became obvious 7 days, reached a peak 14 days, and still remained at a higher level at 21 days after MCAO. MVD of treated group was significantly higher than that of ischemia control group at each time point ($P < 0.05$, see Fig. 2).

EDS Treatment Enhanced Astrocyte Activation

Seven days after MCAO, GFAP immunoreactive cells began to increase, dark staining, slightly thicker and longer processes, indicating slightly activation; 14 days after MCAO, GFAP immunoreactive cells around the cerebral infarct reached a peak, with substantially increased cell size and more and longer processes, showing the morphology of activated astrocytes; 21 days after the ischemia, GFAP immunoreactive cells still remained a large population, slightly less than the population on day 14. Compared to ischemia control group, GFAP immunoreactive cells of EDS treated group had more obvious increase, darker staining and more and longer processes (see Fig. 3). The area of GFAP immunoreactive cells of treated group were compared with

Fig. 1 Neurological evaluation after MCAO in 0, 1, 7, 14 and 21 days. There was a significant difference between ischemia control group and EDS treated group t at 14 and 21 days. n = 6 in each group. *:$P < 0.05$

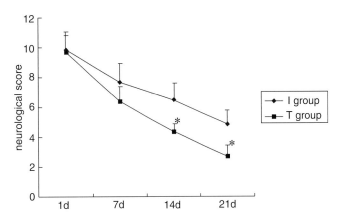

Fig. 2 FVIII-R Ag immunohistochemical staining positive vessels around the infarction in 7, 14 and 21 days after MCAO. The sections were immunostained with antibodies against FVIII-R Ag to show microvessel at day 7. (A represents ischemia control group; B represents EDS treated group). Temporal profiles of the density of microvessels (C). n = 6 in each group. Compared with the sham group: #:$P < 0.05$; compared with the ischemia control group; *:$P < 0.05$

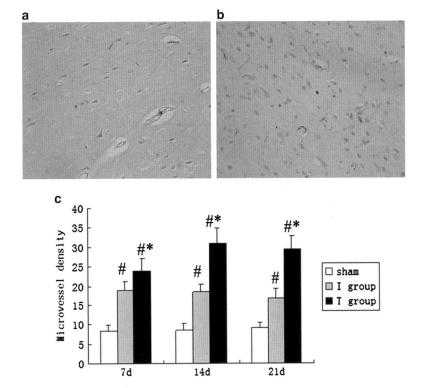

those of ischemia control group, and the difference on each time point was significant (P < 0.05).

Conclusion

We have observed that ecdysterone could alleviate neurological function deficits in the rat MCAO model. Angiogenesis results in the restoration of cerebral blood flow in the ischemia penumbra, which contributes to the long-term functional recovery after stroke. Local blood flow was dramatically dropped after MCAO, and partially restored gradually in up to 21 days or longer [3, 4]. EDS has been reported to upregulate VEGF expression of endothelial cell [5], and can also promote proliferation of cerebral vascular endothelial cells, smooth muscle cells and fibroblasts [6, 7]. In the present study. we have revealed that treatment with EDS after MCAO significantly increased the quantity of factor –VIII positive vessels, indicating that EDS enhanced angiogenesis.

Astrocytes are the most important nerve cells second only to neurons for central nervous system, they account for 40% cells of human central nervous system. They support, protect,

Fig. 3 Activated astrocytes around the infarction in 7, 14 and 21days after MCAO. The sections were immunostained with antibodies against GFAP to show astrocyte at day 7. (A represents ischemia control group; B represents EDS treated group). Temporal profiles of the area of immunoreactive cells for GFAP(C). n = 6 in each group. Compared with the sham group: #:$P < 0.05$; compared with the ischemia control group; #:$P < 0.05$

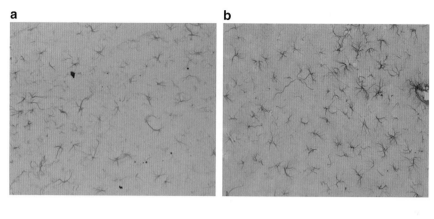

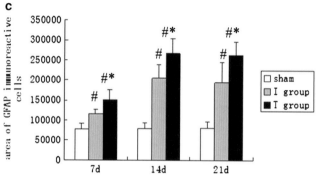

nourish and repair neurons. In addition, astrocyte processes closely surround and support capillary endothelial cells which form blood-brain barrier, they can stabilize new vessels, prevent them from breaking and recessing, and play an important role in maintaining normal structures and functions of capillary [8, 9]. GFAP is used a specific marker of astrocytes. We used GFAP immunohistochemical staining in this study, and observed the changes of astrocytes. It was found in this study that activated astrocytes increased after the ischemia. This finding is similar to what other study has observed [10]. Compared to ischemia control group, GFAP immunoreactive cells of EDS treated group had more obvious increase, darker staining color and more and longer processes at each time point. This indicates that EDS can promote astrocyte activation after ischemia. EDS [11] and VEGF [12] can promote cultured astrocyte proliferation in vitro and also secrete neurotrophic substances which can promote nerve cell survival, axonal regeneration and synapse molding Activated astrocytes after ischemia can stabilize cerebral environment by phagocytizing harmful neurotransmitters [13]; Other studies have also found that astrocytes can provide scaffolding for the exact migration of neurons and their growth cones, guide them to have accurate location, and are also involved in neuron proliferation [14, 15]. Our experiment finds that EDS can promote astrocyte activation after cerebral ischemia; this might benefit injury repair and neurogenesis, and may further promote function recovery.

It is concluded from our study that EDS treatment enhanced angiogenesis and astrocyte activation which could contribute to neurological function recovery.

Acknowledgements This research job is supported by Grant No.30500662, 30800354 from National Science Foundation of China (NSFC) and the Chinese Traditional Medicine Research Project of the "Eleventh Five-Year Plan" of PLA (2006181002).

Conflict of interest statement   We declare that we have no conflict of interest.

References

1. Li J, Qi H, Qi LW, Yi L, Li P. Stimultaneous determination of main phytoecdysones and triterpenoids in Radix Achyranthis Bidentatae by high-performance liquid chromatography with diode array-evaporative light scattering detectors and mass spectrometry. Anal Chim Acta. 2007;596(2):264–72.
2. Luo CX, Zhang YQ, Chi L, Li L, Chen KN. Protective effect and mechanism of ecdysterone on injury of focal cerebral infarct in rats. Med J Nat Def South Chin. 2009;19(2):176–8.
3. Li Y, Lu Z, Keogh CL, Yu SP, Wei L. Erythropoietin-induced neurovascular protection, angiogenesis, and cerebral blood flow restoration after focal ischemia in mice. J Cereb Blood Flow Metab. 2007;27:1043–54.
4. Hoang S, Liauw J, Choi M, Choi M, Guzman RG, Steinberg GK. Netrin-4 enhances angiogenesis and neurologic outcome after cerebral ischemia. J Cereb Blood Flow Metab. 2009;29(2):385–97.

5. Jin J, Huang L, Xiang CQ, Li H, Wu X, Geng JM. Effcets of ecdysterone on collateral formation and expression of VEGF in rat AMI. Chin Pharmac Bul. 2000;16(4):459–61.
6. Chen Z, Zhu G, Zhang JH, Liu Z, Tang WH, Feng H. Ecdysterone-sensitive smooth muscle cell proliferation stimulated by conditioned medium of endothelial cells cultured with bloody cerebrospinal fluid. Acta Neurochir Suppl. 2008;104:183–188.
7. Tang WH, Chen Z, Liu Z, Zhang JH, Xi G, Feng H. The effect of Ecdysterone on cerebral vasospasm following Experimental Subarachnoid Hemorrhage in vitro and in vivo. Neurol Res. 2008;30(6):571–80.
8. Nedergaard M, Dirnagl U. Role of glial cells in cerebral ischemia. Glia 2005;50:281–6.
9. Koehler RC, Gebremedhin D, Harder DR. Role of astrocytes in cerebrovascular regulation. J Appl Physiol. 2006;100(1):307–17.
10. Panickar KS, Norenberg MD. Astrocytes in cerebral ischemic injury: morphological and general considerations. Glia 2005;50:287–98.
11. Kirschenbaum SR, Higgins MR, Tveten M, Tolbert LP. 20-Hydroxyecdysone stimulates proliferation of glial cells in the developing brain of the moth Manduca sexta. J Neurobiol. 1995;28(2):234–47.
12. Krun JM, Mani N, Rosenstein JM. Angiogenic and astroglial responses to vascular endothelial growth factor administration in adult rat brain. Neuroscience 2002;110:589–604.
13. Haydon PG, Carmignoto G. Astrocyte control of synaptic transmission and neurovascular coupling. Physiol Rev. 2006;86(3):1009–31.
14. Mahesh VB, Dhandapani KM, Brann DW. Role of astrocytes in reproduction and neuroprotection. Mol Cell Endocrinol. 2006;246:1–9.
15. Lathia JD, Chigurupati S, Thundyil J, Selvaraj PK, Mughal MR, Woodruff TM, et al. Pivotal role for beta-1 integrin in neurovascular remodeling after ischemic stroke. Exp Neurol. 2010;221(1):107–114.

Bilirubin Oxidation Products Seen Post Subarachnoid Hemorrhage Have Greater Effects on Aged Rat Brain Compared to Young

Joseph F. Clark, Amanda Harm, Ashlie Saffire, Susan J. Biehle, Aigang Lu, and Gail J. Pyne-Geithman

Abstract *Introduction*: We have previously shown that novel oxidation products of Bilirubin, called Bilirubin oxidation products (BOXes), are found in humans and animal models post subarachnoid hemorrhage. We have also proposed that BOXes may play a role in the pathogenesis and clinical complications post SAH. In this study we report on the direct toxicity effects of BOXes on rat brain.

Methods: Identical volumes of either vehicle (normal saline) or BOXes (30 µl of a 20 µM solution) were applied above the dura through a cranial window of young (approximately 7–13 weeks) and aged (approximately 12–18 months) adult male Sprague Dawley rats (Charles River, Wilmington, MA, USA). To determine the extent of BOX-mediated injury, histology and immunocytochemistry were performed at 1, 2, 4, and 7 days post-surgical application of BOXes. We assessed the area of stress gene induction of HSP25/27 and HSP32. Immunohistochemistry was performed using standard avidin-biotin techniques. A monoclonal antibody to HSP25/27 (StressGen, Victoria, British Columbia, Canada), a monoclonal antibody to HSP32/HO-1 (StressGen), and a polyclonal HSP 32/HO-1 antibody were used for the immunocytochemistry.

Results: A single dose of BOXes produced substantial increases in HSP25 and HO-1 in the aged rats at all early time points (≤ 4 days). After 7 days all groups were not significantly different than saline control. Young rats were resistant to BOXes effects compared to saline control with trends towards increased stress gene expression caused by BOXes that did not reach statistical significance.

Conclusion: We conclude from these studies that BOXes have direct effects on stress gene expression of the cortex post single dose application and that this can be seen for several days with apparent resolution at about 7 days. If BOXes are produced at similar levels in patients, the latency and duration of some SAH complications are consistent with these results.

Keywords: Aging · Bilirubin · BOXes · SAH

Introduction

Subarachnoid Hemorrhage (SAH) caused by a ruptured aneurysm occurs in approximately 25 of every 100,000 people per year. Of those that survive the initial bleed, about half develop the devastating and often lethal complication of cerebral vasospasm (CV) [1, 7, 20]. With nearly 30,000 cases of aneurysmal SAH each year in the US [14], that means that nearly 11,000 people in the US suffer from this highly deadly complication every year. This condition can be defined as a pathological constriction of the blood vessels in the brain, with a concomitant inability to relax [17]. The ischemia and infarction that occurs following cerebral vasospasm can be attributed to the pathological vasoconstriction of these cerebral vessels [5, 6, 10, 21].

Blood products have been implicated in the pathogenesis of cerebral vasospasm. Extracts of cerebral spinal fluid from SAH (CSF$_{SAH}$) patients with vasospasm have been reported to be vasoactive, and molecules contained within the CSF$_{SAH}$ have been proposed to be the cause of cerebral vasospasm [2, 3, 6, 8, 13, 15, 16, 21, 22]. We have recently reported on the *in vivo* vasospasm of blood vessels caused by breakdown products of bilirubin [4]. These Bilirubin Oxidation products (BOXes) have been found to be present in the CSF of vasospastic patients (CSF$_V$), and the time

J.F. Clark, A. Harm, A. Saffire, S.J. Biehle and A. Lu
Department of Neurology, University of Cincinnati, PO Box 670536, Cincinnati, OH 45267-0536, USA

G.J. Pyne-Geithman (✉)
Director, Mayfield Neurovascular Research, Department of Neurosurgery, University of Cincinnati, 231 Albert Sabin Way, 4301 MSB, Cincinnati, OH 45267-0517, USA
e-mail: pynegj@ucmail.uc.edu

course of their production is consistent with the time course of CV development [4, 8].

There is extensive study of the oxidations (including per-oxidations) of unsaturated lipids and proteins in biological systems, including the resultant compounds produced. The oxidation of (un-conjugated) bilirubin has largely focused on the degradation of bilirubin between the pyrroles, with little discussion concerning putative biological activity of the products of bilirubin oxidation. We recently reported on a new family of bilirubin oxidation products (BOXes) found in CSF following subarachnoid hemorrhage (SAH) that may be involved in cerebral vasospasm. BOXes are photolabile and are vasoactive *in vivo* and *in vitro*.

There is a growing body of literature suggesting that BOXes may play a role in the complications and pathogenesis seen post SAH. However many of the previous reports on BOXes in vivo focused on the vascular effects without a detailed examination of the effects on the brain. Further previous studies used only young animals when SAH affects people of all ages. Therefore in this paper, we set out to assess the effects of a single application of BOXes on rat brains over several age groups and the time course where those effects were observed. We report intense and sustained effects of BOXes on stress gene expression and that this effect is exacerbated in aged rats.

Methods

Animals

Male Sprague Dawley rats (Charles River, Wilmington, MA, USA) were used. The young group weighed 200–400 g (approximately 7–13 weeks). The aged group weighed 700+ grams (approximately 12–18 months). All surgical procedures were performed according to the National Institutes of Health Guide for the Care and Use of Laboratory Animals, and were approved by the University of Cincinnati Animal Care and Use Committee.

BOXes Preparation

Peroxidation of bilirubin was used to produce BOXes as described previously [8]. We have chosen to use the combination of the BOXes (BOX A, BOX B, and methyl-vinyl-maleimide) as produced by peroxidation of bilirubin because we believe that this is likely to be the most clinically relevant mixture of compounds present in the patients causing vasospasm.

Spectrophotometric Analysis

A Molecular Devices (Sunnyvale, CA) SpectraMax M5 spectrophotometer was used for these analyses. Each sample was scanned between 280 and 500 nm, and a peak at 320 nm was clearly discernable. This is the wavelength at which both BOX A and B absorb [8]. The absorbance at 320 nm was plotted against concentration of BOXes, and the resulting relationship was subjected to linear regression (R = 0.998). These observations produced a molar extinction coefficient (ε) of 6,852 for BOX A and B.

We standardized the doses applied to the rats according to our previous methods [9] and used these doses in this study. Typically, the dose [9] of BOXes solution was 20 µM, consistent with perihematomal BOXes concentrations found in rat and pig models [23].

Surgical Methods

Animals were anesthetized with 2.5% isoflurane with 70% nitrous oxide and 27.5% oxygen. It was administered via a nose cone to ensure deep sedation, as verified by an absence of hind- and forelimb pain reflexes, as well as the absence of corneal reflexes. Normal, non-labored breathing was maintained throughout the surgery. Temperature was monitored and maintained at 37 ± 0.2 °C by use of a heating pad.

Cranial Window

Anesthetized rats were placed in a stereotaxic frame (Kopf Instruments Tujunga, CA, USA). After a dorsal scalp incision and blunt dissection to remove loose connective tissue, a cranial window was produced beginning 1 mm lateral to bregma using aseptic technique. A 3-mm-wide (extending from 1 to 4 mm lateral to bregma) by 5-mm (extending from 2.5 mm anterior to 2.5 mm posterior to bregma) window was created and the surface vessels visualized making sure the dura was still intact. A standardized volume and concentration of BOXes (30 µL of a 20 µM solution) or vehicle (0.9% saline) was applied to the surface of the dura [4]. Using the Axiovision software (Carl Zeiss Inc., Thornwood, NY, USA), images were acquired before the addition of the BOXes or saline, and then 30 min post-application. After exposure to BOXes or vehicle for 15 min, the window was flushed with saline and absorbed with cotton. Cranial windows were temporarily closed by suturing the scalp and EMLA cream was applied for pain management after surgery and as needed thereafter. Animals were allowed to recover on a warming pad with constant monitoring until fully recovered from the anesthesia, after which they were returned to their home cages.

Time Dependence

In order to test time dependence of injury, the rats were allowed to recover for 1, 2, 4 or 7 days following initial surgery. At these time points, rats were anesthetized again with isoflurane and euthanized with ketamine (100 mg/kg), xylazine (20 mg/kg), and heparin intraperitoneally. The animals were perfused with 0.9% saline and 4% paraformaldehyde in 0.1-mol/L phosphate buffer through the ascending aorta. After perfusion brains were rapidly removed and placed in 30% sucrose in 0.1-mol/L phosphate buffer until they were sectioned for immunohistochemistry.

Immunohistochemistry

Immunohistochemistry was performed using standard avidin-biotin techniques. [18, 19]. A monoclonal antibody to HSP25/27 (StressGen, Victoria, British Columbia, Canada), a monoclonal antibody to HSP32/HO-1 (StressGen), and a polyclonal HSP 32/HO-1 antibody [18] were used for the immunocytochemistry. Briefly, 50-µm sections were cut on a sliding microtome. These sections were incubated with blocking buffer containing 2% goat serum, 0.1% bovine serum albumin, and 0.3% Triton X-100 in 0.1-mol/L phosphate buffer. They were then incubated with the antibodies (HSP25/27 at 1:2,000 and HO-1 at 1:8,000) overnight at room temperature. The next day they were washed with phosphate buffered saline and incubated with a biotinylated goat anti-mouse secondary antibody (Vector, Burlingame, CA, USA) for 2 h. After additional phosphate-buffered saline washes, they were incubated in Vectastain Elite ABC kit using the immunoperoxidase system (Vector) for 112 h. Sigma Fast diaminobenzidine tablets (Sigma, St. Louis, MO, USA) were added after three more phosphate-buffered saline washes to visualize the protein. Sections were washed three times, mounted, dried, and covered with glass cover slips.

Results

Immunohistochemistry and Heat Shock Protein Expression

BOXes and saline control both induce HSP25/27 as late as day 7, with BOXes treated rats exhibiting a higher level of expression. HSP 25 can be indicative of protein processing and/or degradation, therefore these results support a general response to the surgery, with exacerbation of this disruption in the BOXes treated group.

In Fig. 1, however, we see HO-1 expression in young rats treated with either vehicle or BOXes. HO-1 is a stress gene (HSP-32) that is expressed in order to facilitate degradation of heme to biliverdin. Its expression can be indicative of hemorrhage or response to hemorrhage and was evident in

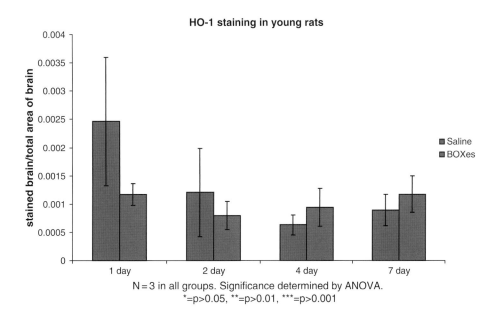

Fig. 1 Young rats exposed to BOXes or Saline showed a significant increase in HO-1 expression in the control group compared to a relative inhibition of expression in the BOXes group on day 1. After day 2 there was no significant difference between groups throughout the next 6 days post BOXes application

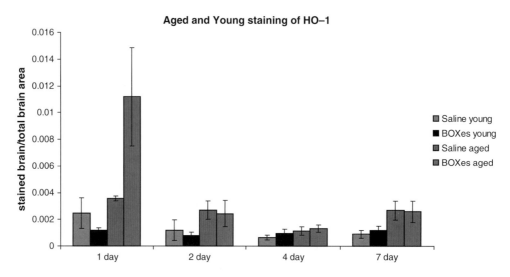

Fig. 2 In the aged rats there is a substantial and significant increase in HO-1 expression induced on day 1 in the BOXes group with an inhibition in the young rats exposed to BOXes for 1 day. After 1 day aged and young rats exhibited similar and not stastically different HO-1 expression in BOXes and saline groups

Fig. 3 BOXes produced a significant and sustained expression of HSP-25 at all time points tested in the aged rats. The young rats had less expression of HSP-25 at all time points and for BOXes as well as saline treated animals, at all time points tested compared to aged rats

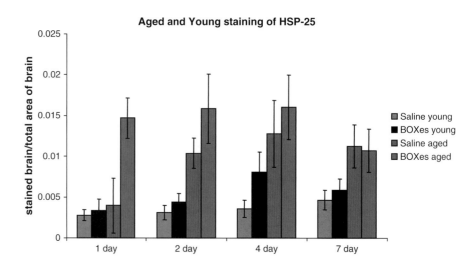

all groups. We observed a significant decrease in HO-1 expression at the early time points post BOXes administration compared to saline control with no differences at the later time points.

Of particular interest we found that in the aged rats, saline and BOXes both had significantly exacerbated effects. This is summarized in Figs. 2 and 3 where we see young and aged rat responses to BOXes. While aged and young rats had different responses, all groups had returned to similar values (BOXes vs saline control) at 7 days.

In Fig. 4 we see two representative histological images of rat brain from the cortex of aged rats post saline and post BOXes respectively at 2 days demonstrating the HSP-25 expression seen. BOXes induce significantly greater expression of stress gene compared to saline controls.

Conclusion

In this paper we report that a single application of BOXes significantly increases stress gene expression in the brains of rats, and that increased expression is sustained for up to 4 days, normalizing to control levels at 7 days. This was the case for HSP-25 in young and aged animals. The intensity of the response was significantly more pronounced in aged rats compared to young rats.

We also observed a significantly greater mortality rate for the aged rats compared to control rats, data not shown. The mortality tended to occur during and immediately after surgery for BOXes and saline rats. There was no significant difference in mortality between BOXes or saline groups.

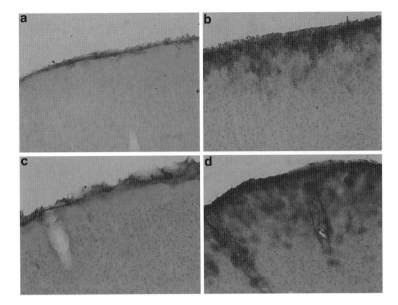

Fig. 4 Representative images of HO-1 (**A**) and HSP-25 (**B**) expression at 1 day in rat cortex.
(**a**) Saline sham in young rat.
(**b**) Boxes treatment in young rat.
(**c**) Saline sham in aged rat.
(**d**) Boxes treatment in aged rat

We believe that it is relevant that BOXes effects are so pronounced and prolonged as to have effects on brain stress gene expression 4 days post application. This, we suggest, is consistent with the sustained pathogenesis seen post SAH putatively caused by the toxic metabolites found in the CSF [11]. It is noteworthy that in the young animals BOXes had less activation of HO-1 compared to saline controls at 1 day and that there was no significant effects seen with HO-1 after that in the young animals. This is indicative of a controlled response to BOXes in the young, where BOXes may be inhibiting hemoxygenase induction because of its prominence in the degradative pathway for bilirubin; it may act as a feedback inhibitor. Further, despite BOXes being a heme metabolite, they are more a hemeoxygenase product (indirectly) therefore the induction of HO-1 is not surprising [12]. In the aged rat brain however the first day post application of BOXes there is a substantial and significant induction of HO-1 that resolves to saline control levels at day 2. It is unclear if the aged brain is responding to BOXes as a heme metabolite or simply as a stress gene response. Nonetheless it is interesting that HSP-25 is significantly elevated at 24 h and remains elevated for 4 days in the aged rat. This potent and sustained response may be a response to the stress of the surgery compounded with the effects of BOXes.

We are confident that the BOXes are having a toxic-like effect on the rats. In previous cell culture studies we have already reported that BOXes are not lethal to cells but act on signaling cascades in tissue [9]. Therefore it is suggested that our results are consistent with a pathologic mechanism of BOXes contributing to the results we report here. They are not likely killing cells or acting as pro-oxidants. Such supposition is based on previous studies using cell culture [9].

In conclusion BOXes have a significantly greater early stimulation of HSP-25 in all groups and act as an apparent negative feedback to inhibit HO-1 expression at 1 day. Aged rats had a significantly greater mortality as well as more pronounced BOXes effects. BOXes also have specific prolonged temporal effects on rat brain consistent with a stress inducing state based on stress gene expression. This effect lasts for about 4 days with apparent resolution by 7 days. Taken together we conclude that BOXes, when present in the CSF of SAH patients, could contribute to complications and pathology seen in these patients. Future studies targeted at understanding the mechanisms of action for BOXes may prove to be useful in treating patients with vasospasm post SAH.

Acknowledgements This work was supported by NS050569, EB007954, and NS042308.

The authors thank and acknowledge the assistance of the late William L. Wurster.

Disclosure:
JFC is co-founder of Xanthostat diagnostics; a company involved in developing and testing diagnostic devices. Xanthostat was not a sponsor of this research nor anticipating obtaining IP from this work.

JFC is a named inventor on IP associated with BOXes. This IP is owned by the Medical Research Council in England.

References

1. Adams HJ, Kassell N, Torner J, Haley EJ. Predicting cerebral ischemia after aneurysmal subarachnoid hemorrhage: influences of clinical condition. Neurology 1987;37:1586–91.
2. Cadoux-Hudson T, Pyne G, Clark J. Subarachnoid hemorrhage induced cerebral vasospasm: a subcellular perspective on the control of tension. Emerg Ther Targets. 1999;3:439–52.

3. Cadoux-Hudson T, Pyne G, Domingo Z, Clark J. The stimulation of vascular smooth muscle oxidative metabolism by CSF from subarachnoid hemorrhage patients increases with Fisher and WFNS grades. Acta Neurochir. 2001;143:65–72.
4. Clark J, Reilly M, Sharp F. Oxidation of bilirubin produces compounds that cause prolonged vasospasm of rat cerebral vessels: a contributor to subarachnoid hemorrhage-induced vasospasm. J Cereb Blood Flow Metab. 2002;22:472–78.
5. Dietrich H, Dacey R. Molecular keys to the problems of cerebral vasospasm. Neurosurgery 2000;46:517–30.
6. Findlay J, Macdonald R, Weir B. Current concepts of pathophysiology and management of cerebral vasospasm following aneurysmal subarachnoid hemorrhage. Cerebrovasc Brain Metab Rev 1991;3:336–61.
7. Kassell N, Drake C. Timing of aneurysm surgery. Neurosurgery 1982;10:514–19.
8. Kranc K, Pyne G, Tao L, Claridge T, Harris D, Cadoux-Hudson T, et al. Oxidative degradation of bilirubin produces vasoactive compounds. Eur J Biochem. 2000;267:7094–101.
9. Lyons MA, Shukla R, Zhang K, Pyne GJ, Singh M, Biehle SJ, et al. Increase of metabolic activity and disruption of normal contractile protein distribution by bilirubin oxidation products in vascular smooth-muscle cells. J Neurosurg. 2004;100:505–11.
10. Macdonald R, Weir B, Runzer T, Grace M, Findlay J, Saito K, et al. Etiology of cerebral vasospasm in primates. J Neurosurg. 1991;75:415–24.
11. Macdonald RL, Marton LS, Andrus PK, Hall ED, Johns L, Sajdak M. Time course of production of hydroxyl free radical after subarachnoid hemorrhage in dogs. Life Sci. 2004;75:979–89.
12. Matz PG, Massa SM, Weinstein PR, Turner C, Panter SS, Sharp FR. Focal hyperexpression of hemeoxygenase-1 protein and messenger RNA in rat brain caused by cellular stress following subarachnoid injections of lysed blood. J Neurosurg. 1996;85:892–900.
13. Mayberg M. Cerebral vasospasm. Neurosurg Clin N Am. 1998;9:615–27.
14. Mayberg M, Batjer H, Dacey R, Diringer M, Haley EJ, Heros R, et al. Guidlelines for the Management of Aneurysmal Subarachnoid Hemorrhage. A Statement for Helathcare Professionals from a Special Writing Group of the Stroke Council, American Heart Association. Circulation 1994;90:2592–605.
15. Pyne G, Cadoux-Hudson T, Clark J. Cerebrospinal fluid from subarachnoid hemorrhage patients causes excessive oxidative metabolism compared to vascular smooth muscle force generation. Acta Neurochir. 2001;143:59–62.
16. Pyne G, Cadoux-Hudson T, Clark J. Magnesium protection against in vitro cerebral vasospasm after subarachnoid hemorrhage. Br J Neurosurg. 2001,15:409–15.
17. Pyne-Geithman GJ, Clark JF. Vascular smooth muscle function: The physiology and pathology of vasoconstriction. Pathophysiology 2005;12:35–45.
18. Turner C, Bergeron M, Matz P, Zegna A, Noble L, Panter S, et al. Heme oxygenase-1 protein is induced in glia throughout brain by subarachnoid hemoglobin. J Cereb Blood Flow Metab. 1998;18:257–73.
19. Turner C, Panter S, Sharp F. Anti-oxidants prevent focal rat brain injury as assessed by induction of heat shock proteins (HSP70, HO-1/HSP32, HSP47) following subarachnoid injections of lysed blood. Brain Res Mol Brain Res. 1999;65:87–102.
20. Weir B, Grace M, Hansen J, Rothberg C. Time course of vasospasm in man. J Neurosurg. 1978;48:173–78.
21. Weir B, Macdonald R, Stoodley M. Etiology of cerebral vasospasm. Acta Neurochir Suppl. 1999;72:27–46.
22. Zhang H, Weir B, Macdonald R, Marton L, Solenski N, Kwan A, et al. Mechanisms of [Ca++]i elevation induced by erythrocyte components in endothelial cells. J Pharmacol Exp Ther. 1996;277:1501–09.
23. Clark JF, Loftspring M, Wurster WL, Beiler S, Beiler C, Wagner KR, Pyne-Geithman GJ. Bilirubin oxidation products, oxidative stress, and intracerebral hemorrhage. PMID:19066073. Acta Neurochir Suppl. 2008;105:7–12.

Preliminary Results of an ICP-Controlled Subarachnoid Hemorrhage Rabbit Model for the Study of Delayed Cerebral Vasospasm

Serge Marbacher, Camillo Sherif, Volker Neuschmelting, Janine-Ai Schläppi, Jukka Takala, Stephan Jakob, and Javier Fandino

Abstract *Introduction*: Intracisternal blood injection is the most common applied experimental subarachoid bleeding technique in rabbits. The model comprises examiner-dependent variables and does not closely represent the human pathophysiological sequelae of ruptured cerebral aneurysm. The degree of achieved delayed cerebral vasospasm (DCVS) in this model is often mild. The aim of this study was to characterize and evaluate the feasibility of a clinically more relevant experimental SAH in vivo model. SAH was performed by arterial blood shunting from the subclavian artery into the great cerebral cistern. A total of five experiments were performed. Intracranial pressure (ICP), arterial blood pressure, heart rate, arterial blood gas analysis, and neurological status were monitored throughout the experiments. SAH induced vasoconstriction of the basilar artery was $52.1 \pm 3.4\%$ on day 3 compared to baseline ($P < 0.05$). Post-mortem gross examination of the brain showed massive blood clot accumulation around the brainstem and ventral surface of the brain. The novel technique offers an examiner independent SAH induction and triggers high degrees of delayed cerebral vasospasm. The severity of vasospasm attained offers a unique opportunity to evaluate future therapeutic treatment options.

Keywords Cerebral aneurysm · Delayed cerebral vasospasm · Model · Rabbit · Subarachnoid hemorrhage

S. Marbacher (✉), C. Sherif, V. Neuschmelting, J.-A. Schläppi, J. Takala, S. Jakob, and J. Fandino
Department of of Intensive Care Medicine, Bern University Hospital and University of Bern, Bern, Switzerland
e-mail: serge.marbacher@ksa.ch

Introduction

Blood injection into the cisterna magna is the standard way for SAH induction in rabbits [1, 2, 4]. Single injection of autologous arterial blood results in mild vasospasm on day 3, whereas additional blood injection postpone peak onset to day 7 with debated enhancement of DCVS [5, 6]. The attained degree of vasospasm is crucial in evaluating the effectiveness of potential treatment after SAH. The achieved mild degree of vasospasm of the cisterna magna blood injection model may have contributed to the fact that numerous therapeutic procedures appeared to relieve experimentally induced vasospasm while they were ineffective when used clinically. Furthermore, the way how autologous arterial blood is injected into the subarachnoid space influences the behavior of the model in each experiment. In order to overcome these drawbacks, we aimed to establish an examiner-independent SAH rabbit model that triggers moderate to severe DCVS.

Methods

In five adult female New Zealand rabbits weighing 3.0–4.6 kg experimental SAH was performed as described below. The protocol of this study was reviewed and approved by the Swiss Institutional Animal Care and Use Committee as meeting the Swiss guidelines for laboratory animal use (approval #109/07).

Anaesthesia, Clinical Observation, and Sacrifice

Induction of general anesthesia was performed by subcutaneous administration of ketamine and xylazine. Neurological status was graded at 6, 12, 24, 48, and 72 h post SAH according to the four-point grading system reported previously [3]. Euthanasia was performed after the follow-up angiography on day 3 post-SAH induction by intraarterial bolus injection of sodium thiopenthal.

Angiography

Digital subtraction angiography (DSA) was performed on day 0 prior to SAH and on day 3 post SAH. The rabbit's left or right subclavian artery was microsurgically exposed and cannulated using a 5.5-french pediatric three-lumen central venous. DSA was performed by intra-arterial bolus injection of non-ionic Iopamidol. Images of the vertebrobasilar system were obtained using a rapid sequential angiographic technique. Measurement of each vessel was performed three times in a blinded fashion using the automatic measurement tool of the ImagePro Discovery® analysis software, and mean values were determined.

SAH Induction and Monitoring

Following baseline DSA on day 0, a 22G × 40 mm spinal access needle was inserted into the cisterna magna transcutaneously. Correct positioning of the needle was determined by successful aspiration of cerebrospinal fluid. The spinal access needle in the cisterna magna was connected to the previously catheterized subclavian artery via blood-filled pressure monitoring tubing. Arterial blood gas status ($PaCO_2$, PaO_2) was analyzed before angiography. Standard cardiovascular monitoring (arterial blood pressure, heart rate) was performed with a Datex S5 Monitor throughout the experiments. The intracranial pressure (ICP) catheter tip was placed over a sealed burr hole in the frontal cortex and pressures were continuously monitored using a Camino multiparameter monitor. SAH was initiated by opening the blood shunt to let blood streaming into the atlantooccipital cistern under arterial pressure.

Gross Examination of Brain

Perfusion-fixation was carried out at room temperature with 200 ml of 0.1M phosphate-buffered solution followed by 200 ml fixative. Immediately after euthanasia, the brains were removed from the skull and the basal and hemispheric surfaces observed and photographed to identify accumulated blood clots and distribution of subarachnoidal blood.

Statistical Methods

Values were expressed as mean ± SD. Statistical significance between baseline and follow-up values were compared using student's paired t-test. Neurological scores were analyzed using a repeated measures 2-way analysis of variance (ANOVA). P value < 0.05 was considered significant.

Results

The animals did not differ significantly in $PaCO_2$, PaO_2, mean arterial blood pressure or heart rate at baseline (Day 0) and follow-up (Day 3) measurements (Table 1). All rabbits showed progressive aggravation of neurological deficits on day 1–3 (Fig. 1).

Table 1 Measurements of physiological parameters

Time point	n	$PaCO_2$ (mmHg)	PaO_2 (mmHg)	MABP (mmHg)	HR (bpm)
Day 0	5	53 ± 3	49 ± 7	66 ± 11	165 ± 16
Day 3	5	47 ± 4	53 ± 1	56 ± 6	177 ± 22

Values were expressed as mean ± SD
PaCO₂ arterial carbon dioxide pressure, *PaO₂* arterial oxide pressure, *MABP* mean arterial blood pressure, *HR* heart rate, *bpm* beats per minute

Angiographic Measurements

Induced vasoconstriction of the basilar artery 3 days after SAH was 52.1 ± 3.4% (range: 43.3–66.7%; n = 5; P < 0.05) (Fig. 2).

ICP Measurements

During experimental SAH, ICP rose to diastolic arterial blood pressure within minutes (Fig. 3).

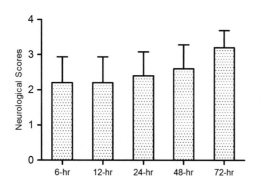

Fig. 1 Neurological status. All rabbits developed progressive neurological deficits after SAH

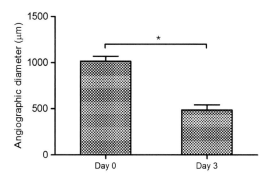

Fig. 2 Induced vasoconstriction of the basilar artery. Bar graph shows significant (*P < 0.05 vs. day 0) basilar artery spasm on day 3 after experimental SAH induction via arterial blood shunt

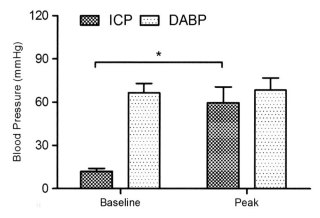

Fig. 3 ICP increase during experimental SAH. Significant increase of ICP was noted within minutes after SAH induction (*P < 0.5 baseline vs. peak). ICP rose close to diastolic arterial blood pressure

Gross Examination of Brain

All brains showed extensive coagulated old dissolved subarachnoid blood in the basal cisterns especially around the circle of Willis, interpeduncular fossa and ventral surface of the brain stem.

Conclusion

This study demonstrates that examiner independent and readily applied SAH induction via arterial blood results in significant transient ICP elevation and triggers moderate to severe DCVS. The provoked neurological deficits are enhanced when compared to previous reported models [1, 5].

Acknowledgements This study was supported by the Department of Intensive Care Medicine, Inselspital, University of Bern, Bern, Switzerland and the Research Fund from the Cantonal Hospital Aarau, Aarau, Switzerland.

We express our gratitude to Hans-Ruedi Widmer, PhD and Angelique Ducray, PhD, Department of Neurosurgery, University Hospital and University of Bern, Bern, Switzerland for their technical laboratory support.

We thank Daniel Mettler, D.V.M., Max Müller, D.V.M., Mr. Daniel Zalokar, and Olgica Beslac, Experimental Surgical Institute, Department of Clinical Research, University Hospital Bern, Bern, Switzerland for their skilful management of animal care, anaesthesia, and operative assistance.

Conflict of interest statement We declare that we have no conflict of interest.

References

1. Baker KF, Zervas NT, Pile-Spellman J, Vacanti FX, Miller D. Angiographic evidence of basilar artery constriction in the rabbit: a new model of vasospasm. Surg Neurol. 1987;27:107–12
2. Chan RC, Durity FA, Thompson GB, Nugent RA, Kendall M. The role of the prostacyclin-thromboxane system in cerebral vasospasm following induced subarachnoid hemorrhage in the rabbit. J Neurosurg. 1984;61:1120–28
3. Endo S, Branson PJ, Alksne JF. Experimental model of symptomatic vasospasm in rabbits. Stroke 1988;19:1420–25
4. Liszczak TM, Black PM, Tzouras A, Foley L, Zervas NT. Morphological changes of the basilar artery, ventricles, and choroid plexus after experimental SAH. J Neurosurg. 1984;61:486–93
5. Spallone A, Pastore FS. Cerebral vasospasm in a double-injection model in rabbit. Surg Neurol. 1989;32:408–17
6. Zhou ML, Shi JX, Zhu JQ, Hang CH, Mao L, Chen KF, et al. Comparison between one- and two-hemorrhage models of cerebral vasospasm in rabbits. J Neurosci Methods. 2007;159:318–24

PKGIα Inhibits the Proliferation of Cerebral Arterial Smooth Muscle Cell Induced by Oxyhemoglobin After Subarachnoid Hemorrhage[1]

Chunxia Luo, Bin Yi, Zhi Chen, Weihua Tang, Yujie Chen, Rong Hu, Zhi Liu, Hua Feng, and John H. Zhang

Abstract The purpose of the present study was to observe the proliferation of cerebral arterial smooth muscle cell (CASMC) induced by oxyhemoglobin (Oxyhb) and interfered by Adenovirus-mediate-PKGI (Ad-PKGI), and to investigate the potential regulative role of the PKGI gene in the molecule mechanism of cerebral vasospasm (CVS) after Subarachnoid hemorrhage (SAH). Tissue-sticking method was used for primary cultured rat CASMCs. Semi-quantitative reverse transcription and polymerase chain reaction (RT-PCR) and western blot were used to examine the PKGI mRNA and protein expressions after CASMC were transfected by Ad-PKG. The proliferation of CASMCs was determined by MTT assay and ^{3}H-TdR incorporation. Ad-PKGI could be transfected into CASMCS and highly express. Oxyhemoglobin could stimulate the proliferation of CASMC; the value of ^{3}H-TdR incorporation and the absorbance value of MTT increased and could block up after CASMC was transfected by Ad-PKG. The results suggested that the PKG signaling pathway might play an important role in CVS after SAH, and the PKG gene might be a target point of gene therapy.

Keywords Cerebral arterial smooth muscle cells (CAMSCs) · Cerebral vasospasm (CVS) · Oxyhemoglobin (Oxyhb) · Protein kinase G (PKG) · Subarachnoid hemorrhage (SAH)

C. Luo, Z. Chen, W. Tang, Y. Chen, R. Hu, Z. Liu, and H. Feng (✉)
Department of Neurosurgery, Southwest Hospital, Third Military Medical University, Gaotanyan 30, Chongqing 400038, People's Republic of China
e-mail: fenghua8888@yahoo.com.cn

B. Yi
Department of Anesthesiology, Southwest Hospital, Third Military Medical University, Gaota nyan 30, Chongqing 400038, People's Republic of China

J.H. Zhang
Department of Neurosurgery, Loma Linda University Medical Center, Loma Linda CA, USA

Introduction

The molecule mechanism of secondary chronic cerebral vasospasm (CVS) after Subarachnoid hemorrhage (SAH) is of great research interest. It has been reported in previous studies that the rat SAH model established via simulation by bloody cerebrospinal fluid (BCSF) shows significant cerebral arterial smooth muscle cell (CASMC) proliferation and migration [1], while its regulatory mechanism has not been identified yet. The cGMP-dependent protein kinase or Protein Kinase G (PKG) is a serine/threonine-specific protein kinase that is activated by cGMP. It phosphorylates a number of biologically important targets and is implicated in the regulation of smooth muscle relaxation, platelet function, sperm metabolism, cell division, and nucleic acid synthesis. Two PKG genes, coding for PKG type I (PKG-I) and type II (PKG-II), have been identified in mammals. The N-terminus of PKG-I is encoded by two alternatively spliced exons that specify for the PKGI and PKGIβ isoforms. PKGIβ is activated at tenfold higher cGMP concentrations than PKGI. Our initial study found that PKGI suppresses the proliferation and migration of VSMC through inhibiting contractile VSMC from being synthetic, and might play a key regulative role in proliferation and migration of vessel smooth muscle cells (VSMCs) [2]. This study investigates the role of PKG in proliferation and migration of CASMC in CVS after SAH, with the aim to provide new ideas for the molecule mechanism and prevention of CVS.

Materials and Methods

Reagents and Instruments

Oxyhemoglobin (sigma), low glucose Dullbecco's modified Eagle's medium (EMEM) (PAA, USA), D-Hanks solution

---

[1]Chunxia Luo and Bin Yi contributed equally to this study

(hyclone, USA), rabbit polyclonal anti-phosphorylated protein of PKGIin rat (NeoMarkers, USA), adenovirus PKGIa (Ad-PKGIa), produced by Chinese Military Respiratory Institute of Xinqiao Hospital, affiliated with Third Military Medical University [3], AMV reverse transcriptase (Promega, USA), Taq DNA polymerase, Oligo (dT), and dNTP (Beijing Dingguo Biological Technology Development Co., Ltd, China), and analytical chemical were purchased from Alpha Imager Gel Imaging System (Alpha Innotech, USA).

Culturing and Grouping of CASMC

SD rats in this study were purchased from the Animal Center of Third Military Medical University, and their weight was about 180–220 g. The cerebral arterial smooth muscle cell (CASMC) in rats had primary culture, transfer culture, purification and identification [4]. CASMCs of 4–6 generations were used in this study.

Inoculated CASMC of the same concentration ($10^6/cm^2$) was divided into the physical saline control group (group N), Oxyhb group (group B), physical saline transfection group (group AN), Oxyhb empty vector group (group KB), and Oxyhb transfection group (group AB). When cells covered about 80% of the area of the bottle bottom, 0.1% fetal bovine serum DMEM was added to replace the original medium. After 24 h of synchronous growth, CASMCs would have proper treatment. Oxyhb was treated with 1 μmol/L concentration [4].

Examination of PKG mRNA and Protein Expression After CMSMC was Transfected by Ad-PKG

5×10^6 CASMCs were taken in each group. Total RNA in the Tripure kit was chosen to perform RT-PCR, with GAPDH as an endogenous reference. PKG gene primer and reaction conditions were the same as our previous study [2]. After amplification, 10 μl PCR product was taken for electrophoresis in 1.5% agarose gel. Alpha Imager scanned the gray scale and read the absorbance value (A) of each strip. The absorbance value ratio of PKG to GAPDH (APKG/AGAPDH) was analyzed. The experiment was repeated 4 times.

The size of the phosphorylated protein of PKG was 60 KD. Western blot was performed as described previously [2]. It was first developed in color in DAB reagent and scanned and stored using the gel imaging system; optical density of the hybrid zone was measured with Alpha Imager, and the protein level on the strip was analyzed. The experiment was repeated 4 times.

^{3}H-TdR Incorporation Test

After cells in each group were digested, we made each group of solution into a cell suspension, counted the cell number, and adjusted the cell concentration to 2×10^4/ml. We inoculated each group of cells on a 96-well plate. Each phase had three wells. We treated the cells with relevant procedures for 12 h, added 1 μCi^{3}H-TdR (1 μCi/well) into each well, continued the culture for 6 h. We then discarded the medium, stopped the incorporation with cold PBS solution, added 0.25% trypsin to digest cells and made them separate from the cell wall, gathered cells on a glass fiber filter with multi-head harvester, washed the cells with physical saline 3 times, stabilized them with 10% trichloroacetic acid, decolorized them with absolute ethanol, dried them for 30 min at 80°C, transferred cells into scintillation fluid, and counted them in a liquid scintillation counter (counts/min, cpm).

MTT Assay

We inoculated 10^3–10^4 cells of each well into a 96-well plate, with the volume of each well being 200 μl, 5 wells for each experiment condition. We placed the plate in 5% CO_2 and cultured for 24 h. We treated each group with specific treatments, continued to have another 24 h culture, replaced the medium with a serum-free medium, added 20 μl MTT solution (5 mg/ml), and inoculated for 4 h at 37°C. We then carefully sucked away and discarded the supernatant in each well. We added 150 μl DMSO into each well and made crystals fully dissolved through 10 min of oscillation. We measured absorbance value of each well using the ELISA reader, with 490 nm to test wavelength and 280 nm as the reference wavelength. We set zero in the blank control well. We then plotted a cell growth curve with time as the lateral-axis and absorbance value (A) as the longitudinal axis.

Statistical Analysis

Data were expressed as mean ± SE. Multiple comparisons were evaluated using one-way ANOVA and significant differences between the 2 groups were analyzed by Tukey's test. A Student's t-test was performed on the two experimental groups. Differences were considered significant if the p value was <0.05.

Results

PKG Transcriptional Level and Protein Expression After CMSMC was Transfected by Ad-PKG

Prior to transfection, PKG transcriptional level and protein expression was low in CASMC; 24 h after CASMC was transfected by Ad-PKG, PKG transcriptional level saw a significant increase (P < 0.05) and PKG phosphorylated protein level also had significant growth (P < 0.05), this indicated that PKG gene can have an effective expression in CASMC after CASMC is transected by Ad-PKG (Table 1).

^{3}H-TdR Incorporation Test

With stimulation by Oxyhb, the ^{3}H-TdR incorporation value had significant growth compared to the control group (P < 0.05). With tranfection by Ad-PKG, the ^{3}H-TdR incorporation value of group AN decreased when compared to group N, while the difference was not statistically significant; and the difference between group KB and group B was not statistically significant either (P > 0.05). After transfected by Ad-PKG and stimulated by Oxyhb, the ^{3}H-TdR incorporation value of group AB did increase, but not obviously like group KB; and it had a significant difference when compared to group B (P < 0.05) (Fig. 1).

MTT Assay

Stimulated by Oxyhb, the absorbance value of group B had a significant increase compared to group N (P < 0.05); the absorbance difference between group KB and group B was not statistically significant (P > 0.05); the absorbance value of group AN did not have any significant difference when compared to that of group N; the absorbance difference between group AB and group B was statistically significant (P < 0.05) (Fig. 2).

Conclusion

The molecule mechanism of CVS after SAH has not been fully identified. It is controversial whether CVS is caused by continuous and active contraction of VSMC or organic stenosis as result of structural damage to vessel wall and VSMC proliferation [5]. Previous studies mainly focus on the reasons that lead to continuous and active contraction of VSMC and signal transduction pathway that modulates smooth muscle contraction, while medical treatment for over contraction of VSMC can only improve CVS in the early stage or to a certain extent, but cannot alleviate serious CVS or CVS in the end-stage. Results of these studies [6] and our

Table 1 PKG mRNA and phosphorylated protein expressions in CASMCs transfected by Ad-PKG as determined by RT-PCR and Western blot ($\bar{x} \pm S$, %, n = 3)

	PKG mRNA	Phosphorylated protein
Untransfected group	37.23 ± 9.13	72.54 ± 12.58
Empty vector group	38.79 ± 11.44	76.33 ± 14.26
Transfected group	86.37 ± 13.15[a]	187.21 ± 23.47[a]

[a] p < 0.05 compared with the untransfected and empty vector groups

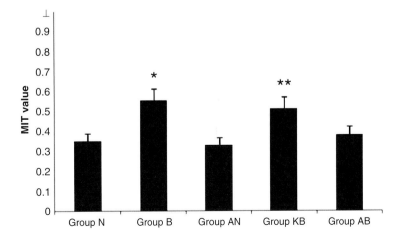

Fig. 1 The MTT assay is used to quantitate CASMC proliferation in different groups. *p<0.05 compared with group N. **p<0.05 compared with group AN and AB

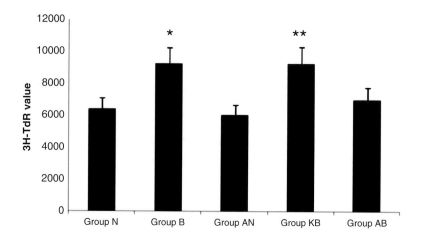

Fig. 2 The ^{3}H-TdR value is used to quantitate CASMC proliferation in different groups. *p<0.05 compared with group N. **p<0.05 compared with group AN and AB

initial studies [7, 8] show that the proliferation and migration of CASMC may play an important role in the hardly irreversible pathogenesis of CVS, and is one of the basic pathophysiological changes of CVS. It is urgent to have further study and targeted interventions on VSMC proliferation following SAH.

PKG can be either soluble cytoplasm I or membrane-bound II. Studies in recent years show that PKG pathway plays an important regulative role in the phenotype of VSMC [9, 10]. Activated PKG has effects on many substrates, including vasodilator-stimulated phosphoprotein (VASP), myosin light chain kinase (MLCK), Rho family, HSP27, Maxi-k channel, and MAPK, so it can control the phenotype of VSMC by modulating the balance of intracellular phosphorylation and dephosphorylation, function of protein G and the skeleton protein system [11, 12]. Through inhibiting expression of PKG, VSMC can turn into synthetic VSMC, which can undergo proliferation and migration, i.e. the major pathological change of CVS. These study results show that the PKG gene might play an important regulative effect in proliferation and migration of CASMC. It might be a target point for gene therapy in the future and deserves in-depth study. It has been found in our study that PKG transcriptional level and protein expression was low in CASMC; after CASMC was transfected by Ad-PKG, PKG transcriptional level and protein expression saw significant increase (P < 0.05), this showed that Ad-PKG can effectively transfect CASMC and highly express the PKG gene in CASMC.

The ^{3}H-TdR incorporation test found that when stimulated by Oxyhb, ^{3}H-TdR incorporation had a great increase with a significant difference compared to the control group (P < 0.05). Transfected by Ad-PKG, ^{3}H-TdR incorporation of group AN was less than that of the control group, while the difference was not statistically significant. After being transfected by Ad-PKG and stimulated by Oxyhb, the ^{3}H-TdR incorporation value of group AB did increase, but not obviously like group KB; and it had a significant difference when compared to group B (P < 0.05). The results of this study suggest that with stimulation by Oxyhb, CASMC has more DNA synthesis and obvious proliferation; the proliferation can be inhibited by Ad-PKG transfection, i.e. PKG gene expression can inhibit Oxyhb from stimulating CASMC proliferation. In the MTT test, we found that with stimulation by Oxyhb, the absorbance value of group B had a great increase with a significant difference when compared to group N (P < 0.05). The absorbance value difference between Group AN and group N was not significant, and the difference between group AB and group B was significant (P < 0.05). The study results suggest that with stimulation by Oxyhb, the number of CASMC had growth and this indicated obvious proliferation of CASMC; however, the proliferation can be significantly suppressed by Ad-PKG transfection. The findings of the study show that the PKG signaling pathway might play an important regulative role in proliferation and migration of CASMC in CVS after SAH. However, the upstream regulatory gene and down-stream target gene of this pathway have not been identified yet, and further study should be performed in this direction.

PKG is a non-secretory protein inherent in cell expression, so study methods are generally gene knock-out and transfection (infection) by transgenic animal and exogenous gene. For CASMC, it is more economical, simple, and effective to introduce the exogenous PKG gene with adenovirus as a vector [13]. Both ^{3}H-TdR incorporation and the MTT method were used to test CASMC proliferation in this study, and more accurate and persuasive results were yielded.

In conclusion, the PKG gene plays an important regulative role in the molecule mechanism of CVS after SAH, and can be used as a target point of gene therapy.

Acknowledgements This research job is supported by Grant No. 30700347, 30500662, 30772224 and 30801186 from the National Science Foundation of China (NSFC) and Grant No.2007BB5045 from the Natural Science Foundation of Chongqing, China.

Conflict of interest statement We declare that we have no conflict of interest.

References

1. Borel CO, McKee A, Parra A, Haglund MM, Solan A, Prabhakar V, et al. Possible role for vascular cell proliferation in cerebral vasospasm after subarachnoid hemorrhage. Stroke 2003;34(2):427–33.
2. Yi B, Lu JY, Qian GS, Bai L, Wang GS, Zhao Y. Changes of Cell Phenotype and PKGIa Expression in Pulmonary Arterial Smooth Muscle Cells Induced by Hypoxia. Mil Med J South China. 2008;22(5):27–9.
3. Yi B, Lu JY, Bai L, Wang GS, Qian GS. Establishment and identification of recombinant adenovirus vector in human wild PKGIa gene. Acad J Second Mil Med Univ J. 2009;30(1):69–72.
4. Tang WH, Zhu G, Zhang JH, Chen Z, Liu Z, Feng H. The effect of Oxyhemoglobin on the proliferation and migration of cultured vascular smooth muscle cells. Acta Neurochir Suppl. 2008;104:197–203.
5. Zhang ZD, Macdonald RL. Contribution of the remodeling response to cerebral vasospasm. Neurol Res. 2006;28(7):713–20.
6. Macdonald RL, Pluta RM, Zhang JH. Cerebral vasospasm after subarachnoid hemorrhage: the emerging revolution. Nat Clin Pract Neurol. 2007;3(5):256–63.
7. Tang WH, Chen Z, Liu Z, Zhang JH, Xi G, Feng H. The effect of ecdysterone on cerebral vasospasm following experimental subarachnoid hemorrhage in vitro and in vivo. Neurol Res. 2008;30 (6):571–80.
8. Chen Z, Zhu G, Zhang JH, Liu Z, Tang WH, Feng H. Ecdysterone-sensitive smooth muscle cell proliferation stimulated by conditioned medium of endothelial cells cultured with bloody cerebrospinal fluid. Acta Neurochir Suppl. 2008;104:183–88.
9. Negash S, Narasimhan SR, Zhou W, Liu J, Wei FL, Tian J, Raj JU. Role of cGMP-dependent protein kinase in regulation of pulmonary vascular smooth muscle cell adhesion and migration: Effect of hypoxia. Am J Physiol Heart Circ Physiol. 2009;297(1):H304–12.
10. Lukowski R, Weinmeister P, Bernhard D, Feil S, Gotthardt M, Herz J, et al. Role of smooth muscle cGMP/cGKI signaling in murine vascular restenosis. Arterioscler Thromb Vasc Biol. 2008;28(7):1244–50.
11. Shih CD. Activation of nitric oxide/cGMP/PKG signaling cascade mediates antihypertensive effects of muntingia calabura in anesthetized spontaneously hypertensive rats. Am J Chin Med. 2009;37(6):1045–58.
12. Li M, Sun X, Li Z, Liu Y. Inhibition of cGMP phosphodiesterase 5 suppresses serotonin signalling in pulmonary artery smooth muscles cells. Pharmacol Res. 2009;59(5):312–18.
13. Casteel DE, Zhang T, Zhuang S, Pilz RB. cGMP-dependent protein kinase anchoring by IRAG regulates its nuclear translocation and transcriptional activity. Cell Signal. 2008;20(7):1392–99.

Characteristics of In Vivo Animal Models of Delayed Cerebral Vasospasm

Serge Marbacher, Javier Fandino, and Neil Kitchen

Abstract Animal models provide a basis for clarifying the complex pathogenesis of delayed cerebral vasospasm (DVCS) and for screening of potential therapeutic approaches. The aim of this work was to identify and analyze the most consistent and feasible models and their characteristics for each animal. An online search of the MEDLINE PubMed and EMBASE medical databases (1969 to week 21 of 2007) was performed using the key words "mice", "rat", "rabbit", "canine", and "primate" in combination with "subarachnoid hemorrhage", "model", and "vasospasm". Seven techniques were mainly used to induce experimental subarachnoid hemorrhage in closed and open cranium approaches. Among the great number of experimental SAH methods and associated parameters only a fistful reliable models can be identified and recommended for experimental work in mice, rats, rabbits, dogs and nonhuman primates.

Keywords: Animal model · delayed cerebral vasospasm · Subarachnoid hemorrhage

Introduction

Symptomatic delayed cerebral vasospasm (DCVS) develops in approximately 30% of patients sustaining ruptured aneurysm and is the leading potentially treatable cause of death and disability after subarachnoid hemorrhage (SAH) [5]. Despite awareness of the entity for almost half a century, the exact cause of DCVS remains cryptic. The absence of satisfactory prevention or efficacious therapy of DCVS has resulted in intensive research efforts. Many animal models have been designed to address the complex pathogenesis of DCVS and to evaluate potential treatment modalities.

In order to closely mimic the human situation after SAH, many different bleeding techniques have been proposed and applied in the mouse, rat, rabbit, dog, primate, cat, pig, and goat animal models. The diverse SAH techniques, blood volumes, and chosen time points of measuring DCVS influence the findings to a great extent. The arbitrary use of experimental parameters can lead to results of uncertain relevance. The inconsistency of published findings is the most controversial issue in vasospasm research today [12].

Methods

The literature was searched to identify basic animal models of experimental SAH, their refinements/modifications, and studies conducted applying these models. We searched the MEDLINE PubMed and EMBASE medical databases up to 2007 (week 21) using the key words "mouse", "rat", "rabbit", "canine", "primate", "cat", "pig", and "goat" in combination with "subarachnoid hemorrhage" and "vasospasm". The search was automatically restricted to animals by using the MEDLINE PubMed limit "animals".

We considered in vivo experimental mouse, rat, rabbit, cat, dog, pig, goat, and nonhuman primate SAH studies and models investigating DCVS in large cerebral arteries. In vitro experiments, studies on small cerebral or extracranial vessels, as well as studies with agents causing vasoconstriction other than whole blood were not evaluated.

Results

Murine. Three mouse models were identified and nine experimental studies were included in the analysis. Seven studies used endovascular puncture to induce experimental

S. Marbacher (✉), J. Fandino, and N. Kitchen
Department of Neurosurgery, Cantonal Hospital Aarau, 5000 Aarau, Switzerland
e-mail: serge.marbacher@ksa.ch

SAH and two studies were performed using intracisternal blood injection. The endovascular puncture model leads to DCVS with 20% [4] to 62% [9] of cerebral artery constriction. The preliminary studies focusing on the time course after experimental SAH via endovascular puncture revealed an initial phase of constriction within the first 24 h and a second phase peaking on day 3, followed by nearly complete restitution of the arterial diameter after 1 week [4, 7].

Rat. 83% of all studies are based on intracisternal blood injection (67% single intracisternal blood injection and 16% double intracisternal blood injection). 60% of single-injection experiments used 0.3 ml autologous arterial blood and 56% of double-injection experiments used 2 × 0.3 ml. In most of the settings (68%) the time delay between the two injections was 48 h. The use of 0.3 ml results in DCVS with vessel narrowing ranging from 19 [8] to 29% [6] and the use of two times 0.3 ml results in DCVS with vessel narrowing of up to 47% [10]. 12% of all studies have been reported on the basis of endovascular vessel puncturing. After single injection chronic vasoconstriction occurs on day 2 after SAH. In the rat double-hemorrhage model, investigations showed maximal arterial constriction on day 7.

Rabbit. 98% (including 14% of multiple injections) of all performed experimental DCVS research in the rabbit is based on intracisternal blood injection. The most common volumes of constant and weight-adapted injections in the single hemorrhage model were found to be 3 ml (45%) and 1 ml/kg (48%), respectively. These quantities yielded DCVS with vessel narrowing ranging from 19 [1] to 55% [2] in the single-hemorrhage model. Each research group working with the double-hemorrhage model applied a different constant or weight-adapted blood volume. The single hemorrhage model showed maximal narrowing 3 days after SAH. The double injection method generates a slightly more delayed onset of vasospasm, with a peak onset between day 4 and day 6 after initial hemorrhage.

Canine. Intracisternal blood injection techniques accounted for 97% of all DCVS experiments performed in dogs. 90% of performed studies used a double cisterna magna injection. The most common applied constant blood amount was 2 × 4 ml (46%) followed by 2 × 5 ml (26%). The most popular weight-adapted injections were 0.4 ml/kg (35%) and 0.5 ml/kg (37%). Over 95% of all angiographic studies were within the range of 45% [11] to 66% [3] of arterial vasoconstriction compared to baseline values. 17 experiments (68%) revealed maximal narrowing on day seven after initial SAH.

Primate. Thirteen primate models were identified and 95 experimental studies were included in the analysis. For the last 12 years craniotomy and blood clot placement has been the only method used in monkeys. The most commonly applied amount of blood is 5 ml (42%), followed by 3 ml (10%). Intracisternal blood injection was performed until 1996, and accounts for 22% of all DCVS experiments performed in nonhuman primates. Seven studies revealed maximal vessel narrowing on day seven after craniotomy and arterial blood clot placement.

Table 1 Animal models of delayed cerebral vasospasm

Animal	SAH technique	Blood amount	DCVS peak	Vasospasm
Mouse	Endovascular puncture	Various	Day 3	20–62%
Rat	Single hemorrhage	0.3 ml	Day 2	19–29%
	Double hemorrhage[b]	0.3 ml + 0.3 ml	Day 7[a]	28–47%
Rabbit	Single hemorrhage	3 ml or 1 ml/kg	Day 3	19–55%
	Double hemorrhage[b]	Not established	Day 5[a]	Not established
Dog	Double hemorrhage[b]	2 × 4–5 ml or 0.4–0.5 ml/kg	Day 7[a]	45–66%
Primate	Blood clot placement	5 ml	Day 7[a]	32–52%

Summary of most consistent experimental SAH techniques, blood amount and DCVS. Peak onset
SAH subarachnoid hemorrhage, *DCVS* delayed cerebral vasospasm, *ml* milliliters of autologous arterial blood
[a]The first blood injection is considered on day 0
[b]Time delay between two injections is 48 h

Conclusion

Among the great number of experimental SAH methods and associated parameters only a fistful reliable and consistent models can be identified and recommended for experimental work in mice, rats, rabbits, dogs and nonhuman primates (Table 1). Implementation of more standardized experimental techniques could increase the comparability among laboratories, facilitate interpretation of achieved results, and increase the relevance of future experimental studies.

Acknowledgements We express our gratitude to the staff of the Rockefeller Medical Library, UCL Institute of Neurology and National Hospital for Neurology and Neurosurgery, Queen Square, London, UK for their professional assistance in literature search and document delivery. No funds were or will be received for this study.

Conflict of interest statement We declare that we have no conflict of interest.

References

1. Ahmad I, Imaizumi S, Shimizu H, Kaminuma T, Ochiai N, Tajima M, Yoshimoto T. Development of calcitonin gene-related peptide slow-release tablet implanted in CSF space for prevention of cerebral vasospasm after experimental subarachnoid haemorrhage. Acta Neurochir (Wien). 1996;138:1230–40
2. Chan RC, Durity FA, Thompson GB, Nugent RA, Kendall M The role of the p rostacyclin-thromboxane system in cerebral vasospasm following induced subarachnoid hemorrhage in the rabbit. J Neurosurg. 1984;61:1120–28
3. Chyatte D Prevention of chronic cerebral vasospasm in dogs with ibuprofen and high-dose methylprednisolone. Stroke 1989;20:1021–26
4. Kamii H, Kato I, Kinouchi H, Chan PH, Epstein CJ, Akabane A, Okamoto H, Yoshimoto T Amelioration of vasospasm after subarachnoid hemorrhage in transgenic mice overexpressing CuZn-superoxide dismutase. Stroke 199930:867–71; discussion 872
5. Kassell NF, Torner JC, Haley EC, Jr., Jane JA, Adams HP, Kongable GL. The International Cooperative Study on the Timing of Aneurysm Surgery. Part 1: Overall management results. J Neurosurg. 1990;73:18–36
6. Kemaloglu S, Ozkan U, Yilmaz F, Ak E, Acemoglu H, Olmez G, Simsek R, Bakir A. Preventive effects of intracisternal alphatochopherol on cerebral vasospasm in experimental subarachnoid haemorrhage. Yonsei Med J. 2003;44:955–960
7. Lin CL, Calisaneller T, Ukita N, Dumont AS, Kassell NF, Lee KS A murine model of subarachnoid hemorrhage-induced cerebral vasospasm. J Neurosci Methods. 2003;123:89–97
8. Lin CL, Su YF, Dumont AS, Shih HC, Lieu AS, Howng SL, Lee KS, Kwan AL The effect of an adenosine A1 receptor agonist in the treatment of experimental subarachnoid hemorrhage-induced cerebrovasospasm. Acta Neurochir (Wien). 2006;148:873–79; discussion 879
9. McGirt MJ, Parra A, Sheng H, Higuchi Y, Oury TD, Laskowitz DT, Pearlstein RD, Warner DS Attenuation of cerebral vasospasm after subarachnoid hemorrhage in mice overexpressing extracellular superoxide dismutase. Stroke 2002;33:2317–23
10. Vatter H, Weidauer S, Konczalla J, Dettmann E, Zimmermann M, Raabe A, Preibisch C, Zanella FE, Seifert V Time course in the development of cerebral vasospasm after experimental subarachnoid hemorrhage: clinical and neuroradiological assessment of the rat double hemorrhage model. Neurosurgery 2006;58:1190–97; discussion 1190–1197
11. Zhou C, Yamaguchi M, Kusaka G, Schonholz C, Nanda A, Zhang JH Caspase nhibitors prevent endothelial apoptosis and cerebral vasospasm in dog model of experimental subarachnoid hemorrhage. J Cereb Blood Flow Metab. 2004;24:419–31
12. Zubkov AY, Nanda A, Zhang JH Signal transduction pathways in cerebral vasospasm. Pathophysiology. 2003;9:47–61

Endothelin Related Pathophysiology in Cerebral Vasospasm: What Happens to the Cerebral Vessels?

Hartmut Vatter, Jürgen Konczalla, and Volker Seifert

Abstract The central role of Endothelin (ET) in the development of cerebral vasospasm (CVS) after subarachnoid hemorrhage (SAH) is supported by several investigations. These investigations provided, furthermore, that changes of the ET-receptor expression and function in the wall of the cerebral arteries are a considerable factor for the development of CVS. The biological activity of ET-1 is mediated by two receptor subtypes, named ET(A) and ET(B). Under physiological conditions the dominant vasocontractile effect of ET-1 is mediated by ET(A)-receptors on smooth muscle cells (SMC), which is attenuated by an ET(B)-receptor dependent release of nitric oxide (NO) from endothelial cells (EC). In the physiological cerebrovasculature ECs express exclusively ET(B)- and SMCs only ET(A)-receptors. In case of CVS an increased expression of the ET(B)-receptor could be detected in cerebral vessels. However, the loss of the vasodilative and the missing of a vasocontractile ET(B)-receptor mediated effect was demonstrated. Therefore, any ET(B)-receptor mediated vasoactivity seems to be lost in case of CVS and the biological impact of the increased expression remains unclear so far. The ET(A)-receptor expression seems to be not increased during the development of CVS. Therefore, the proven increase of the ET-dependent vasocontractility seems to be rather by the loss of the ET(B)-receptor mediated effect than by an increased ET(A)-receptor activity. In spite of the more significant changes of the ET(B)-receptor expression the pathophysiological effect of ET, namely the vasoconstriction, seems to be exclusively mediated by the ET(A)-receptor. Therefore, tailored approaches for the treatment of CVS remain to be ET(A)-receptor selective antagonists.

Keywords Cerebral vasospasm · Contraction · Endothelin · Endothelium · Relaxation · Subarachnoid hemorrhage · Vascular smooth muscle cell

Introduction

Cerebral vasospasm (CVS) is one of the substantial causes for delayed neurological deficits, which are responsible for the high morbidity and mortality of the patients suffering from aneurysmal subarachnoid hemorrhage (SAH) [1, 2]. Several observations support the concept that Endothelin (ET) is an important factor in the pathophysiological cascade leading to CVS. These observations include the extremely potent and long-lasting contractile effect of ET-1 on cerebral vessels [3–5], the close correlation between levels of ET-1 and ET-3 in the cerebrospinal fluid (CSF) of patients after SAH developing CVS [6], and the effectiveness of ET receptor antagonists in the prevention and treatment of CVS in animal models [4, 7] and recently in clinical trials [8, 9]. Furthermore, experimental investigations demonstrated that the cerebrovasculature itself seems to be not only the target of increased ET levels but also involved in the pathologically altered ET system in case of CVS [3–5, 10]. Pathophysiological changes of the ET metabolism, receptor expression and function were observed in several cardiovascular diseases [11, 12], which may be, at least in part, transferable the development of CVS after SAH.

Besides a de novo or increased synthesis and release of ET by Endothelial cells (EC), smooth muscle cells (SMC) or invading leucocytes inside the adventitia, changes of the ET-receptor expression and function in the wall of the cerebral arteries could be a potential factor for the development of CVS [3–5, 10] (Table 1). The aim of the present review was, therefore, to investigate the data from the literature supporting the pathophysiological relevance of changes inside the cerebral vessel wall for the development of CVS.

H. Vatter (✉), J. Konczalla, and V. Seifert
Department of Neurosurgery, Center of Clinical Neurosciences, Johann Wolfgang Goethe University, Frankfurt am Main, Germany
e-mail: H.Vatter@em.uni-frankfurt.de

Table 1 Potential changes of the ET metabolism during the development of CVS

	Endothelium	Smooth muscle cells
ET synthesis	Increased	De novo
ET(A)-receptor	De novo expression	Increased expression; enhanced vasoconstriction
ET(B)-receptor	Changed expression; loss of vasorelaxation	De novo expression; de novo vasoconstriction

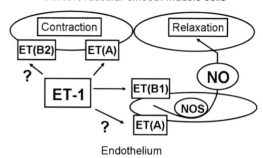

Fig. 1 Effect of ET in the vessel wall of the cerebrovasculature. The dominant vasocontractile effect of ET-1 is mediated by the ET(A)-receptor on the SMCs. This effect is attenuated by an ET(B)-receptor dependent release of nitric oxide (NO) from the endothelium by stimulation of the NO-synthase (NOS) under physiological conditions. This effect is lost during the development of CVS. The expression and the functional significance of an ET(B)-receptor on SMCs and an ET(A)-receptor on ECs after SAH is unclear at present

Increased Endothelin Synthesis

Inside the vessel wall of the cerbrovasculature EC is the main source for ET under physiological conditions [3]. Stimulation by various substances like noradrenaline, serotonin, angiotensin II, bradykinin, interleukin-1, dopamine, oxyhemoglobin, thrombin or transforming growth factor β was demonstrated to result in an increased synthesis and release of ET-1 by these cells [10–12]. Furthermore, a decreased blood flow leading to reduced shear forces in the endothelium results in an increase of the ET-1 expression [10]. On the mRNA level the transcription of ET-1 was neither significantly increased for ET-1 nor for ET-3 in the middle cerebral artery in a SAH model in monkeys [13]. However, the content of ET-1 in the canine basilar artery was about 50% higher after experimental SAH [14, 15]. Furthermore, the level of the pre-cursor peptide big ET-1 was even doubled compared to the controls [14]. Regarding the localisation of the release a significant increase of ET-1 could be detected in the endothelial layer and the adventitia of the basilar artery in a canine SAH model [16]. Accordingly, there are convincing data supporting an increased synthesis and release of ET-1 inside the wall of cerebral arteries by the endothelium. A further source for the ET content inside the adventitia are probably inflammatory cells invading the adventitia after SAH, which was reviewed in detail elsewhere [17]. However, a significant synthesis and release of ETs from SMC in an autocrine manner is not supported by data from the literature.

Changes of the ET Receptors

The biological activity of ET-1 is mediated by two receptor subtypes, named ET(A) and ET(B) [18]. In cerebral vessels under physiological conditions the dominant vasocontractile effect of ET-1 is exclusively mediated by ET(A)-receptors on SMCs, which is attenuated by an ET(B)-receptor dependent release of nitric oxide (NO) from ECs. In the physiological cerebrovasculature ECs express exclusively ET(B)- and SMCs only ET(A)-receptors [3, 18–20]. Possible pathophysiological changes of ET-receptors leading to CVS are summarized in Fig. 1. These changes could consist of an increased expression or effect of the ET(A)-receptor on SMCs or its de novo expression inside the endothelium. Similarly, a de novo expression of a contractile ET(B)-receptor on SMCs or the morphological and/or functional injury of its vasorelaxant effect on the ECs would be consistent with an enhanced contractility resulting in CVS.

The levels of the ET(A)-receptor mRNA in the middle cerebral artery were approximately threefold higher compared to the ET(B)-receptor in a monkey model but not significantly changed by artificial SAH. In contrast ET(B)-receptor mRNA was still lower than for the ET(A)-receptor but significantly increased after SAH [13]. Accordingly, a constant ET(A)-receptor mRNA level could be detected after SAH in a rat model, whereas the ET(B)-receptor mRNA increased by a factor between 2 and 8 [21]. Therefore, the main changes after SAH (at least on the transcription level) seem to affect the ET(B)-receptor, even though the ET(A)-receptor content remains to be quantitatively higher.

ET(A)-Receptor Expression and Function After SAH

Receptor binding essays did not show any significant quantitative change in ET(A)-receptor expression after SAH in the monkey model mentioned above, which is in good correlation with the unchanged mRNA levels [13]. Consistently, in a rat SAH model the ET(A)-receptor immunoreactivity in the SMC-layer was not significantly enhanced in case of CVS.

However, a significant ET(A)-receptor immunostaining in the endothelium was observed in this investigation [22].

The characterization of the ET(A)-receptor mediated effect is complicated by the fact that selective ET(A)-receptor agonists are not available so far. Several investigations demonstrated an enhanced contractile effect of ET-1 on cerebral vessels after SAH, which consists mainly of a leftwards shift of the concentration effect curve (CEC) indicating a higher sensitivity to the compound [21–23]. These results would be consistent with an increased ET(A)-receptor transduction, an additional de novo ET(B)-receptor mediated contraction, or the loss of the ET(B)-receptor dependent vasorelaxation. However, the leftwards shift of the CECs was quantitatively similar to the observation in physiological vessels without endothelial function [22, 23], which supports the loss of the ET(B)-receptor dependent vasorelaxation. Furthermore, the enhanced contraction could be inhibited by a selective ET(A)-receptor antagonist in a competitive fashion [22], which was comparable to the inhibition on the physiological cerebrovasculature [19]. Therefore, the morphological and functional data indicate, that neither the expression nor the function of the ET(A)-receptor on cerebrovascular SMC is significantly altered after SAH.

The morphological correlate and the functional significance of the ET(A)-receptor immunoreactivity inside the endothelium after SAH [22] remains unclear, so far. This observation may be explained by leucocytes invading the endothelium [17] or an expression by ECs. In fact an ET(A)-receptor mediated increased permeability of the cerebrovascular endothelium was reported previously [24]. Furthermore, a proliferative stimulus on the ECs could be initiated by activation of these ET(A)-receptors [11, 12]. However, their significance during CVS after SAH is not investigated so far. Therefore, the present data are in good correlation, that the relevant vasocontraction leading to CVS is in the main part ET(A)-receptor dependent in spite of only minor alterations of the ET(A)-receptor expression and function inside the vessel wall.

Alteration of the ET(B)-Receptor

The de novo expression of a contractile ET(B)-receptor on cerebrovascular SMCs could be one explanation for the enhanced contractile effect of ET-1 on cerebral vessels after SAH as discussed above [21–23]. Accordingly, an enhanced ET(B)-receptor immunoreactivity in the cerebral vessel wall was observed 3–48 h after artificial SAH in a single hemorrhage model in the rat, which seems to be in both EC and SMC [23]. However, this observation is in some discrepancy to the receptor binding essays in the monkey model mentioned above. In spite of altered mRNA levels no significant change in the ET(B)-receptor expression after SAH could be detected and the receptors were limited to the endothelium [13]. Similarly, a significant ET(B)-receptor expression could only be observed inside the endothelium in a rat double SAH model, which was not different compared to the control group [25]. Functional investigation in the rat double SAH model demonstrated that activation of the ET(B)-receptor by the selective agonist sarafotoxin S6c did not induce any contraction in cerebral vessels with or without endothelial function [25, 26]. Therefore, there are no convincing data supporting the existence of a contractile ET(B)-receptor in case of delayed CVS. However, the vasorelaxant potency of sarafotoxin S6c on the cerebrovasculature was significantly reduced after experimental SAH in a time dependent manner [25, 26]. This observation strongly suggests the loss of the ET(B)-receptor relaxation during the development of CVS after SAH.

The data regarding an altered expression of the ET(B)-receptor in ECs or SMCs after SAH are, therefore, inconclusive at present. Accordingly, only speculations can be made on the functional significance of such receptors, which could mediate proliferative stimuli on SMC [12] or may be involved in the clearence of ET-1 from the CSF [27]. However, there is good evidence that ET(B)-receptor dependent vasomotor effects are lost during the development of CVS.

Conclusion

Taken together the changes of the ET metabolism during the development of CVS inside the wall of the cerebrovasculature consists of an increased synthesis, which seems to be performed by ECs and invading leucocytes inside the adventitia. The ET(A)-receptor transcription, expression and function in the SMCs seems to be not significantly changed after SAH. However, the contractile effect leading to CVS is mainly mediated by the ET(A)-receptor. The ET(B)-receptor dependent vasorelaxation seems to be lost in case of CVS. In spite of some inconclusive observations of an ET(B)-receptor expression on SMCs no data supports the existence of an ET(B)-receptor dependent vasocontraction after SAH.

Conflict of interest statement We declare that we have no conflict of interest.

References

1. Bederson JB, Connolly ES Jr, Batjer HH, Dacey RG, Dion JE, Diringer MN, et al. Guidelines for the management of aneurysmal subarachnoid hemorrhage: a statement for healthcare professionals

from a special writing group of the Stroke Council, American Heart Association. Stroke 2009;40:994–1025.
2. Raabe A, Beck J, Berkefeld J, Deinsberger W, Meixensberger J, Schmiedek P, et al. [Recommendations for the management of patients with aneurysmal subarachnoid hemorrhage]. Zentralbl Neurochir. 2005;66:79–91.
3. Salom JB, Torregrosa G, Alborch E. Endothelins and the cerebral circulation. Cerebrovasc Brain Metab Rev. 1995;7:131–52.
4. Vatter H, Zimmermann M, Seifert V, Schilling L. Experimental approaches to evaluate endothelin-A receptor antagonists. Methods Find Exp Clin Pharmacol. 2004;26:277–86.
5. Zimmermann M, Seifert V. Endothelin and subarachnoid hemorrhage: an overview. Neurosurgery 1998;43:863–75.
6. Seifert V, Loffler BM, Zimmermann M, Roux S, Stolke D. Endothelin concentrations in patients with aneurysmal subarachnoid hemorrhage. Correlation with cerebral vasospasm, delayed ischemic neurological deficits, and volume of hematoma. J Neurosurg. 1995;82:55–62.
7. Chow M, Dumont AS, Kassell NF. Endothelin receptor antagonists and cerebral vasospasm: an update. Neurosurgery 2002;51:1333–41.
8. Macdonald RL, Kakarieka A, Mayer S, Pasqualin A, Ruefenacht D, Schmiedek P, et al. Prevention of cerebral vasospasm after aneurysmal subarachnoid hemorrhage with clazosentan, an endothelin receptor antagonist. 2006.
9. Vajkoczy P, Meyer B, Weidauer S, Raabe A, Thome C, Ringel F, et al. Clazosentan (AXV-034343), a selective endothelin A receptor antagonist, in the prevention of cerebral vasospasm following severe aneurysmal subarachnoid hemorrhage: results of a randomized, double-blind, placebo-controlled, multicenter phase IIa study. J Neurosurg. 2005;103:9–17.
10. Miyauchi T, Masaki T. Pathophysiology of endothelin in the cardiovascular system. Annu Rev Physiol. 1999;61:391–415.
11. Böhm F, Pernow J. The importance of endothelin-1 for vascular dysfunction in cardiovascular disease. Cardiovasc Res. 2007 Oct 1;76(1):8–18.
12. Schiffrin EL. Vascular endothelin in hypertension. Vascul Pharmacol. 2005;43:19–29.
13. Hino A, Tokuyama Y, Kobayashi M, Yano M, Weir B, Takeda J, et al. Increased expression of endothelin B receptor mRNA following subarachnoid hemorrhage in monkeys. J Cereb Blood Flow Metab. 1996;16:688–97.
14. Roux S, Loffler BM, Gray GA, Sprecher U, Clozel M, Clozel JP. The role of endothelin in experimental cerebral vasospasm. Neurosurgery 1995;37:78–85.
15. Yamaura I, Tani E, Maeda Y, Minami N, Shindo H. Endothelin-1 of canine basilar artery in vasospasm. J Neurosurg. 1992;76:99–105.
16. Hirose H, Ide K, Sasaki T, Takahashi R, Kobayashi M, Ikemoto F, et al. The role of endothelin and nitric oxide in modulation of normal and spastic cerebral vascular tone in the dog. Eur J Pharmacol. 1995;277:77–87.
17. Dumont AS, Dumont RJ, Chow MM, Lin CL, Calisaneller T, Ley KF, et al. Cerebral vasospasm after subarachnoid hemorrhage: putative role of inflammation. Neurosurgery 2003;53:123–33; discussion 133–125.
18. Rubanyi GM, Polokoff MA. Endothelins: molecular biology, biochemistry, pharmacology, physiology, and pathophysiology. Pharmacol Rev. 1994;46:325–415.
19. Vatter H, Zimmermann M, Tesanovic V, Raabe A, Schilling L, Seifert V. Cerebrovascular characterization of clazosentan, the first nonpeptide endothelin receptor antagonist clinically effective for the treatment of cerebral vasospasm. Part I: inhibitory effect on endothelin(A) receptor-mediated contraction. J Neurosurg. 2005;102:1101–7.
20. Vatter H, Zimmermann M, Tesanovic V, Raabe A, Seifert V, Schilling L. Cerebrovascular characterization of clazosentan, the first nonpeptide endothelin receptor antagonist shown to be clinically effective for the treatment of cerebral vasospasm. Part II: effect on endothelin(B) receptor-mediated relaxation. J Neurosurg. 2005;102:1108–14.
21. Hansen-Schwartz J, Hoel NL, Zhou M, Xu CB, Svendgaard NA, Edvinsson L. Subarachnoid hemorrhage enhances endothelin receptor expression and function in rat cerebral arteries. Neurosurgery 2003;52:1188–94.
22. Vatter H, Konczalla J, Weidauer S, Preibisch C, Zimmermann M, Raabe A, et al. Effect of delayed cerebral vasospasm on cerebrovascular endothelin A receptor expression and function. J Neurosurg. 2007;107:121–7.
23. Ansar S, Vikman P, Nielsen M, Edvinsson L. Cerebrovascular ETB, 5-HT1B, and AT1 receptor upregulation correlates with reduction in regional CBF after subarachnoid hemorrhage. Am J Physiol Heart Circ Physiol. 2007;293:H3750–58.
24. Stanimirovic DB, Bertrand N, McCarron R, Uematsu S, Spatz M. Arachidonic acid release and permeability changes induced by endothelins in human cerebromicrovascular endothelium. Acta Neurochir Suppl (Wien). 1994;60:71–5.
25. Vatter H, Konczalla J, Weidauer S, Preibisch C, Raabe A, Zimmermann M, et al. Characterization of the endothelin-B receptor expression and vasomotor function during experimental cerebral vasospasm. Neurosurgery 2007;60:1100–8.
26. Konczalla J, Vatter H, Weidauer S, Raabe A, Seifert V. Alteration of the cerebrovascular function of endothelin B receptor after subarachnoidal hemorrhage in the rat. Exp Biol Med (Maywood). 2006;231:1064–8.
27. D'Orleans-Juste P, Labonte J, Bkaily G, Choufani S, Plante M, Honore JC. Function of the endothelin(B) receptor in cardiovascular physiology and pathophysiology. Pharmacol Ther. 2002;95:221–38.

Expression and Role of COMT in a Rat Subarachnoid Hemorrhage Model

Zhaohui He, Xiaochuan Sun, Zongduo Guo, and John H. Zhang

Abstract *Objective*: The present study aimed to investigate the expression of COMT mRNA and protein and detect the plasma content of catecholamine (CA), the diameter and thickness of the basilar artery in the early stage of subarachnoid hemorrhage (SAH) to explore the role of COMT in SAH.

Methods: SAH was induced by injection of nonheparinized autologous arterial blood into the chiasmatic cistern. RT-PCR and Western blotting were used to detect the mRNA and protein levels of COMT in the rat striatum at different time points (6, 12, 24, 48, and 72 h after SAH). High performance liquid chromatography was performed to detect plasma CA. With HE staining, the basilar artery diameter and its thickness were measured.

Results: Compared with the normal group and sham group, the increased expression of mRNA and protein of COMT began at 6 h after SAH($P < 0.01$), which peaked at 12 h ($P < 0.01$); it began to drop 24 h after SAH ($P < 0.01$). However, 48 h after SAH, the level of COMT (mRNA and protein) was still higher than that of the normal group ($P < 0.01$). Three days after SAH, the expression of COMT nearly reached normal levels ($P > 0.05$). For rats undergoing SAH, plasma CA began to increase 6 h after injury, which reached a maximum at 24 h after SAH, and then started to drop. Three days later, it still remained elevated compared with that of the normal group and sham group ($P < 0.01$). The most marked contraction and increased wall thickness of the basilar artery were found at 24 h after SAH ($P < 0.01$), which at least lasted for 2 days ($P < 0.01$), and 72 h after injury, the diameter and thickness of the basilar artery almost reached normal levels ($P > 0.05$).

Conclusion: (1) SAH could induce the expression of COMT in the rat striatum in the early stage. (2) Plasma CA levels were significantly elevated in the early stage of SAH accompanied by cerebrovascular vasospasm (CVS). (3) In the early stage of SAH, increased plasma and CVS may be associated with the insufficient increase and persistence of COMT expression.

Keywords Cerebral vasospasm · COMT · Subarachnoid hemorrhage

Introduction

Cerebral vasospasm (CVS) after subarachnoid hemorrhage (SAH) frequently results in severe cerebral ischemia and other brain injuries and is the main cause of aneurysm-related death or disability. Numerous studies have found that CVS after subarachnoid hemorrhage is associated with derangements in the metabolism of catecholamine (CA). Catechol-O-methyltransferase (COMT) is a rate-limiting enzyme in the degradation of CA. However, there have been no previous reports on the association of COMT and derangements in the metabolisms of CA after SAH. In the present study, we investigated the expression of COMT after SAH and explored the mechanisms for the development of CVS following SAH in rats.

Materials and Methods

Animals and Experimental Groups

A total of 66 rats were randomized into three groups, the normal group (n = 6), sham group (n = 30), and SAH group (n = 30). Rats in the sham group and SAH group were

Z. He, X. Sun (✉), and Z. Guo
Department of Neurosurgery, First Affiliated Hospital of Chongqing Medical University, Chongqing, People's Republic of China
e-mail: sunxch1445@gmail.com

J.H. Zhang
Department of Neurosurgery, Loma Linda University, Loma Linda, CA, USA

sacrificed at five different time points such as 6, 12, 24, 48, and 72 h (n = 6 rats for each time point). Rats in the sham group only received drilling and cannulation. The SAH group was administered with 0.15 ml/100 g body weight of autologous arterial blood.

Induction of SAH

According to the model described previously [1] reported, the rats were anesthetized intraperitoneally with 1% chloral hydrate (40 mg/kg). Aseptic techniques were used in the surgery. The right femoral artery was exposed and indwelling ligature was made. The animals were fixed in a stereotaxic frame to maintain the head in the horizontal position. A mid sagittal incision was made and after the periosteum was bluntly dissected, a hole with a diameter of 1 mm was drilled with an electric dental drill 5 mm anterior to the bregma and 3 mm from the mid sagittal line. The dura mater was carefully punctured and a PE10 fine cannula was advanced close to the subarachnoid space at the anterior cranial fossa to the circle of Willise, and the depth of the cannula was 1 cm in depth. After the presence of the cannula in the subarachnoid space was confirmed by the flowing out of colorless cerebrospinal fluid through the connecting syringe, blood was withdrawn from the femoral artery and 0.3 ml (0.15 ml/100 g body weight) of nonheparinized autologous arterial blood was slowly injected into the subarachnoid space within 30 s. Then, the cannula was removed and the hole in the skull was closed with tissue glue followed by suturing of the incision. The rats were maintained in a head down position for 30 min.

Collection of Samples for HE Staining

Three rats from each group were sacrificed after anesthesia intraperitoneally with 3.5% chloral hydrate (1 ml/100 g body weight) at predetermined time points for HE staining. After the chest was opened and the ascending aorta was cannulated, rapid flushing with normal saline was carried out followed by infusion of 400 ml 4% formaldehyde/0.1M PBS solution (4°C, pH 7.4). After the skull was opened, brain tissues and the brain stem (along with the basilar artery) was removed and then fixed in 4% formaldehyde/0.1M PBS solution at 4°C for 24 h followed by dehydration and embedding with paraffin.

Collection of Samples for High Performance Liquid Chromatography (HPLC), RT-PCR and Western Blot Analysis

Three rats from each group were decapitated after anesthesia intraperitoneally with 3.5% chloral hydrate (1 ml/100 g body weight) at preset time points for high performance liquid chromatography (HPLC), RT-PCR, and Western blotting. Blood was withdrawn and after centrifugation plasma was stored at −80°C for HPLC. After the skull was opened, the striatum was rapidly removed and snap frozen in liquid nitrogen and stored at −80°C for RT-PCR and Western blotting.

Reverse Transcription Polymerase Chain Reaction

The sequences of the primers for COMT and the internal reference GAPDH were from the published rat cDNA sequences in the NCBI Gene Bank (Synthesized by Shanghai Sangon Biological Engineering Technology & Service Limited Company). The concentration of primers was 10 μmol/L (Table 1).

Total RNA was extracted using Trizol reagents and the purity and concentration of RNA was determined. RT-PCR reaction system: 5 × RT Buffer, 4 μl; Oligo(Dt), 1.0 μl; dNTP mix(10 mmol/l), 2 μl; RNase Inhibitor (40 U/μl), 0.5 μl; RNA Ace, 0.5 μl; RNase Free dH$_2$O, 2 μl. Five microliter of PCR product in 1 μl of loading buffer was used for agarose gel electrophoresis (5 V/cm for 2 h) and were visualized under UV light. The absolute integrated optical density (IOD) of each band was determined using the GEL-PRO gel image analysis system and semi-quantitatively analyzed.

Western Blot Analysis

Brain tissues (100 mg) were homogenized in a homogenizer containing liquid nitrogen and were incubated with 0.5–1 ml of lysis buffer (Tris-HCL 50 mmoL/L PH 7.4, Nacl 150 mmoL/L, NP-40 and Triton-x-100 1%, EDTA 1 mmoL/L, PMSF 1 mmoL/L and 3 protease inhibitor) for 20–30 min on ice. Then, the lysate was mixed with loading buffer (1:1) for incubation at 100°C for 3–5 min. The mixture was centrifuged at 12,000 rpm (13,400 × g) for 15 min (4°C). The supernatant was obtained and its protein concen-

Table 1 The sequences of the primers for COMT and the internal reference GAPDH

Gene	Forward primer	Reverse primer	Length (BP)
COMT	5′CCTCCTCCTGCTCTTGCGACAC 3′	5′CTTTCGCGTCACCCACATTCA 3′	230
GAPDH	5′ACCCATCACCATCTTCCAGGAG 3′	5′GAAGGGGCGGAGATGATGAC 3′	159

tration was determined using the BCA method. The samples were aliquoted and stored at 80°C. Fifteen percent resolving gel and 5% stacking gel were prepared, and 80 μg of protein was resolved by sodium dodecyl sulfate polyacrylamide gel electrophoresis (SDS–PAGE) at 80 V through the stacking gel and at 120 V through the separating gel. After the gel transfer system was properly set up, electrophoretic transfer was performed at 100 V for 2 h. Then, the NC membrane was blocked with blocking buffer (non-fat milk, 0.5 g; TBS, 10 ml) for 2 h under continuous shaking at RT followed by three rinses with TBST for 10 min each. Primary antibody against COMT was appropriately diluted (1:700) and incubated with the membrane for 2 h under shaking at RT followed by three rinses with TBST (10 min × 3). Subsequently, the membrane was incubated with the goat anti-rabbit secondary antibody (1:700) for 2 h under shaking at RT followed by three rinses with TBST (10 min × 3). Then, developing solution was prepared by mixing solution A and B in a 1:1 ratio (PIERCE, Use 0.125 ml Working Solution per cm^2 of membrane)and a gel imaging system and Quangtity one software were used to analyze the results. β-actin was used as control.

Detection of CA with HPLC (Electrochemistry Method)

One milliliter of plasma was mixed with 0.1% perchloric acid and the mixture then was centrifuged at 3,500 rmp for 5 min. The supernatant was obtained, which then was mixed with 2 ml of H$_2$O, 2 ml of Tris HCl and 40 mg of aluminium sesquioxide for 5 min followed by centrifugation at 3,500 rmp for 5 min. The supernatant was removed and the pellet was rinsed twice with 2 ml of H$_2$O. Finally, the pellet was mixed with 100 ml 0.1 mol/l HCl and vortexed briefly, which was subsequently centrifuged at 3,500 rmp for 5 min. The supernatant (20 μl) was obtained for analysis. HPLC (ESA CoulArray 5600A) and MD-150 column were used; the mobile phase was 60 mM NaH$_2$PO$_2$, 1.5 mM sodium caprylyl sulfonate, 50 μM EDTA, 9% acetonitrile (pH 3.5). The voltage was −100 mV for channel 1, 50 mV for channel 2 and 250 mV for channel 3.

Morphological Analysis and Measurement of the Diameter and Wall Thickness of the Basilar Artery

The tissues were consecutively cut into 5 μm sections for HE staining. Paraffin sections were routinely deparaffined with xylene and gradient dehydration with alcohol was performed. Then, the sections were stained with alum hematoxylin for 8 min followed by treatment with 2% hydrochloride alcohol for several seconds. Subsequently, the sections were counterstained with 0.5–1% eosin for 3 min followed by gradient dehydration with alcohol for 6 min. Treatment with xylene for 5 min and the sections were covered with cover slip using neutral balsam. The maximal and minimal internal diameters of the basilar artery were measured microscopically as described by Oruckqptan et al. [2] (×100). The thickness of the basilar artery wall was measured under a higher magnification (×400): Thickness of the basilar artery wall = thickness$_{intima}$ + thickness$_{tunica\ media}$.

Statistical Analysis

Data were presented as Mean ± SD, all the measurement data were statistically analyzed using SPSS 13.0 software (SPSS, USA), Statistical analysis was performed using variance analysis; $P < 0.05$ was considered statistically significant.

Results

The Expression of COMT mRNA

The COMT mRNA content in the rat striatum of different groups was as follows: (1) Normal group: COMT-mRNA was observed. (2) Sham group: 6 h after sham surgery, the expression of COMT mRNA began to increase, which reached a maximum 24 h after injury and subsequently decreased. However, no significant difference was noted ($P > 0.05$). (3) SAH group: Compared with the other two groups, the expression of COMT mRNA in the rat striatum of the SAH group was significantly increased 6 h after surgery ($P < 0.01$) and peaked 12 h after injury ($P < 0.01$) followed by a decrease at 24 h after injury ($P < 0.01$). However, the COMT mRNA content was still higher at 48 h after SAH ($P < 0.01$) compared with that of the normal group and sham group at the corresponding time points. It nearly reached the normal level 72 h after injury and no significant difference was observed between the SAH group and the normal group or sham group at this time point ($P > 0.05$) (Fig. 1).

The Expression of COMT Protein

The expression of COMT protein in the rat striatum of different groups was as follows: (1) Normal group: COMT was expressed. (2) Sham group: the expression of COMT began to increase 6 h after surgery and reached a maximum

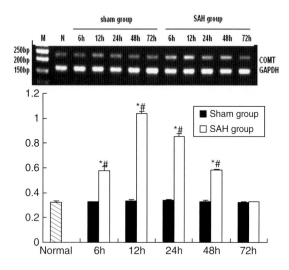

Fig. 1 Compared with normal and sham groups, COMT-mRNA expression in SAH group was significantly increased 6 h after surgery and peaked 12 h after injury followed by a decrease at 24 h after injury, it was still higher at 48 h after SAH and nearly reached the normal level 72 h after injury. (n = 3 for each group, *: P < 0.01 vs. control group; #: P < 0.01 vs. sham operation group)

at 24 h after injury, which then decreased. However, no significant difference was found in the expression of COMT between the sham group and normal group at the corresponding time points (P > 0.05). (3) SAH group: Compared with that of the normal group and sham group, the expression of COMT in the SAH group began to increase as early as 6 h after injury (P < 0.01) and peaked 12 h after SAH (P < 0.01) followed by a decrease 24 h after injury (P < 0.01). However, 48 h after SAH, the expression of COMT was still higher than that in the sham group and normal group (P < 0.01). At 72 h after SAH, the expression of COMT nearly reached the normal level, which was not different from that in the normal group and sham group at the same time points (P > 0.05) (Fig. 2).

The Content of Plasma CA

The plasma content of norepinephrine (NE), epinephrine (E) and dopamine (DA) started to increase 6 h after surgery and reached a maximum at 24 h. Then they gradually decreased. However, significant difference was not noted in these parameters between the normal group and sham group (P > 0.05). In the SAH group, the plasma content of NE, E and DA increased 6 h after surgery and peaked 24 h after injury, which then gradually decreased. However, 72 h after SAH, they were still at a higher level than that of the normal group and sham group at the corresponding time points. Significant difference was observed between the SAH group and the

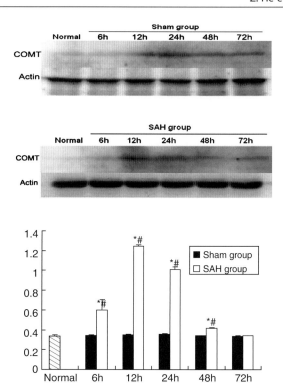

Fig. 2 Compared with normal and sham groups, COMT protein expression in SAH group began to increase as early as 6 h after surgery and peaked 12 h after SAH followed by a decrease at 24 h after injury, it was still higher at 48 h after SAH and nearly reached the normal level 72 h after injury. (n = 3 for each group, *:P < 0.01 vs. control group; #: P < 0.01 vs. sham operation group)

sham group or the normal group at different time points (P < 0.01) (Fig. 3).

Morphology and Measurements of Basilar Artery

(1) Normal group: the intima of the basilar artery was smooth and no fold was found in the internal elastic membrane. The smooth muscle cells were orderly arranged and the adventitia were thin. (2) Sham group: no significant difference was found between the normal group and sham group in the morphology, diameter, and wall thickness of the basilar artery (P > 0.05). (3) SAH group: Compared with that of the normal group and sham group, the diameter of the basilar artery started to decrease and the wall thickness increased 6 h after SAH. However, no difference was found among these groups (P > 0.05). Twelve hours after SAH, the diameter of the basilar artery continued to decline and the wall thickness of the artery further increased, which became more evident 24 h after injury (P < 0.01) and lasted until 48 h after injury

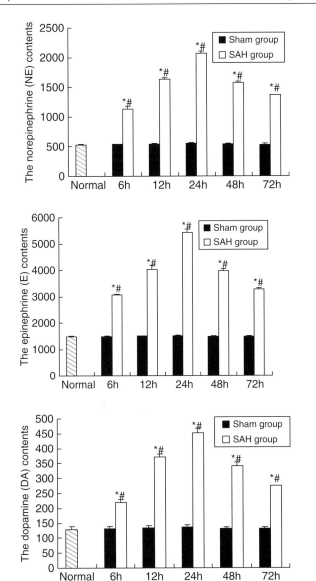

Fig. 3 In the SAH group, the plasma content of NE, E and DA increased 6 h after surgery and peaked 24 h after injury, which then gradually decreased. However, 72 h after SAH, they were still at a higher level than that of the normal group and sham group at the corresponding time points. (n = 3 for each group, *: P < 0.01 vs. control group; #: P < 0.01 vs. sham operation group)

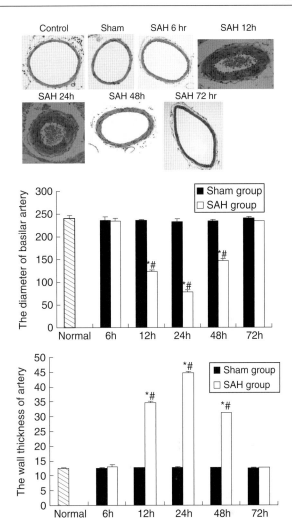

Fig. 4 Compared with normal group and sham group, the diameter of the basilar artery started to decrease and the wall thickness increased 6 h after SAH, 12 h after SAH, the diameter of basilar artery continued to decline and the wall thickness of artery further increased, which became more evident 24 h after injury and lasted until 48 h after injury, At 72 h after SAH, the diameter and wall thickness of the basilar artery were almost normal in size. (n = 3 for each group, *: P < 0.01 vs. control group; #: P < 0.01 vs. sham operation group)

(P < 0.01). At 72 h after SAH, the diameter and wall thickness of the basilar artery were almost normal in size (P > 0.05) (Fig. 4).

Conclusion

CVS after aneurysmal subarachnoid hemorrhage frequently causes severe cerebral ischemia and other brain damages. It is the predominant cause of death or disability by aneurysm rupture [3, 4]. According to the statistics, the mortality of patients with SAH is extremely high in the early stage: approximately 12% of patients die before treatment and 25% of patients with SAH die within 24 h after the onset of SAH [5].

"Dual-phase phenomenon" has been observed in CVS after SAH: early (acute) CVS and delayed (chronic) CVS [6]. Once delayed CVS occurs after SAH, damages to the vessel wall and brain tissues have become irreversible and the spasmodic vessels have lost the ability to dilate in response to vasodilators [6]. To date, no completely effective therapeutic interventions are available to alleviate delayed CVS and attenuate the extent of brain injury caused by delayed CVS. A significant portion of patients with SAH fail to recover from neurological dysfunction or even succumb to the disease [7, 8]. Early CVS affects the occurrence and development of delayed CVS [9]. It has been observed that early brain injury (EBI) after SAH is the main cause of death induced by SAH. However, no pathological changes are noted in vascular smooth muscles in the early stage of CVS when vasodilators are still effective. Therefore, the mechanisms by which vasoconstriction occurs in the early stage of SAH and subsequent EBI have recently become a focus of many research efforts.

CA is a metabolite with extensive biological activities [10–13]. Numerous studies have found that the production of CA is dramatically increased after SAH and it could induce CVS by (a) its vasoactive effects [14]; (b) induction of calcium overload in neurons [15]; (c) induction of apoptosis [16, 17]; (d) promoting the production of free radicals [18]; and (e) increasing the toxic effects of excitatory amino acids [19].

In the metabolic pathway of CA, the tyrosine hydroxylase (TH) and dopamine-β-hydroxylase (DβH) are the main rate-limiting enzymes in the synthesis of CA. Recent studies indicated that the expression of TH in rat hippocampus significantly increased 7–24 h after transient forebrain ischemia in a time dependent manner [20]. After traumatic brain injury, the expression and activity of TH and the content of DA and NE were dramatically increased [21]. Therefore, it has been postulated that the increased activity of TH was closely related with the increased content of CA after cerebral ischemia and traumatic brain injury. Clinical investigations suggested that the activity of DβH in the peripheral blood was markedly elevated after SAH and reached a maximum at 48 h after injury, which then gradually decreased within 2 weeks [22]. Recent studies indicated that the content of DβH in the hypothalamus and brainstem of rabbits with SAH was significantly elevated when compared with that of the control group and the basilar artery spasm was more severe than that in the control group [23]. The results also suggested a positive correlation between the severity of basilar artery spasm and the content of DβH in the hypothalamus and brainstem. Thus, DβH may play an important role in the pathogenesis of CVS after SAH.

COMT is a rate-limiting enzyme in the degradation of CA. Under the catalysis of magnesium, the enzyme introduces a methyl group to CA, which is donated by S-adenosyl methionine (SAM) to produce 3-methoxy-4-hydroxy derivatives resulting in the activation of CA or inactivation of toxic effects of CA [24].

Based on the analysis of the metabolic pathway of CA, the activity of COMT may be associated with the content of CA. Increased activity may lead to elevated inactivation of CA, reducing the severity of CVS. Other studies found that the expression of COMT was markedly decreased at different time points after pulmonary embolism, implying a decreased degradation of CA. Regional high concentration of CA may promote the contraction of pulmonary vessels, resulting in reactive pulmonary hypertension [25]. Three to fourteen days after controlled cortical impact injury, the expression of COMT continuously increased, which was postulated to be associated with cognitive dysfunction and sluggishness [26]. To date, no studies have reported the relationship between the expression of COMT and the content of CA or CVS after SAH, and further studies are required.

Studies found that neurons in the striatum and prefrontal cortex are the main cells expressing COMT. The expression of COMT in neurons was higher than that in glial cells [27]. In the present study, we targeted the striatum to explore the expression of COMT.

Our study indicated that, compared with the normal group and sham group, the mRNA and protein expression of COMT began to increase at as early as 6 h after SAH ($P < 0.01$) and reached a maximum at 12 h ($P < 0.01$) followed by a decrease 24 h after injury ($P < 0.01$). The mRNA and protein expression of COMT remained at a high level 2 days after SAH when compared with that of the normal group and sham group at the corresponding time points ($P < 0.01$). Three days after SAH, the mRNA and protein expression of COMT nearly reached normal levels and no significant difference was observed when compared with the normal group and sham group at the same time point ($P > 0.05$). In the case of CA, it increased 6 h after SAH and reached the peak level 24 h after injury followed by a gradual decrease. However, the content of CA was still higher than that of the normal group and sham group at the corresponding time points. Significant difference was noted in the content of CA between the SAH group and the normal group or sham group at any time point ($P < 0.01$). Compared with the normal group and sham group, the basilar artery started to contract and the wall thickness of the artery increased 6 h after SAH. However, no significant difference was found ($P > 0.05$). Twelve hours after SAH, the contraction and increased thickness of the artery wall were aggravated, which was the most marked at 24 h after SAH ($P < 0.01$). Three days after SAH, the diameter and thickness nearly returned to normal levels ($P > 0.05$).

The present study suggested that SAH could induce the expression of COMT in rat striatum accompanied by CVS and increased CA. On the basis of the metabolic pathway of CA, we postulated that increased COMT levels promoted the degradation of CA. However, COMT overexpression could not completely degrade CA, which was substantially produced. Therefore, the severity of CVS at the early stage of SAH was not effectively resolved. Although elevated COMT levels after SAH played a role in the reduction of the severity of CVS in the early stage of SAH, its neuroprotective effects were insufficient. Fortunately, the irreversible damage to the vessels and the brain was not observed in the early stage of SAH during which vasodilator was applicable. Thus, the early stage of SAH may be a critical time point. We postulated that treatments that would increase the expression of COMT in the early stage of SAH may promote the degradation of CA and reduce the content of CA in the blood, leading to the reduction of CVS and the severity of EBI after SAH. These treatments may also delay or block the occurrence of and development into chronic CVS and improve the prognosis in patients with SAH.

Acknowledgement Financial support from the Nature Science Funds of Chongqing Science and Technology Committee (CSTC, 2008BB5219) is gratefully acknowledged.

Conflict of Interest Statement We declare that we have no conflict of interest.

References

1. Ansar S, Svendgaard NA, Edvinsson L. Neurokinin-1 receptor antagonism in a rat model of subarachnoid hemorrhage: prevention of upregulation of contractile ETB and 5-HT1B receptors and cerebral blood flow reduction. J Neurosurg. 2007;106(5):881–6.
2. Oruckaptan HH, Caner HH, Kilinc K, Ozgen T. No apparent role for neutrophils and neutrophil-derived myeloperoxidase in experimental subarachnoid haemorrhage and vasospasm: a preliminary study. Acta Neurochir (Wien). 2000;142(1):83–90.
3. Ferro JM, Canhão P, Peralta R. Update on subarachnoid haemorrhage. J Neurol. 2008;255(4):465–79.
4. Brisman JL, Eskridge JM, Newell DW. Neurointerventional treatment of vasospasm. Neurol Res. 2006;28(7):769–76.
5. Mayberg MR. Cerebral vasospasm. Neurosurg Clin N Am. 1998;9:615–27.
6. Shen Jian-Kang JK. The pathogenesis of cerebral vasospasm and its prevention and treatment. Int Cerebrovas Dis. 2006;14(7):481–93.
7. Otten ML, Mocco J, Connolly ES Jr, Solomon RA. A review of medical treatments of cerebral vasospasm. Neurol Res. 2008;30(5):444.
8. Cahill J, Zhang JH. Subarachnoid hemorrhage: is it time for a new direction? Stroke 2009;40(3 Suppl):S86–87.
9. Broderick JP, Brott TG, Duldner JE, Tomsick T, Leach A. Initial and recurrent bleeding are the major causes of death following subarachnoid hemorrhage. Stroke 1994;25(7):1342.
10. Solomon RA, McCormack BM, Lovitz RN, Swift DM, Hegemann MT. Elevation of brain norepinephrine concentration after experimental subarachnoid hemorrhage. Neurosurgery 1986;19(3):363–6.
11. McCormack BM, Swift DM, Hegemann MT, Solomon RA. Increased norepinephrine synthesis in the cerebral hemispheres of rats following subarachnoid hemorrhage. Brain Res. 1986;382(2):395–8.
12. Dilraj A, Botha JH, Rambiritch V, Miller R, van Dellen JR. Levels of catecholamine in plasma and cerebrospinal fluid in aneurysmal subarachnoid hemorrhage. Neurosurgery 1992;31(1):42–50.
13. Naredi S, Lambert G, Edén E, Zäll S, Runnerstam M, Rydenhag B, Friberg P. Increased sympathetic nervous activity in patients with nontraumatic subarachnoid hemorrhage. Stroke 2000;31:901–6.
14. Magnoni MS, Kobayashi H, Frattola L, Spano PF, Trabucchi M. Effect of common carotid occlusion on beta advenergic receptor function in cerebral microvessels. Stroke 1985;16(3):505–10.
15. Chung YH, Shin CM, Kim MJ, Cha CI. Enhanced expression of L-type Ca2+ channels in reactive astrocytes after ischemic injury in rats. Neurosci Lett. 2002;302(2):93–9.
16. Meguro T, Chen B, Lancon J, Zhang JH. Oxyhemoglobin induces caspase-mediated cell death in cerebral endothelial cells. J Neurochem. 2001;77(4):1128–35.
17. Meguro T, Chen B, Parent AD, Zhang JH. Caspase inhibitors attenuate oxyhemoglobin - induced apoptosis in endothelial cells. Stroke 2001;32(2): 561–6.
18. Delbarre B, Delbarre G, Rochat C, Calinon F. Effect of piribedil, a D-2 dopaminergic agonist, on dopamine, amino acid, and free radicals in gerbil brain after cerebral ischemia. Mol Chem Neuropathol. 1995;26(1):43–55.
19. Furukawa N, Arai N, Goshima Y, Miyamae T, Ohshima E, Suzuki F, et al. Endogenously released DOPA is a causal factor for glutamate release and resultant delayed neuronal cell death by transient ischemia in rat striata. J Neurochem. 2001;76(3):815–23.
20. Miyazaki H, Ono T, Okuma Y, Nagashima K, Nomura Y. Glial cell line-derived neurotrophic factor modulates ischemia-induced tyrosine hydroxylase expression in rat hippocampus. Eur J Neurosci. 2000;12(6):2032–8.
21. Kobori N, Clifton GL, Dash PK. Enhanced catecholamine synthesis in the prefrontal cortex after traumatic brain injury: implications for prefrontal dysfunction. J Neurotrauma. 2006;23(7):1094–102.
22. Abe N, Tominaga S, Ohta H, Kawakami H, Tagawa K, Suzuki T, et al. Changes in plasma dopamine-beta-hydroxylase activity in patients with acute subarachnoid hemorrhage. No To Shinkei. 1979;31(8):771–7.
23. Kovacic S, Bunc G, Ravnik J. Correspondence between the time course of cerebral vasospasm and the level of cerebral dopamine-beta-hydroxylase in rabbits. Auton Neurosci. 2006;130(1–2):28–31.
24. Männistö PT, Kaakkola S. Catechol-O-methyltransferase (COMT): biochemistry molecular biology, pharmacology, and clinical efficacy of the new selective COMT inhibitors. Pharmacol Rev. 1999;51(4):594–622.
25. Li S, Liu A, Ti X, Que H, Yang S, Zhang X, et al. Expression changes of metabolism-related enzymes in the lung tissues of rats with pulmonary embolism. Journal of Xi an Jiaotong University (Medical Sciences). 2006;27(6):529–32.
26. Redell JB, Dash PK. Traumatic brain injury stimulates hippocampal catechol-O-methyltransferase expression in microglia. Neurosci Lett. 2007;413(1):36–41.
27. Shirakawa T, Abe M, Oshima S, Mitome M, Oguchi H. Neuronal expression of catechol-O-methyltransferase mRNA in neonatal rat suprachiasmatic nucleus. Neuroreport 2004;15(87):1243–39.

Section VI: Clinical Manifestations of Subarachnoid Hemorrhage

Monitoring of the Inflammatory Response After Aneurysmal Subarachnoid Haemorrhage in the Clinical Setting: Review of Literature and Report of Preliminary Clinical Experience

C. Muroi, S. Mink, M. Seule, D. Bellut, J. Fandino, and E. Keller

Abstract *Background:* Clinical and experimental studies showed a marked inflammatory response in aneurysmal subarachnoid haemorrhage (SAH), and it has been proposed to play a key role in the development of cerebral vasospasm (CVS). Inflammatory response and occurrence of CVS may represent a common pathogenic pathway allowing point of care diagnostics of CVS. Therefore, monitoring of the inflammatory response might be useful in the daily clinical setting of an ICU. The aim of the current report is to give a summary about factors contributing to the complex pathophysiology of inflammatory response in SAH and to discuss possible monitoring modalities.

Methods: Review and analysis of the existing literature and definition of own study protocols.

Results: In cerebrospinal fluid, interleukin (IL)-6 has been found to be significantly higher in patients with CVS during the peri-vasospasm period. While systemic inflammatory response syndrome, high C-reactive protein levels and leukocyte counts has been linked with the occurrence of CVS, less has been reported about cytokines levels in the jugular bulb of the internal jugular vein and in the peripheral blood. Preliminary evaluation of own data suggests, that IL-6 values in the peripheral blood and the arterio-jugular differences of IL-6 are increased with the inflammatory response after SAH.

Conclusion: Monitoring of the inflammatory response, in particular IL-6, might be a useful tool for the daily clinical management of patients with SAH and CVS.

Keywords Cerebral vasospasm · Inflammatory response · Interleukin-6 · Subarachnoid haemorrhage

C. Muroi (✉)
Neurocritical Care Unit, University Hospital Zurich, Zurich, Switzerland
Department of Neurosurgery, Kantonsspital Aarau, Aarau, Switzerland
e-mail: carl.muroi@ksa.ch

D. Bellut
Department of Neurosurgery, University Hospital Zurich, Switzerland

S. Mink and E. Keller
Neurocritical Care Unit, University Hospital Zurich, Zurich, Switzerland

M. Seule
Neurocritical Care Unit, University Hospital Zurich, Zurich, Switzerland
Department of Neurosurgery, Kantonsspital St. Gallen, St. Gallen, Switzerland

J. Fandino
Department of Neurosurgery, Kantonsspital Aarau, Aarau, Switzerland

Introduction

Neuroinflammation has been proposed to play a key role in the development of cerebral vasospasm (CVS) in aneurysmal subarachnoid haemorrhage (SAH) [6, 9, 44, 49]. The more, an attenuation of CVS could be achieved by suppression of inflammatory components in experimental studies. These findings suggest that inflammatory response and occurrence of CVS represent a common pathogenic pathway. Therefore its monitoring might be useful in the daily clinical setting. The aim of the current report is (1) to give a short summary about factors contributing to the complex pathophysiology of inflammatory response in SAH and CVS, (2) to discuss possible monitoring modalities including own preliminary clinical experience.

SAH and Inflammatory Response, an Overview

There is increasing evidence that local inflammation of the central nervous system (CNS) is related to severity of illness, clinical outcome and occurrence of CVS [9, 49]. By the presence of a blood clot in the subarachnoid space and by

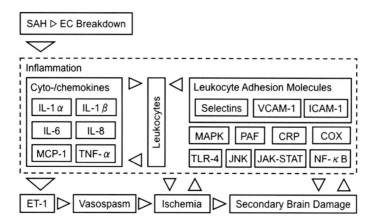

Fig. 1 Diagram showing inflammatory components, which has been reported in clinical and/or laboratory studies as contributors to the inflammatory response after SAH. *EC* erythrocyte; *IL* interleukin; *MCP* monocyte chemotactant protein; *TNF* tumor necrosis factor; *VCAM* vascular cell adhesion molecule; *ICAM* intracellular cell adhesion molecule; *MAPK* mitogen-activated protein kinase; *PAF* platelet-activating factor; *CRP* C-reactive proteine; *COX* cyclooxygenase; *TLR* toll-like receptor; *JNK* C-Jun N-terminal kinase; *JAK-STAT* Janus kinase-signal transducer and activator of transcription; *NF* nuclear factor; *ET* endothelin

the breakdown of erythrocytes, a complex series of cellular and molecular events is elicited triggering as well a local inflammatory response in the CNS as a systemic inflammatory response. Factors which are reported to contribute to the complex pathophysiology of inflammatory response after SAH are shown in Fig. 1. In the acute stages adhesion molecules are expressed, leading to leukocyte adherence at the endothelium with subsequent migration and activation. Capture and rolling are mediated primary by the selectins (L-, P- and E-selectins). Firm adhesion and diapedesis relies heavily on intracellular adhesion molecule (ICAM)-1 and vascular cell adhesion molecules (VCAM)-1 [9]. VCAM-1, ICAM-1, P- and E-selectin were found to be elevated as well in the cerebrospinal fluid (CSF) as in the serum of patients with SAH. To a certain extent, positive correlations with development of CVS could be observed [17, 21, 25, 30, 36, 43, 47]. Anti-adhesion strategies by blocking ICAM-1 or E-selectin showed a marked decrease of CVS in experimental studies [3, 5, 23, 39]. Leukocytes are critical constituents of the inflammatory response in terms of elaboration and propagation. Leukocytes produce a host of factors, especially cytokines, which further activate and propagate immune responses [51]. Some of the cytokines found to be related with development of CVS after SAH include tumour necrosis (TNF)-α, interleukin (IL)-1β, IL-1α, IL-6 and IL-8 [9, 10, 49]. In several clinical studies increased levels of these cytokines were found in the CSF of patients with SAH [13, 18, 19, 22, 27, 31, 32, 40, 51]. In particular high levels of IL-6 in the CSF have been linked with the occurrence of CVS and outcome [10, 13, 22, 27, 40]. In experimental studies, intracisteral IL-6 injection induced CVS and neutralizing IL-6 by antibodies showed a reduction of CVS [4, 40]. IL-6 is a pleiotropic cytokine and acts as an acute phase reactant [20]. Two best-described actions of IL-6 are triggering acute phase protein production by hepatocytes and mononuclear leukocyte activation. IL-6 may promote CVS by the involvement of cycloxigenase activation and/or activation of inflammatory cells to produce endothelin (ET)-1. However the exact mechanism how IL-6 may induce CVS is unclear. ET-1 can be declared as the primary suspect in the development and propagation of CVS [6, 9, 24, 49]. Levels of ET-1 are increased in CSF and serum in patients with SAH in close correlation with the development of CVS [11, 16, 50]. In a phase 2b randomized trial, a selective endothelin receptor antagonist significantly decreased CVS in a dose-dependent manner and showed a trend for reduction in CVS-related morbidity/mortality in patients with SAH [24]. The exact mechanism of ET-1 release and its origin is unclear. Substances that appear to stimulate ET-1 release include haemoglobin and inflammatory cytokines among others. Fassbender et al. showed that activated mononuclear cells in the CSF of patients with SAH produced ET-1 in parallel with inflammatory cytokines [11]. The fact that ET-1 production occurs by activated leukocytes with accompanying inflammatory response is suggestive that inflammatory response and occurrence of CVS by ET-1 release represent a common pathogenic pathway [9]. In more recent experimental studies, a couple of signal transduction pathways or transcription factors in the inflammatory cascade were found to be involved in the development of CVS [38, 41, 48, 53, 55, 56]. These factors contribute to the understanding of the pathophysiology and development of anti-inflammatory strategies. Less has been reported about the role of systemic IL-6 levels. Increased serum IL-6 levels among other inflammatory cytokines were found, however the levels were much lower compared to those in the CSF [7, 10, 18, 27, 31]. Therefore, inflammatory cytokines in the CSF, in particular IL-6, are assumed to be produced locally

Table 1 Overview of selected clinical studies with potential predictive inflammatory markers

Study (reference)	Parameter	Time of sampling	Criterion CVS	Results[a]
Fassbender et al. [10] (n = 35)	IL-6, TNF-α, IL-1β in CSF	d1–3, 5, 7, 9, 11	TCD > 210 cm/s	IL-6 higher d2, 3, 5, 9, 11; IL-1β higher on d2; TNF-α on d9[b]
Fountas et al. [12] (n = 41)	CRP in CSF and serum	Day 0–3, 5, 7, 9 after admission	Angio	Mean CRP higher in CSF and serum[b]
Gaeatni et al. [13] (n = 41)	IL-6, IL-8, MCP-1, E-Selectin in CSF	At time of surgery, n = 14 < 72h, n = 17 > d10	DIND + TCD > 160 cm/s + angio	IL-6 higher (only in patients with surgery <72 h): 2,520.7 ± 1,170.6 vs. 916.4 ± 382.2 pg/ml
Hirashima et al. [15] (n = 21)	IL-6, IL-1β, TNF-α, PAF in the jugular bulb	D0–4, d5–9, d10–14	DIND	PAF higher d5–9: 807 ± 815 vs. 111 ± 77 pg/ml[c]
Kim et al. [19] (n = 77)	MCP-1 in CSF and serum	D0–14	Angio	mean MCP-1 in CSF higher only in patients with H&H III: 3.66 ± 0.12 vs. 3.24 ± 0.16 log ng/ml
Kubo et al. [21] (n = 33)	ICAM-1, VCAM-1, E-selectin, P-selectin, hsCRP in serum	Day 0 and 7	DIND	ICAM-1 higher d0: 189.2 ± 67.4 vs. 96 ± 32.4 ng/ml; VCAM-1 higher d0: 381.3 ± 129.1 vs. 276 ± 89.4 ng/ml; hsCRP higher d0,7: 7,252.6 ± 10,115.9 vs. 363.6 ± 178.3, 34,651.5 ± 43,932.3 vs. 2,016 ± 929.3 ng/ml[c]
Kwon et al. [22] (n = 19)	IL-6, TNF-α, IL-1β in CSF	D0	Ischemia in CT d14 after SAH	IL-6 higher: 1207.20 ± 629.14 vs. 363.82 ± 544.45 pg/ml[c]
McGirt et al. [28] (n = 224)	Lc count systemic	n.a. (retrospective)	Angio, TCD > 180 cm/s or DIND	Higher peak Lc count <d5; largest difference d3; peak of 15 x 1,000 / ul with 3.3x increase in likelihood
Mocco et al. [30] (n = 158)	ICAM-1 in serum	On alternate day until day 12 after admission	TCD > 200 cm/s	Significant mean rate of rise in the peri-CVS period[b]
Niikawa et al. [35] 1997 (n = 103)	Lc and platelet counts systemic	D0–21 (retrospective)	n.a.	Lc count higher d3–5, 6–8, 9–11, 12–14: 11.8 ± 4.5 vs. 9.7 ± 3.8, 10.2 ± 3.1 vs. 8.4 ± 2.6, 10.8 ± 4.2 vs. 8.2 ± 2.9, 10.9 ± 4.5 vs. 8.8 ± 3.4[c]; platelet counts higher d0-21
Nissen et al. [36] (n = 36)	ICAM-1, VCAM-1, PECAM, E-selectin, P-selectin, L-selectin in serum	On alternate day until discharge	DIND + TCD > 120 cm/s	P-selectin higher: 149.5 ± 17.0 vs. 112.9 ± 8.1 ng/ml; L-selectin higher: 897.9 ± 53.6 vs. 633.8 ± 93.7 ng/ml
Osuka et al. [41] (n = 24)	IL-6, IL-8, IL-1β in CSF and serum	Day 0–3, 5, 7, 11, 14 after admission	n.a.	IL-6 in CSF higher at d5, 7; IL-8 in CSF higher d5[b]
Polin et al. [43] (n = 17)	E-selectin, ICAM-1, VCAM-1, L-selectin in CSF	D0,1 or 3	Angio	E-selectin higher: 19.86 ± 17.68 vs. 1.77 ± 0.93 ng/ml
Roethoerl et al. [46] (n = 88)	Lc count and CRP systemic	D1–8 (retrospective)	DIND	CRP higher d5, 6, 7, 8: 147.35 vs. 106.09, 160.75 vs. 104.75, 141.61 vs. 82.50, 123.25 vs. 69.30 mg/l; Lc count higher d4, 5, 6, 7: 12.98 vs. 10.39, 12.00 vs. 9.81, 12.23 vs. 9.31, 12.01 vs. 9.46 × 1,000/ul[d]
Roethoerl et al. [47] (n = 15)	ICAM-1, VCAM-1 in serum and CSF	Admisson to d9	TCD > 120 cm/s	Significant correlation between secondary increase of ICAM-1 and VCAM-1 and increased TCD[b]

n number of patients; *IL* interleukin; *TNF* tumor necrosis factor; *CSF* cerebrospinal fluid; *d* days after SAH; *SAH* aneurysmal subarachnoid haemorrhage; *TCD* transcranial Doppler sonography; *MCP* monocyte chemotactant protein; *PAF* platelet activating factor; *angio* angiography; *DIND* delayed ischemic neurological deficit; *CRP* C-reactive protein; *CVS* cerebral vasospasm; *ICAM* intracellular adhesion molecule; *VCAM* vascular cell adhesion molecule; *hs* high sensitivity; *H&H* Hunt and Hess grade; *Lc* Leukocyte; *n.a.* information not available; *PECAM* platelet-endothelial adhesion molecule

[a]Results with statistical significance only, values given as mean ±SEM
[b]No absolute values indicated
[c]Values given as mean ±SD
[d]SEM or SD not indicated

within the CNS. The origin and impact of systemic inflammatory cytokines in SAH is unclear. They might originate from the CNS through a disrupted blood-brain barrier and/or reflect a systemic inflammatory response. Naredei et al. evaluated the correlation between sympathetic activation and the systemic inflammatory response by sampling norepinephrine kinetic determination and measurement of inflammatory cytokines, including IL-6. The results showed a pronounced activation of sympathetic nervous system and inflammatory systems with a lack of significant association between them [33]. Systemic inflammatory response is a well-known phenomenon in several types of brain insults. Although the prognostic significance of systemic leukocytosis and fever in the outcome of patients with SAH has been recognized earlier [26, 34, 37, 42, 52], the relationship between systemic inflammatory response and occurrence of CVS is a relatively new observation. The prognostic significance of leukocytosis in the outcome has been already described in 1974 [34]. Further studies revealed increased serum leukocyte counts in patients who developed CVS [35, 52] and McGirt et al. described leukocytosis to be an independent risk factor for CVS [28]. Systemic inflammatory response syndrome (SIRS) [1], defined by a combination of clinical features, occurs in relation to a variety of severe clinical conditions including SAH. Patients with SIRS had significantly more CVS in the course than patients without SIRS [8, 54]. C-reactive protein (CRP) is a prototypical acute phase protein, highly sensitive (but less specific) for inflammatory response, produced by hepatocytes in response to IL-6 stimulus [20]. Clinical studies showed significant higher CRP levels in patients with CVS [12, 21, 46].

Monitoring of the Inflammatory Response in a Clinical Setting, Possible Modalities

The possible monitoring modalities are (1) Assessment of clinical parameters defining SIRS, (2) measurement of inflammatory markers in the CSF, (3) in the jugular bulb of the internal jugular vein and (4) in the peripheral blood. The assessment of SIRS is simple, however various different pathological conditions might make the assessment and interpretation of these variables difficult. Selected clinical studies concerning the measurement of inflammatory components are summarized in Table 1. Based on the literature, IL-6 in the CSF might be the most useful parameter. A point-of-care test for IL-6 in CSF using a lateral flow immunoassay chip-test has been recently described, allowing a bedside IL-6 measurement within 20 min [7]. However there is neither a cut-off value nor a reference range for IL-6 in the CSF defined yet. Further, patients with SAH may not always have CSF drainages in the pre- and peri-CVS period for sampling. Jugular blood oxymetry and the arterio-jugular lactate difference have been proposed as indicators of cerebral ischemia and prognosis [2, 14, 45]. Its sensitivities to detect focal cerebral ischemia by CVS may be limited. However measurement of inflammatory parameters from blood samples taken in the jugular bulb might be a useful tool [15, 29]. Reviewing the literature less is reported on inflammatory markers in the systemic blood. Given the fact that not all patients have a ventricular drainage, spinal tap and/or jugular bulb catheter, measurement of inflammatory cytokines in the peripheral blood would be the most practical approach. Own preliminary examinations show the practicability of daily monitoring of IL-6 levels in the peripheral and jugular venous blood for clinical use with indices for a specific course during the CVS phase. The secondary rise might be more distinctive in patients with CVS. Elevated arterio-jugular difference of IL-6 might be related with positive lactate indices later on. These patients may suffer from ischemia due to CVS.

Conclusion

Inflammatory response after SAH seems to represent a common pathogenic pathway with the occurrence of CVS. Reviewing the literature, monitoring of the compartmental inflammation of the CNS seems to be valuable, in particular measurement of IL-6. Since SIRS has been linked to the occurrence of CVS, monitoring of systemic inflammatory markers might be of interest. At the Neurocritical Care Unit, University Hospital Zurich, a study is going on with daily measurements of IL-6 in the peripheral and jugular venous blood to identify a characteristic pattern to detect CVS early before delayed ischemic neurological deficits are manifest.

Conflict of Interest Statement We declare that we have no conflict of interest.

References

1. American College of Chest Physicians/Society of Critical Care Medicine Consensus Conference. Definitions for sepsis and organ failure and guidelines for the use of innovative therapies in sepsis. Crit Care Med. 1992;20:864–74.
2. Artru F, Dailler F, Burel E, Bodonian C, Grousson S, Convert J, et al. Assessment of jugular blood oxygen and lactate indices for detection of cerebral ischemia and prognosis. J Neurosurg Anesthesiol. 2004;16:226–31.
3. Bavbek M, Polin R, Kwan AL, Arthur AS, Kassell NF, Lee KS. Monoclonal antibodies against ICAM-1 and CD18 attenuate cerebral vasospasm after experimental subarachnoid hemorrhage in rabbits. Stroke 1998;29:1930–5; discussion 1935–1936.

4. Bowman G, Dixit S, Bonneau RH, Chinchilli VM, Cockroft KM. Neutralizing antibody against interleukin-6 attenuates posthemorrhagic vasospasm in the rat femoral artery model. Neurosurgery 2004;54:719–25; discussion 725–16.
5. Clatterbuck RE, Gailloud P, Ogata L, Gebremariam A, Dietsch GN, Murphy KJ, et al. Prevention of cerebral vasospasm by a humanized anti-CD11/CD18 monoclonal antibody administered after experimental subarachnoid hemorrhage in nonhuman primates. J Neurosurg. 2003;99:376–82.
6. Crowley RW, Medel R, Kassell NF, Dumont AS. New insights into the causes and therapy of cerebral vasospasm following subarachnoid hemorrhage. Drug Discov Today. 2008;13:254–60.
7. Dengler J, Schefold JC, Graetz D, Meisel C, Splettstosser G, Volk HD, et al. Point-of-care testing for interleukin-6 in cerebro spinal fluid (CSF) after subarachnoid haemorrhage. Med Sci Monit. 2008;14:BR265–8.
8. Dhar R, Diringer MN. The burden of the systemic inflammatory response predicts vasospasm and outcome after subarachnoid hemorrhage. Neurocrit Care. 2008;8:404–12.
9. Dumont AS, Dumont RJ, Chow MM, Lin CL, Calisaneller T, Ley KF, et al. Cerebral vasospasm after subarachnoid hemorrhage: putative role of inflammation. Neurosurgery 2003;53:123–33.
10. Fassbender K, Hodapp B, Rossol S, Bertsch T, Schmeck J, Schutt S, et al. Inflammatory cytokines in subarachnoid haemorrhage: association with abnormal blood flow velocities in basal cerebral arteries. J Neurol Neurosurg Psychiatry. 2001;70:534–7.
11. Fassbender K, Hodapp B, Rossol S, Bertsch T, Schmeck J, Schutt S, et al. Endothelin-1 in subarachnoid hemorrhage: An acute-phase reactant produced by cerebrospinal fluid leukocytes. Stroke 2000;31:2971–5.
12. Fountas KN, Tasiou A, Kapsalaki EZ, Paterakis KN, Grigorian AA, Lee GP, et al. Serum and cerebrospinal fluid C-reactive protein levels as predictors of vasospasm in aneurysmal subarachnoid hemorrhage. Clinical article. Neurosurg Focus. 2009;26:E22.
13. Gaetani P, Tartara F, Pignatti P, Tancioni F, Rodriguez y Baena R, De Benedetti F. Cisternal CSF levels of cytokines after subarachnoid hemorrhage. Neurol Res. 1998;20:337–42.
14. Heran NS, Hentschel SJ, Toyota BD. Jugular bulb oximetry for prediction of vasospasm following subarachnoid hemorrhage. Can J Neurol Sci. 2004;31:80–6.
15. Hirashima Y, Nakamura S, Endo S, Kuwayama N, Naruse Y, Takaku A. Elevation of platelet activating factor, inflammatory cytokines, and coagulation factors in the internal jugular vein of patients with subarachnoid hemorrhage. Neurochem Res. 1997;22:1249–55.
16. Juvela S. Plasma endothelin concentrations after aneurysmal subarachnoid hemorrhage. J Neurosurg. 2000;92:390–400.
17. Kaynar MY, Tanriverdi T, Kafadar AM, Kacira T, Uzun H, Aydin S, et al. Detection of soluble intercellular adhesion molecule-1 and vascular cell adhesion molecule-1 in both cerebrospinal fluid and serum of patients after aneurysmal subarachnoid hemorrhage. J Neurosurg. 2004;101:1030–6.
18. Kikuchi T, Okuda Y, Kaito N, Abe T. Cytokine production in cerebrospinal fluid after subarachnoid haemorrhage. Neurol Res. 1995;17:106–8.
19. Kim GH, Kellner CP, Hahn DK, Desantis BM, Musabbir M, Starke RM, et al. Monocyte chemoattractant protein-1 predicts outcome and vasospasm following aneurysmal subarachnoid hemorrhage. J Neurosurg. 2008;109:38–43.
20. Kishimoto T. The biology of interleukin-6. Blood 1989;74:1–10.
21. Kubo Y, Ogasawara K, Kakino S, Kashimura H, Tomitsuka N, Sugawara A, et al. Serum inflammatory adhesion molecules and high-sensitivity C-reactive protein correlates with delayed ischemic neurologic deficits after subarachnoid hemorrhage. Surg Neurol. 2008;69:592–6; discussion 596.
22. Kwon KY, Jeon BC. Cytokine levels in cerebrospinal fluid and delayed ischemic deficits in patients with aneurysmal subarachnoid hemorrhage. J Korean Med Sci. 2001;16:774–80.
23. Lin CL, Dumont AS, Calisaneller T, Kwan AL, Hwong SL, Lee KS. Monoclonal antibody against E selectin attenuates subarachnoid hemorrhage-induced cerebral vasospasm. Surg Neurol. 2005;64:201–5; discussion 205–6.
24. Macdonald RL, Kassell NF, Mayer S, Ruefenacht D, Schmiedek P, Weidauer S, et al., : Conscious-Investigators. Clazosentan to overcome neurological ischemia and infarction occurring after subarachnoid hemorrhage (CONSCIOUS-1): randomized, double-blind, placebo-controlled phase 2 dose-finding trial. Stroke 2008;39:3015–21.
25. Mack WJ, Mocco J, Hoh DJ, Huang J, Choudhri TF, Kreiter KT, et al. Outcome prediction with serum intercellular adhesion molecule-1 levels after aneurysmal subarachnoid hemorrhage. J Neurosurg. 2002;96:71–5.
26. Maiuri F, Gallicchio B, Donati P, Carandente M. The blood leukocyte count and its prognostic significance in subarachnoid hemorrhage. J Neurosurg Sci. 1987;31:45–8.
27. Mathiesen T, Andersson B, Loftenius A, von Holst H. Increased interleukin-6 levels in cerebrospinal fluid following subarachnoid hemorrhage. J Neurosurg. 1993;78:562–7.
28. McGirt MJ, Mavropoulos JC, McGirt L, Alexander MJ, Friedman AH, Laskowitz DT, et al. Leukocytosis as an independent risk factor for cerebral vasospasm following aneurysmal subarachnoid hemorrhage. J Neurosurg. 2003;98:1222–6.
29. Menon DK, Day D, Kuc RE, Downie AJ, Chatfield DA, Davenport AP. Arteriojugular endothelin-1 gradients in aneurysmal subarachnoid haemorrhage. Clin Sci (Lond). 2002;103(Suppl 48):399S–403S.
30. Mocco J, Mack WJ, Kim GH, Lozier AP, Laufer I, Kreiter KT, et al. Rise in serum soluble intercellular adhesion molecule-1 levels with vasospasm following aneurysmal subarachnoid hemorrhage. J Neurosurg. 2002;97:537–41.
31. Muroi C, Frei K, El Beltagy M, Cesnulis E, Yonekawa Y, Keller E. Combined therapeutic hypothermia and barbiturate coma reduces interleukin-6 in the cerebrospinal fluid after aneurysmal subarachnoid hemorrhage. J Neurosurg Anesthesiol. 2008;20:193–8.
32. Nam DH, Kim JS, Hong SC, Lee WH, Lee JI, Shin HJ, et al. Expression of interleukin-1 beta in lipopolysaccharide stimulated monocytes derived from patients with aneurysmal subarachnoid hemorrhage is correlated with cerebral vasospasm. Neurosci Lett. 2001;312:41–4.
33. Naredi S, Lambert G, Friberg P, Zall S, Eden E, Rydenhag B, et al. Sympathetic activation and inflammatory response in patients with subarachnoid haemorrhage. Intensive Care Med. 2006;32:1955–61.
34. Neil-Dwyer G, Cruickshank J. The blood leukocyte count and its prognostic significance in subarachnoid hemorrhage. Brain 1974;97:79–86.
35. Niikawa S, Hara S, Ohe N, Miwa Y, Ohkuma A. Correlation between blood parameters and symptomatic vasospasm in subarachnoid hemorrhage patients. Neurol Med Chir (Tokyo). 1997;37:881–4; discussion 884–5.
36. Nissen JJ, Mantle D, Gregson B, Mendelow AD. Serum concentration of adhesion molecules in patients with delayed ischaemic neurological deficit after aneurysmal subarachnoid haemorrhage: the immunoglobulin and selectin superfamilies. J Neurol Neurosurg Psychiatry. 2001;71:329–33.
37. Oliveira-Filho J, Ezzeddine MA, Segal AZ, Buonanno FS, Chang Y, Ogilvy CS, et al. Fever in subarachnoid hemorrhage: relationship to vasospasm and outcome. Neurology 2001;56:1299–304.
38. Ono S, Date I, Onoda K, Shiota T, Ohmoto T, Ninomiya Y, et al. Decoy administration of NF-kappaB into the subarachnoid space for cerebral angiopathy. Hum Gene Ther. 1998;9:1003–11.

39. Oshiro EM, Hoffman PA, Dietsch GN, Watts MC, Pardoll DM, Tamargo RJ. Inhibition of experimental vasospasm with anti-intercellular adhesion molecule-1 monoclonal antibody in rats. Stroke 1997;28:2031–7; discussion 2037–8.
40. Osuka K, Suzuki Y, Tanazawa T, Hattori K, Yamamoto N, Takayasu M, et al. Interleukin-6 and development of vasospasm after subarachnoid haemorrhage. Acta Neurochir (Wien). 1998;140:943–51.
41. Osuka K, Watanabe Y, Yamauchi K, Nakazawa A, Usuda N, Tokuda M, et al. Activation of the JAK-STAT signaling pathway in the rat basilar artery after subarachnoid hemorrhage. Brain Res. 2006;1072:1–7.
42. Parkinson D, Stephensen S. Leukocytosis and subarachnoid hemorrhage. Surg Neurol. 1984;21:132–4.
43. Polin RS, Bavbek M, Shaffrey ME, Billups K, Bogaev CA, Kassell NF, et al. Detection of soluble E-selectin, ICAM-1, VCAM-1 and L-selectin in the cerebrospinal fluid of patients after subarachnoid hemorrhage. J Neurosurg. 1998;89:559–67.
44. Provencio JJ, Vora N. Subarachnoid hemorrhage and inflammation: bench to bedside and back. Semin Neurol. 2005;25:435–44.
45. Robertson CS, Narayan RK, Gokaslan ZL, Pahwa R, Grossman RG, Caram P Jr, et al. Cerebral arteriovenous oxygen difference as an estimate of cerebral blood flow in comatose patients. J Neurosurg. 1989;70:222–30.
46. Rothoerl RD, Axmann C, Pina AL, Woertgen C, Brawanski A. Possible role of the C-reactive protein and white blood cell count in the pathogenesis of cerebral vasospasm following aneurysmal subarachnoid hemorrhage. J Neurosurg Anesthesiol. 2006;18:68–72.
47. Rothoerl RD, Schebesch KM, Kubitza M, Woertgen C, Brawanski A, Pina AL. ICAM-1 and VCAM-1 expression following aneurysmal subarachnoid hemorrhage and their possible role in the pathophysiology of subsequent ischemic deficits. Cerebrovasc Dis. 2006;22:143–9.
48. Sasaki T, Kasuya H, Onda H, Sasahara A, Goto S, Hori T, et al. Role of p38 mitogen-activated protein kinase on cerebral vasospasm after subarachnoid hemorrhage. Stroke 2004;35:1466–70.
49. Sercombe R, Tran Dinh YR, Gomis P. Cerebrovascular inflammation following subarachnoid hemorrhage. Jpn J Pharmacol. 2002;88:227–49.
50. Suzuki R, Masaoka H, Hirata Y, Marumo F, Isotani E, Hirakawa K. The role of endothelin-1 in the origin of cerebral vasospasm in patients with aneurysmal subarachnoid hemorrhage. J Neurosurg. 1992;77:96–100.
51. Takizawa T, Tada T, Kitazawa K, Tanaka Y, Hongo K, Kameko M, et al. Inflammatory cytokine cascade released by leukocytes in cerebrospinal fluid after subarachnoid hemorrhage. Neurol Res. 2001;23:724–30.
52. Weir B, Disney L, Grace M, Roberts P. Daily trends in white blood cell count and temperature after subarachnoid hemorrhage from aneurysm. Neurosurgery 1989;25:161–5.
53. Yatsushige H, Yamaguchi M, Zhou C, Calvert JW, Zhang JH. Role of c-Jun N-terminal kinase in cerebral vasospasm after experimental subarachnoid hemorrhage. Stroke 2005;36:1538–43.
54. Yoshimoto Y, Tanaka Y, Hoya K. Acute systemic inflammatory response syndrome in subarachnoid hemorrhage. Stroke 2001;32:1989–93.
55. Zhou ML, Shi JX, Hang CH, Cheng HL, Qi XP, Mao L, et al. Potential contribution of nuclear factor-kappaB to cerebral vasospasm after experimental subarachnoid hemorrhage in rabbits. J Cereb Blood Flow Metab. 2007;27:1583–92.
56. Zhou ML, Wu W, Ding YS, Zhang FF, Hang CH, Wang HD, et al. Expression of Toll-like receptor 4 in the basilar artery after experimental subarachnoid hemorrhage in rabbits: a preliminary study. Brain Res. 2007;1173:110–16.

Perimesencephalic Subarachnoid Hemorrhage: Risk Factors, Clinical Presentations, and Outcome

Yuhan Kong, John H. Zhang, and Xinyue Qin

Abstract *Background:* Perimesencephalic nonaneurysmal subarachnoid hemorrhage (PNSH) appears to have an origin and natural history distinct from aneurysm rupture. However, the risk factors and complications of this pattern are still in debate. We performed a study with goals of comparing PNSH risk factors and clinical presentations with other sorts of spontaneous subarachnoid hemorrhages (SAH) and exhibit the PNSH outcome and prognosis.

Methods: Retrospective review of patients who experienced SAH between May 2006 and July 2008 in the First Affiliated Hospital of Chongqing Medical University was undertaken. Patients were categorized as perimesencephalic nonaneurysmal subarachnoid hemorrhage (PNSH), nonperimesencephalic nonaneurysmal subarachnoid hemorrhage (NPNSH), aneurismal subarachnoid hemorrhage (ASH), and uncertain SAH of which the patterns were not clear. The possible risk factors and clinical presentations within the three groups were used to proceed for statistical analysis.

Results: A total of 159 residents were identified. Among of them, 12 patients had the perimesencephalic pattern. Patients with PNSH showed less likelihood with the female ($P = 0.029$), alcohol consumption ($P = 0.033$), hypertensive ($P = 0.005$), diabetes ($P = 0.013$) or hyperlipidemia ($P = 0.034$) when compared with aneurismal SAH. The clinical presentations of this pattern showed less conscious disturbance ($P = 0.004$), vomiting ($P = 0.005$), or poor Hunt & Hess Grade ($P = 0.003$). There was one death among PNSH patients during 12 months mean follow-up.

Conclusions: Patients with PNSH present better clinical course than other forms of SAH, which could assist the diagnosis of this pattern. The moderate clinical course may suggest clinician apt to exclude aneurysm rupture. However, similar presents in remaining nonaneurysmal subarachnoid hemorrhage might suggest benign entities in other forms of nonaneurysmal subarachnoid hemorrhage.

Keywords Clinical presentations · Perimesencephalic subarachnoid hemorrhage (PNSH) · Risk factors

Introduction

Perimesencephalic subarachnoid hemorrhage (PNSH) is described as a benign entity of SAH for which computed tomographic (CT) imaging is characteristic, and the clinical course is much better than that of patients with aneurysmal subarachnoid hemorrhage [1]. In previous studies, patients with a perimesencephalic nonaneurysmal subarachnoid hemorrhage (PNSH) are not at risk for rebleeding in the earlier period after the initial bleeding and associated with an almost invariably excellent prognosis. Most of these patients recovered to their previous status [2–4]. About 21–68% of patients undergoing spontaneous SAH who present no signs of bleeding on a high quality four-vessel digital subtraction angiogram (DSA) are attributed to perimesencephalic pattern [5, 6].

In PNSH, the hemorrhage is confined anterior to the midbrain or pons, with or without extension of blood around the brainstem, into the suprasellar cistern, or into the basal part of the sylvian fissures, and no extension of blood to the anterior interhemispheric fissure and to the lateral sylvian fissure, except for a small amount of blood, with no evidence of intraventricular or intracerebral hemorrhage [7]. In this study, we performed a study with goals of exhibiting PNSH risk factors and clinical presentations with other sorts of spontaneous SAH in our district.

Y. Kong and X. Qin (✉)
Department of Neurology, the First Affiliated Hospital of Chongqing Medical University, Chongqing 400016, People's Republic of China
e-mail: qinxinyue@yahoo.com

J.H. Zhang
Department of Physiology and Pharmacology, Loma Linda University, Loma Linda CA, USA
Department of Neurosurgery, Loma Linda University, Loma Linda CA, USA
Department of Anesthesiology, Loma Linda University, Loma Linda CA, USA

Methods

Patients and Procedure

We reviewed all inpatients suffering from SAH between May 2006 and July 2008 in our hospital. An unenhanced CT scan or magnetic resonance imaging (MRI) was performed within 72 h after the onset in all cases. 64MDCT-angiography or DSA was performed once SAH diagnosis was defined. We collected information concerning the patients' demographics (age and sex) and clinical data (previous medical history, history of craniocerebral trauma, vital signs, severity and location of headache, neurological symptoms and signs). The severity of SAH was evaluated using the Hunt & Hess grading system [8].

Patients were categorized as perimesencephalic nonaneurysmal subarachnoid hemorrhage (PNSH), nonperimesencephalic nonaneurysmal subarachnoid hemorrhage (NPNSH), aneurismal subarachnoid hemorrhage (ASH), and uncertain SAH of which with technically defective angiographic results (without angiographic findings). Outcome was assessed in patients with PNSH at discharge from our hospital according to the Glasgow outcome scale (GOS) [9]. The Karnofsky Performance Scale Index [10] was used to assess the prognosis in PNSH patients. Traumatic SAH was excluded. We also excluded patients whose clinical data were not available.

Statistic Analysis

Clinical and demographic characteristics of PNSH patients were compared to other categories of SAH patients using Chi-squared test or Fisher's exact test (when cells have expected count <5) for categorical variables and Student's t-test for continuous variables.

Results

Of all the 159 cases that fulfilled the inclusion criteria, 112 patients with positive representation for SAH underwent both 64MDCT-angiography and DSA. 25 patients underwent only computed tomographic angiography (CTA). Seven patents rejected to perform angiography. 14 patients died of respiratory and circulatory failure, some of which combined with other diseases such as diabetes, uremia or hepatic inadequacy. Among the remaining cases, 96 had aneurysm rupture, 19 had nonaneurysmal hemorrhage but not of PNSH pattern, and 12 had PNSH. In the 32 cases who did not perform DSA, there was one negative of vascular lesion through CTA and had hemorrhage possibly in accordance with PNSH by radiographic standards. To avoid false negatives, it was not admitted in PNSH group for analysis.

Risk Factor

Patient demographics among SAH categories are presented in Table 1. Compared with nonaneurysmal SAH, there was no significance between PNSH and nonaneurysmal SAH. Whereas compared with aneurismal SAH, although there was no significance between ages, patients with PNSH

Table 1 Demographics for patients with subarachnoid hemorrhage[a]

	All SAH	PNSH	NPNSH	ASH	Uncertain SAH
Total (%)	159	12(7.5)	19(11.9)	96(60.4)	32(20.1)
Age, mean (range)	55.8(20–89)	49.1(22–73)	50.1(26–72)	55.5(32–73)	61.4(32–89)
Male–female ratio	1:1.1	3:1	2.2:1	1:1.4*	1:1.1
Current smoking[b]	68(42.8)	3(25.0)	7(36.8)	43(44.8)	15(46.9)
Drinker	65(40.9)	2(16.7)	6(31.6)	51(53.1)*	11(34.4)
Hypertensive	97(61.0)	2(16.7)	9(47.4)	65(67.7)**	21(65.6)
Diabetes	24(15.1)	0(0)	2(10.5)	17(17.7)	5(15.6)
COPD/Pulmonary infection	17(10.7)	0(0)	4(21.1)	8(8.3)	5(15.6)
Hyperlipidemia	36(22.6)	0(0)	3(15.8)	29(30.2)*	4(12.5)
Disturbance of blood coagulation	20(12.6)	2(16.7)	3(15.8)	12(12.5)	3(9.4)

Statistical analysis was proceeded between PNSH group and other groups (NPNSH and ASH). There's no significance between PNSH group and NPNSH group. Patients with PNSH were less likely to be female, drinker, hypertensive or hyperlipidemia compared to ASH group

[a]*SAH* subarachnoid hemorrhage, *PNSH* Perimesencephalic nonaneurysmal subarachnoid hemorrhage, *NPNSH* Nonperimesencephalic nonaneurysmal subarachnoid hemorrhage, *ASH* Aneurismal subarachnoid hemorrhage, Uncertain SAH (All cases absence of digital substration angiography)

[b]Current smoking was defined as any smoking within the previous 6 months

*When compared with PNSH, P value <0.05

**When compared with PNSH, P value <0.01

were less likely to be female ($P = 0.029$), alcohol consumption ($P = 0.033$), hypertensive ($P = 0.005$), diabetes ($P = 0.013$) or hyperlipidemia ($P = 0.034$).

Clinical Presentations

The frequency of clinical presentation among patients with PNSH and all other patients with SAH were compared in Table 2. Compared with nonaneurysmal SAH, patients with PNSH were less likely to suffer conscious disturbance ($P = 0.004$), vomiting ($P = 0.005$); when compared with aneurismal SAH, discrepancies were more prominent: conscious disturbance ($P = 0$) or poor Hunt & Hess Grade ($P = 0.003$), with a trend toward less neck rigidity ($P = 0.077$)

Clinical Course of PNSH

As revealed in Table 3, we exhibit details about the admitted patients with PNSH. In our study, these patients showed a low Hunt & Hess grade. There was no patient who died even undergoing with severe chronic renal failure at the same time. Moreover, there was no patient that presented hemiparesis or cranial nerve palsy, and no hydrocephalus occurred. Importantly, rebleeding did not occur, and repeated angiography did not reveal the source of bleeding in all patients. After 2 or 3 weeks, all patients were dismissed without a neurologic deficit (GOS 5). One death occurred among PNSH patients during a mean follow-up of 12 months. However, the cause of death was end-stage renal failure which was unrelated to SAH. The rest patients got 90–100 marks according to Karnofsky Performance Scale Index.

Discussion

Etiological Factor of Perimesencephalic Subarachnoid Hemorrhage

It was first raised by van Gijn et al. [11] in 1985 as a radiographic and exclusionary diagnosis. Since that time, referral-based studies on PNSH have confirmed the favorable prognosis and described it as a benign form of subarachnoid hemorrhage. Yet the etiology of this entity is still uncertain. In last century, researchers have failed to identify any source of hemorrhage in most cases, even with the aid of surgical exploration and autopsy [12]. Canhao et al. [13] postulated that cause of bleeding could be a minimal arterial leak from small perforating arteries in their subarachnoid course before entering the brainstem. This was supported by Maarten G. Lansberg a few years later. [14]. But venous origin is proposed as the most likely cause of perimesencephalic SAH [15, 16]. In recent years, Amjad Shad et al. [17] proposed that hypertensive venous rupture secondary to venous sinus stenosis as an alternative cause for PNSH. Haruki Yamakawa et al. [18] suggested that failure of longitudinal anastomoses between the primary primitive veins, as well as excessive strenuous exertion including components of the Valsalva maneuver, might be the cause.

Comparison of Prognosis Between PNSH and Others SAH Pattern

Subjects with PNSH had a significantly better in-hospital course (lower incidence of hydrocephalus, angiographic vasospasm) than those with non-PNSH. Rupture of an aneurysm is typically associated with significant morbidity and mortality. Evidence has become available that patients with an aneurysmal subarachnoid hemorrhage have a reduced life expectancy. Patients who survive the rupture of an aneurysm are often faced with a lengthy hospital stay that centers on hemodynamic monitoring, hyperdynamic therapy, and management of hydrocephalus, hyponatremia, and other complications [19]. Patients with aneurysmal subarachnoid hemorrhage are in danger of both new episodes of subarachnoid hemorrhage and cardiovascular disease [20]. But these are very uncommon in perimesencephalic SAH. A relatively large-scale study shows that patients with perimesencephalic

Table 2 Clinical presentations for patients with subarachnoid hemorrhage[a]

Symptoms/signs	PNSH (n = 12)	NPNSH (n = 19)	ASH (n = 96)
Sudden severe headache	12(100)	17(89.5)	87(90.6)
Conscious disturbance	0(0)	9(47.4)*	78(81.3)**
Vomiting	7(58.3)	10(52.6)	62(64.6)
Neck rigidity	8(66.7)	7(36.8)	84(87.5)
Dizziness	2(16.7)	5(26.3)	4(4.2)
Hemiparesis	0(0)	4(21.1)	15(15.6)
Cranial nerve palsies	0(0)	4(21.1)	18(18.8)
Poor Hunt & Hess Grade (4 or 5)	0(0)	2(10.5)	43(49.4)*

Statistical analysis is proceed between PNSH group and other groups (NPNSH and ASH) Patients with PNSH were less likely to suffer conscious disturbance compared to NPNSH group; when compared with aneurismal SAH, patients with PNSH were less likely to suffer conscious disturbance or poor Hunt &Hess Grade, with a trend toward less neck rigidity

[a] *PNSH* perimesencephalic nonaneurysmal subarachnoid hemorrhage; *NPNSH* nonperimesencephalic nonaneurysmal subarachnoid hemorrhage; *ASH* aneurismal subarachnoid hemorrhage

*When compared with PNSH, P value < 0.05

**When compared with PNSH, P value < 0.01

Table 3 PNSH patients' data

Patient No.	Age (year)/sex	Medical history	Presenting signs and symptoms	Hunt & Hess	Bleeding part on CT	DSA and CTA
1	57/F	NA	Thunderclap headache, Neck rigidity	II	Suprasellar cistern, Prepontine cistern	Negative
2	56/M	Smoking, Drinking	Sudden headache, Vomiting, Neck rigidity	I	Prepontine cistern, basal cistern	Negative
3	73/M	Hypertension, chronic renal failure, electrolyte disturbance	Severe thunderclap headaches, Vomiting, dizziness	II	Suprasellar cistern, quadrigeminal cistern, ambient cisterns, basal Sylvian fissure	Negative
4	33/M	Smoking	Sudden headache	I	Lateral Sylvian fissure Suprasellar cistern	Negative
5	63/M	Transient ischemic attack	Sudden headache, vomiting, neck rigidity	I	Suprasellar cistern, lateral Sylvian fissure	Negative
6	37/F	NA	Thunderclap headache, neck rigidity	II	Lateral Sylvius cistern, suprasellar cistern, ambient cisterns, quadrigeminal cistern, anterior interhemispheric fissure	Negative
7	20/M	NA	Sudden headache, febrility, vomiting	I	Basal cistern, prepontine cistern	Negative
8	58/M	Smoking, drinking	Thunderclap headache, neck rigidity	II	Suprasellar cistern, ambient cisterns, quadrigeminal cistern	Negative
9	21/M	NA	Sudden headache	I	Prepontine cistern, basal cistern	Negative
10	54/M	Hypertension, recent leg fracture	Severe headache, vomiting, neck rigidity	I	Suprasellar cistern, prepontine cistern	Negative
11	51/F	NA	Thunderclap headache, dizziness, vomiting, neck rigidity	II	Suprasellar cistern, ambient cisterns, lateral Sylvian fissure	Negative
12	66/M	Tuberculous pleurisy	Acute throbbing, headache, vomiting, neck rigidity	II	Suprasellar cistern, prepontine cistern, ambient cisterns	Negative

CTA computed tomography angiography; *DSA* digital subtraction angiogram; *F* female; *M* male; *NA* data not available

hemorrhage have no excess in mortality compared with the general population. Moreover, even on very long-term follow-up all patients regained independence for activities of daily life and no episodes of rebleeding occurred [21].

For other nonaneurysmal SAH, the incidence, clinical course, and outcome of patients with nonaneurysmal non-perimesencephalic SAH are not well described. In the study of Dong-Hun Kang et al. Nonaneurysmal SAH is categorized as Perimesencephalic non-aneurysmal SAH (PNSH), Diffuse-type non-aneurysmal SAH (DNSH) and Localized-type non-aneurysmal SAH (LNSH). They reported that both the PNSH and non-PNSH groups revealed similarly favorable long-term prognoses, which were confirmed by 3D-CTA at least 3 years after the onset of SAH. They proposed the hypothesis that benign prognosis for both PNSH and non-PNSH patients in limited circumstances [22, 23].

Value of Repeated Angiography

Nowadays, DSA is used as a reference standard to diagnose aneurysms. Some studies suggest that CTA might have a greater sensitivity for finding very small-sized aneurysms. To discover aneurysms of 5 mm or less, Conventional angiography requires ideal projection in order to visualize the aneurysm sac, but this cannot be obtained or is not routinely checked as a part of an aneurysm workup [24, 25]. As in PNSH, several studies have confirmed the high negative predictive value of computed tomographic angiography for aneurysm in patients with this condition and promote CTA alone as a conclusive diagnostic test to rule out aneurysms in patients with the classic perimesencephalic SAH pattern and clinical history [6, 26, 27]. Repeated angiography were considered low yield and superfluous in these patients [28, 29].

However, Topcuoglu et al. [30] assessed the diagnostic yield of imaging tests in 86 patients in whom the initial catheter angiography failed to reveal the cause of SAH. Forty-one of these had n-PMN SAH. In their study, three aneurysms were picked up on second angiography and one on third angiography, all in patients with n-PMN SAH. Repeated imaging studies were not fruitful in diagnosis in patients with PMN SAH. They advocated even a third DSA.

In our opinion, a second angiography is advocated. 64MDCT-angiography is helpful in detecting intracranial aneurysms with the forte of less discomfort and risks for the patients. It can be considered for the first line imaging technique. Because aneurysm rupture occasionally produces a PNSH-like pattern of bleeding [7] and many occult aneurysm scan be detected by repeated angiography, DSA continues to be recommended for those doubtful or negative CTA cases.

Conclusion

In general, our study showed a good clinical presents compared perimesencephalic subarachnoid hemorrhage with other forms of spontaneous subarachnoid hemorrhage. Perimesencephalic pattern might be less likely to affect females and incorporate with other diseases, which is in keeping with previous reports. Our study also showed a moderate clinical presentation which implied patients with this pattern of better outcome. The moderate clinical course may suggest clinician apt to exclude aneurysm rupture. Moreover, few differences of clinical presentation between perimesencephalic pattern and remaining nonaneurysmal subarachnoid hemorrhage suggest that other patterns of nonaneurysmal subarachnoid hemorrhage might be relatively benign entities, too.

Conflict of interest statement We declare that we have no conflict of interest.

References

1. Rinkel GJ, Wijdicks EF, Vermeulen M, Ramos LM, Tanghe HL, Hasan D, et al. Nonaneurysmal perimesencephalic subarachnoid hemorrhage: CT and MR patterns that differ from aneurysmal rupture. AJNR Am J Neuroradiol. 1991;12:829–34.
2. Rinkel GJ, Wijdicks EF, Vermeulen M, Hageman LM, Tans JT, van Gijn J. Outcome in perimesencephalic (nonaneurysmal) subarachnoid hemorrhage: a follow-up study in 37 patients. Neurology 1990;40:1130–2.
3. van Gijn J, Rinkel GJ. Subarachnoid hemorrhage: diagnosis, causes and management. Brain 2001;124(Pt 2):249–78.
4. Greebe P, Rinkel GJ. Life expectancy after perimesencephalic subarachnoid hemorrhage. Stroke 2007;38(4):1222–4.
5. Ildan F, Tuna M, Erman T, Gocer AI, Cetinalp E. Prognosis and prognostic factors in nonaneurysmal perimesencephalic hemorrhage: a follow-up study in 29 patients. Surg Neurol. 2002;57(3):160–5.
6. Kershenovich A, Rappaport ZH, Maimon S. Brain computed tomography angiographic scans as the sole diagnostic examination for excluding aneurysms in patients with perimesencephalic subarachnoid hemorrhage. Neurosurgery 2006;59(4):798–801.
7. Schwartz TH, Solomon RA. Perimesencephalic nonaneurysmal subarachnoid hemorrhage: review of the literature. Neurosurgery 1996;39:433–40.
8. Hunt WE, Hess RM. Surgical risk as related to time of intervention in the repair of intracranial aneurysm. J Neurosurg. 1968;28:14–20.
9. Jennett B, Bond M. Assessment of outcome after severe brain damage: a practical scale. Lancet 1975;1:480–4.
10. de Haan R, Aaronson A, Limburg M, Hewer RL, van Crevel H. Measuring quality of life in stroke. Stroke 1993;24:320–7.
11. van Gijn J, van Dongen KJ, Vermeulen M, Hijdra A. Perimesencephalic hemorrhage: a nonaneurysmal and benign form of subarachnoid hemorrhage. Neurology 1985;35:493–7.
12. Jafar JJ, Weiner HL. Surgery for angiographically occult cerebral aneurysms. J Neurosurg. 1993;79:674–9.
13. Canhao P, Falcao F, Pinho e Melo T, Ferro H, Ferro J. Vascular risk factors for perimesencephalic nonaneurysmal subarachnoid hemorrhage. J Neurol. 1999;246(6):492–6.
14. Maarten G. Lansberg. Concurrent presentation of perimesencephalic subarachnoid hemorrhage and ischemic stroke. J Stroke Cerebrovasc Dis. 2008;17:248–50.
15. Rinkel GJE, Wijdicks EFM, Hasan D, Kienstra GE, Franke CL, Hageman LM, et al. Outcome in patients 295 with subarachnoid hemorrhage and negative angiography according to pattern of hemorrhage on computed tomography. Lancet 1991;338:964–8.
16. Van der Schaaf IC, Velthuis BK, Gouw A, Rinkel GJ. Venous drainage in perimesencephalic hemorrhage. Stroke 2004;35:1614–8.
17. Shad A, Rourke TJ, Hamidian Jahromi A, Green AL. Straight sinus stenosis as a proposed cause of perimesencephalic non-aneurysmal haemorrhage. J Clin Neurosci. 2008;15:839–41.
18. Yamakawa H, Ohe N, Yano H, Yoshimura S, Iwama T. Venous drainage patterns in perimesencephalic nonaneurysmal subarachnoid hemorrhage. Clin Neurol Neurosurg. 2008;110:587–91.
19. Herrmann LL, Zabramski JM. Nonaneurysmal subarachnoid hemorrhage: a review of clinical course and outcome in two hemorrhage patterns. J Neurosci Nurs. 2007;39:135–42.
20. Ronkainen A, Niskanen M, Rinne J, Koivisto T, Hernesniemi J, Vapalahti M. Evidence for excess long-term mortality after treated subarachnoid hemorrhage. Stroke 2001;32:2850–3.
21. Greebe P, Rinkel GJ. Life expectancy after perimesencephalic subarachnoid hemorrhage. Stroke 2007;38:1222–24.
22. Kang DH, Park J, Lee SH, Park SH, Kim YS, Hamm IS. Does non-perimesencephalic type 315 non-aneurysmal subarachnoid hemorrhage have a benign prognosis? J Clin Neurosci. 2009;16:904–8.
23. Gupta SK, Gupta R, Khosla VK, Mohindra S, Chhabra R, Khandelwal N, et al. Nonaneurysmal nonperimesencephalic subarachnoid hemorrhage: is it a benign entity? Surg Neurol. 2009;71:566–72.
24. Dammert S, Krings T, Moller-Hartmann W, Ueffing E, Hans FJ, Willmes K, et al. Detection of intracranial aneurysms with multi-slice CT: comparison with conventional angiography. Neuroradiology 2004;46:427–34.
25. Karamessini MT, Kagadis GC, Petsas T, Karnabatidis D, Konstantinou D, Sakellaropoulos GC, et al. CT angiography with three dimensional techniques for the early diagnosis of intracranial aneurysm: comparison with intra-arterial DSA and the surgical findings. Eur J Radiol. 2004;49:212–23.
26. Ruigrok YM, Rinkel GJ, Buskens E, Velthuis BK, van Gijn J. Perimesencephalic hemorrhage and CT angiography: a decision analysis. Stroke 2000;31:2976–83.
27. Amir K, Zvi HR, Maimon S. Brain computed tomography angiographic scans as the sole diagnostic examination for excluding aneurysms in patients with perimesencephalic subarachnoid hemorrhage. Neurosurgery 2006;59:798–802.
28. Hashimoto H, Iida J, Hironaka Y, Okada M, Sakaki T. Use of spiral computerized tomography angiography in patients with subarachnoid hemorrhage in whom subtraction angiography did not reveal cerebral aneurysms. J Neurosurg. 2000;92:278–83.
29. Huttner HB, Hartmann M, Kohrmann M, Neher M, Stippich C, Hahnel S, et al. Repeated digital substraction angiography after perimesencephalic subarachnoid hemorrhage? J Neuroradiol. 2006;33:87–9.
30. Topcuoglu MA, Ogilvy CS, Carter BS, Buonanno FS, Koroshetz WJ, Singhal AB. Subarachnoid hemorrhage without evident cause on initial angiography studies: diagnostic yield of subsequent angiography and other neuroimaging tests. J Neurosurg. 2003;98:1235–40.

The Relationship Between IL-6 in CSF and Occurrence of Vasospasm After Subarachnoid Hemorrhage

W. Ni, Y.X. Gu, D.L. Song, B. Leng, P.L. Li, and Y. Mao

Abstract *Background:* It is hypothesized that inflammatory response after subarachnoid hemorrhage (SAH) may play a relevant role in the development and maintenance of vasospasm. This research investigated the correlation between IL-6 in cerebrospinal fluid (CSF) after SAH and the occurrence of vasospasm.

Methods: We analyzed both daily clinical manifestation and laboratory data of CSF in 46 patients who suffered from intracranial aneurismal subarachnoid hemorrhage during a period of 14 days, studied the relationship between the development of vasospasm and the quantities of the inflammatory factor, revealing potential power of IL-6 for predicting vasospasm detected by transcranial doppler (TCD).

Results: The incidence of vasospasm developed in 43.5% of the patients, with a mean onset of 6.1 ± 4.6 days after intracranial aneurysm treatment. Patients with vasospasm demonstrated statistically significant higher median values of IL-6$_{CSF}$ on Day 1, 2, 3, 5 and 7 ($P < 0.05$). The cut-off value is settled in 400 pg/ml on Day 3 after treatment. On the other hand, gender, Hunt & Hess scale (H&H) and Fisher scale of CT after SAH were proved to be the correlation factor with vasospasm.

Conclusion: IL-6$_{CSF}$ seems to be a reliable early marker for predicting vasospasm after subarachnoid hemorrhage on Days 3 after treatment before clinical onset.

Keywords Interleukin-6 · Subarachnoid hemorrhage · TCD · Vasospasm

---

W. Ni, Y.X. Gu (✉), D.L. Song, B. Leng, P.L. Li, and Y. Mao (✉)
Department of neurosurgery, Huashan Hospital, Fudan University, Shanghai, People's Republic of China
e-mail: Yingmao168@hotmail.com

Introduction

Vasospasm is one of the most important complications after the incidence of acute intracranial aneurysmal SAH. Several studies have focused on the inflammatory response, which may play a relevant role in the development and maintenance of vasospasm [1–4]. IL-6 is one of the inflammatory factor which has been focused by several randomized control trial [5, 6]. This research evaluated the relationship between IL-6 in cerebrospinal fluid and vasospasm/DCI quantitatively.

Clinical Material and Methods

Patients

Forty-six patients from neurosurgical intensive care unit NICU handled with the aneurysm by endovascular or clipping treatment within 72 h after aneurysmal SAH were enrolled into the research. Twenty-four patients were male; the other 22 patients were female. The range of age were 29–74 years old (54 ± 11 years old on average). Thirty-two patients of this group had smoking history. Hypertension was admitted in 26 patients.

Admission Condition

Forty-six patients were all admitted to Huashan hospital, Shanghai complaining of headache companied with nausea and vomiting. Twenty patients were unconscious or had an unconsciousness history in the course. All the patients were evaluated by Hunt–Hess scale. CT scan which was first time adopt after SAH was evaluated as an important index using Modified Fisher Grade Scale in this research [7]. The entire clinical conclusion was listed in Table 1.

Table 1 Baseline characteristics of patients

	With vasospasm	Without vasospasm	Significance
Mean age ± SD (range)	53 ± 6 year (42–65 year)	54 ± 11 year (29–74 year)	NS
Women	20%	69.20%	Significant (P < 0.01)
Hunt & Hess			Significant (P < 0.01)
1(%)	5(25%)	23(88.5%)	
2(%)	10(50%)	1(3.8%)	
3(%)	0	1(3.8%)	
4(%)	4(20%)	0	
5(%)	1(5%)	1(3.8%)	
Fisher Grade			Significant (P < 0.01)
2(%)	4(20%)	14(53.8%)	
3(%)	9(45%)	11(42.3%)	
4(%)	7(35%)	1(3.8%)	
Operation NS			
Craniotomy	10(50%)	17(65.4%)	
E.V.T	10(50%)	9(34.6%)	
GOS			Significant (P < 0.01)
1(%)	1(5%)	0	
2(%)	1(5%)	1(3.8%)	
3(%)	6(30%)	1(3.8%)	
4(%)	8(40%)	4(15.4%)	
5(%)	4(20%)	20(76.9%)	

Therapeutic Methods

All the patients were given aneurysm treatment in the supra-acute phase. Twenty-three patents among this group underwent aneurysm clipping exclusively, 21 patients accepted endovascular treatment exclusively. One patient receive endovascular treatment companied with aneurysm clipping. One patient underwent hematoma evacuation and cranial decompression after aneurysm embolization.

Test Methods

Lumbar drainage was placed on each patient for shunting of CSF, removing spasmogens that exist in the CSF and reducing the risk of vasospasm [8]. We strictly controlled the drainage height of Lumbar drainage between 15 and 20 cm and the volume around 150 ml, synchronously, collected cerebrospinal fluid about 10 ml at the same time just 1, 2, 3, 5, 7 days after treatment for aneurysm, sent 4 ml for regular and biochemical examination to evacuate the center-infected cases, 6 ml for centrifugation by Thermo (IEC MULTI-RF 84670188) centrifuge at 1,000 rpm/min under 5°C for 15 min, took 4 ml supernatant and sent to 80°C refrigerator for preservation. We used Elisa method (Shanghai Xi Tang Biology Technology Co. Ltd.) to measure the content degree of IL-6 2 months later and explored its relationship with vasospasm according to clinical data. TCD examination was conducted for them through temporal window [9], measuring blood flow velocity of bilateral M2 segment of middle cerebral artery at the same point before surgery, 1–3, 5–7, and 9–14 days after surgery, at the same time observed the occurrence of symptomatic vasospasm.

Result

In our group, the draining volume of lumbar drainage was 146.3 ± 17.5 ml on average. GOS scale was measured in all the discharging patients. Twenty patients were diagnosed as vasospasm among all 46 patients. The average occurrence time of vasospasm is 6.1d ± 4.6 after treatment. Eighteen of these 46 patients had symptoms, occupying 90% of vasospasm patients diagnosed by TCD. Eight patients of 18 vasospasm patients could be found new hypo-dense lesion in CT scan, 12 patients with psychiatric disorders, four patients with motor disability, and two patients with barylalia (Table 1).

We divided them into two subgroups on the criteria of vasospasm. Using Students' T test showed gender is a significant factor for the incidence of vasospasm. Male is in statistically higher risk of vasospasm than female (P < 0.01). On the other hand, using nonparametric test (rank sum test), we confirmed patients who are graded in lower H&H Grade and lower Fisher Scale revealed statistical significance for lower incidence rate of vasospasm than higher grade. Moreover, patients who were afflicted by developing vasospasm should spend more duration staying in hospital (P < 0.05) (Table 1).

Because all values for IL-6$_{CSF}$ are nonparametric distribution, the series of data are presented as the medians including interquartiles and ranges (Tables 2 and 3). The relationships between the median of the IL-6$_{CSF}$ on Days 1–7 for the two subgroups, which were clarified as "with or without vasospasm", were studied using binary logistic regression. Binary logistic regression revealed the value of IL-6 in patients suffering from vasospasm later is significantly higher than non-vasospasm for Day 1, 2, 3, 5, 7 (P = 0.008, 0.001, 0.001, 0.001, 0.001). After treatment, the phenomena of higher volume of IL-6 lasted at least 7 days (Fig. 1).

Next step showed determining cut-off value of IL-6 which can predict vasospasm as it turns out. Figure 2 displayed A.ROC of IL-6 in CSF on Days 1, 2, 3, 5, 7. The receiver operating characteristic of IL-6$_{CSF}$ on Days 1–7 is

Table 2 Time course of serial TCD measurements of patients with subarachnoid hemorrhage (n = 46)

Day Velocity (mm/s)	D-pre	D-1	D-2	D-3	D-5	D-6	D-7	D-9	D-10	D-11	D-12	D-13	D-14
Median TCD	83.3	91.5	93.5	91.3	91.0	93.3	92.0	90.5	89.8	88.0	87.0	84.0	83.5
Q1	66.0	73.9	74.3	78.8	74.0	76.9	73.4	75.9	73.9	73.3	71.8	70.8	70.0
Q3	98.0	108.6	106.9	111.6	113.6	118.3	120.0	118.1	113.5	108.5	107.1	104.5	99.0
Range	49–161	52.5–168	54.5–175	55.5–169	51–165	52.5–160.5	51.5–158.5	53.5–162.5	53.5–153.5	52.5–146	55–126.5	53.5–145.5	55.5–139.5

Table 3 Time course of serial measurements of IL-6 in cerebrospinal fluid (n = 46)

Day Unit(pg/ml)	D-1	D-2	D-3	D-5	D-7
Median	410.405	461.549	408.905	470.027	415.816
Q1	286.495	297.161	281.980	274.729	234.887
Q3	572.765	682.170	675.219	714.999	699.558
Min	101.553	106.969	114.513	124.675	100.690
Max	1,770.282	1,829.697	2,098.440	1,861.639	1,674.570

Table 4 Cut-off values for IL-6 in CSF with relative risk predicting occurrence of vasospasm after subarachnoid hemorrhage and 95% CI

	Relative Risk	Upper	Lower	sensitivity	specificity
Cut-off Day-1 400	3.00	1.31	6.89	75.00%	69.23%
Cut-off Day-2 400	8.25	2.16	31.55	90.00%	76.92%
Cut-off Day-3 200	–	–	–	100.00%	19.23%
Cut-off Day-3 400	7.56	1.98	28.89	90.00%	73.08%
Cut-off Day-3 600	4.71	2.44	9.10	65.00%	96.15%
Cut-off Day-3 800	3.17	1.98	5.06	40.00%	100.00%
Cut-off Day-3 1000	2.63	1.79	3.86	20.00%	100.00%
Cut-off Day-5 400	6.92	1.81	26.43	90.00%	69.23%
Cut-off Day-7 400	5.67	1.92	16.73	85.00%	73.08

shown, with the highest area under the curve for Day 3 of 0.913 (95% CI, 0.058–1.000). So we choose Day 3 to conduct the χ_2 analysis with the cut-off of IL-6 in 400, 600 and 800 pg/ml (Table 4). Finally we found when 400 pg /ml on Day 3 was chosen as the cut-off, the relative risk is increased to 7.56 (95% confidence interval [CI], 1.98–28.89). The positive predictive value is 72%, as the sensitivity is 90%, the specificity is 73.08% (Fig. 2).

Discussion

Post-subarachnoid hemorrhagic vasospasm is the major cause of morbidity and mortality. Many patients are made diagnosis definitely after ischemic syndrome has been severe and the pathogenetic condition is hard to change. How to predict the occurrence of vasospasm is the key point of the therapy for vasospasm. Fisher Scale is regarded as the effective predicting factor in prophase of SAH [10, 11]. The patients in higher Fisher Grade seem to take higher risk of vasospasm. This conclusion was also confirmed in our study.

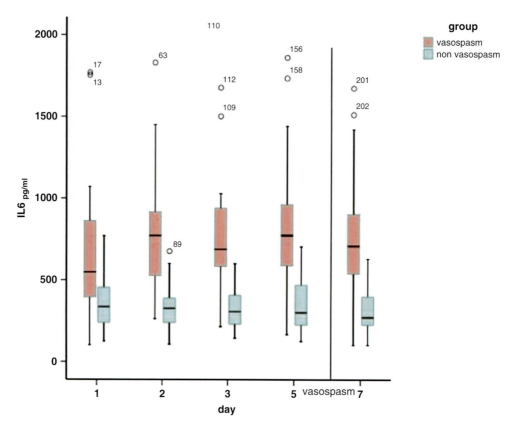

Fig. 1 Box plots of IL-6$_{CSF}$ in picograms per milliliter for patients with (*red boxes*) and without (*blue boxes*) vasospasm. Binary logistic regression revealed a statistically significance effect for Day 1, 2, 3, 5, 7 (P = 0.008, 0.001, 0.001, 0.001, 0.001, respectively)

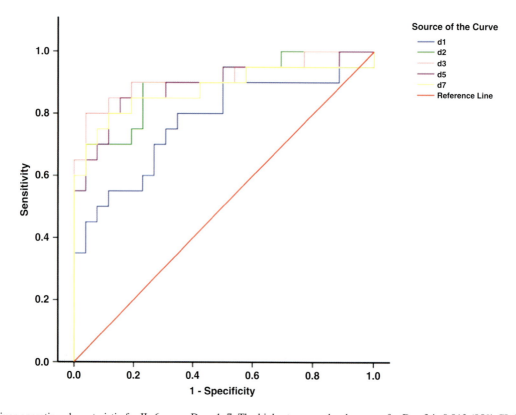

Fig. 2 Receiver operating characteristic for IL-6$_{CSF}$ on Days 1–7. The highest area under the curve for Day 3 is 0.913 (95% CI, 0.058–1.000)

TCD can detect vasospasm before clinical symptoms and give direction for further treatments as a non-invasive, bedside new-type facility reflecting the hemodynamic change in vessels.[7] Although positive predictive value remained low despite the adoption of restrictive criteria for vasospasm [12], TCD is also regarded as an important mean to detect vasospasm before advent of symptoms. Gonzalez used TCD to detect flow velocity of MCA through temporal windows for 68 patients who were confirmed as aneurysmal SAH, the detection rate reach to 81.1% in the symptomatic patients, accordingly 77.2% in those patients suffering vasospasm verdicted by angiogram when selecting 120 cm/s as the cut-off for vasospasm [13].

Past literatures have reported that IL-6 seems to be the potential predictive factor for vasospasm. Schoch et al. analyzed daily clinical data and laboratory tests of the cerebrospinal fluid (CSF) of 64 patients with mostly poor-grade subarachnoid hemorrhage during a period of 14 days and found that IL-6$_{CSF}$ seems to be a reliable early marker for predicting vasospasm after subarachnoid hemorrhage on Days 4 and 5 before clinical onset [5]. Hendryk et.al noted a statistically significant increase concentration of IL-6 in CSF only in the acute phase after SAH (Days 0–3) in patients in poor clinical condition, who are tend to take higher risk of vasospasm and cerebral ischemia later [14]. They considered this increase of ILs level in CSF is probably related to the intensity of the SAH, and secondarily aggravates the vasospasm and ischemic changes in the brain. In our study, 90 patients in good clinical condition in 46 patients, serial measurements of IL-6$_{CSF}$ with SAH also showed that median values of IL-6 $_{CSF}$ in patients developing vasospasm were statistically significantly higher than in patients without vasospasm from the first day after treatment. This result indicated IL-6 in CSF could swiftly increase for predicting vasospasm even if in patients in good clinical condition, concurred with the previous literature which reported that characteristic early responding of IL-6 after subarachnoid hemorrhage. Accordingly significant increase concentration of IL-6 in CSF for predicting vasospasm after acute aneurysmal subarachnoid hemorrhage can be generalized for all the patients regardless of their clinical condition.

The role of the inflammatory reaction to SAH in vasospasm has been studied. Fassbender et.al have proved that the increased secretion of IL-6 is positive correlated with the concentration of Endothelin-1(ET-1) [15]. Some researchers have reported that IL-6 can induce vasospasm by promoting the release of ET-1,motivating the overexpression of Angiotensin II type 1 (AT1) receptor and seems to be the antagonism against some vasodilatings such as prostaglandin I$_2$ [16–18].

We also found that gender may play a considerable role in the course of vasospasm. Although female has predilection for carrying aneurysm, no evidence supported that they take higher risk for aneurysm rupture event. Graf et al. has summarized the clinical data of vasospasm and found no obvious contrast between male (39.2% and female (39.4% in the incidence rate of vasospasm [19]. However, there are studies that reported injecting estradiol to treat with vasospasm can reduce the release of ET-1 and protect the expression of nitric-oxide synthase in normal endothelium to against vasospasm in male rat models of SAH [20, 21].

Through this research and the statistics of clinical data, we move a step forward to validate the increased IL-6 in cerebrospinal fluid can be used to predict cerebral vasospasm. However, because the patient with untreated aneurysm is regarded as the contraindication for lumber puncture, we had to place it after treatment. This observing point for vasospasm may make deflection for each patients taking treatment at the different time after SAH. Meanwhile, although IL-6 increased from the first day after operation, we could not find the fluctuation when vasospasm happened. So the exact power for IL-6$_{CSF}$ influencing on vasospasm remains controversial. Further conclusion depends on large sample randomized, double-blind controlled experiment.

Conclusion

We have found that the quantity contrast of IL-6 between patients with vasospasm and non-vasospasm occurred is statistically significant in the 1, 2, 3, 5, 7 days after treatment. The cut-off value is settled in 400 pg/ml on Day 3 after treatment. Therefore, monitoring value of IL-6 in cerebrospinal fluid on the third day after operation in patients with high Fisher grade is helpful for early diagnosis of vasospasm.

Acknowledgement This study was supported by No. 2006BAI01A12 from the National Key Technology R&D Program and No. 30700864 from the National Natural Science Foundation of China.

Conflict of interest statement We declare that we have no conflict of interest.

References

1. Gallia GL, Tamargo RJ. Leukocyte-endothelial cell interactions in chronic vasospasm after subarachnoid hemorrhage. Neurol Res. 2006;28(7):750–8.
2. Yuhei Y, Yoshihiro T, Katsumi H. Acute systemic inflammatory response syndrome in subarachnoid hemorrhage. Stroke 2001;32: 1989–93.
3. Aaron S, Dumont J, Michael D. Cerebral vasospasm after subarachnoid hemorrhage: putative role of inflammation. Neurosurgery 2003;53:123–35.

4. Sercombe R, Dinh Y, Gomis P. Cerebrovascular inflammation following subarachnoid hemorrhage. Jpn J Pharmacol. 2002;88: 227–49.
5. Schoch B, Regel JP, Wichert M. Analysis of intrathecal interleukin-6 as a potential predictive factor for vasospasm in subarachnoid hemorrhage. Neurosurgery 2007;60:828–36.
6. Dengler J, Schefold JC, Graetz D. Point-of-care testing for interleukin-6 in cerebro spinal fluid (CSF) after subarachnoid haemorrhage. Med Sci Monit. 2008;14:BR265–8.
7. Frontera JA, Claassen J, Schmidt JM, Wartenberg KE, Temes R, Connolly ES Jr, et al. Prediction of symptomatic vasospasm after subarachnoid hemorrhage: the modified fisher scale. Neurosurgery 2006;59(1):21–7; discussion 21–7.
8. Klimo P Jr, Kestle JR, MacDonald JD, Schmidt RH. Marked reduction of cerebral vasospasm with lumbar drainage of cerebrospinal fluid after subarachnoid hemorrhage. J Neurosurg. 2004;100(2):215–24.
9. Rigamonti A, Ackery A, Baker AJ. Transcranial Doppler monitoring in subarachnoid hemorrhage: a critical tool in critical care. Can J Anaesth. 2008;55(2):112–23.
10. Milojević T, Baljozović B, Rakić M. Cerebral vasospasm after subarachnoid hemorrhage. Acta Chir Iugosl. 2008;55:55–60.
11. Holling M, Jeibmann A, Gerss J, Fischer BR, Wassman H, Paulus W, et al. Prognostic value of histopathological findings in aneurysmal subarachnoid hemorrhage. J Neurosurg. 2009;110:487–91.
12. Lee JY, Lee MS, Whang K, Lee JM, Kim SH, Lee SS. Accuracy of transcranial Doppler sonography for predicting cerebral infarction in aneurysmal subarachnoid hemorrhage. J Clin Ultrasound. 2006;34(8):380–4.
13. Gonzalez N, Boscardin W, Glenn T, Vinuela F, Martin NA. Vasospasm probability index: a combination of transcranial doppler velocities, cerebral blood flow, and clinical risk factors to predict cerebral vasospasm after aneurysmal subarachnoid hemorrhage. Neurosurgery 2007;107:1101–12.
14. Hendryk S, Jarzab B, Josko J. Increase of the IL-1 beta and IL-6 levels in CSF in patients with vasospasm following aneurysmal SAH. Neuro Endocrinol Lett. 2004;25:141–7.
15. Fassbender K, Hodapp B, Rossol S, Bertsch T, Schmeck J, Schütt S, et al. Endothelin-1 in subarachnoid hemorrhage:An acute-phase reactant produced by cerebrospinal fluid leukocytes. Stroke 2000;31:2971–5.
16. Boesen E, Sasser J, Saleh M, Potter WA, Woods M, Warner TD, et al. Interleukin-1beta, but not interleukin-6, enhances renal and systemic endothelin production in vivo. Am J Physiol Renal Physiol. 2008;295:F446–53.
17. Wassmann S, Stumpf M, Strehlow K, Schmid A, Schieffer B, Böhm M, et al. Interleukin-6 induces oxidative stress and endothelial dysfunction by overexpression of the angiotensin II type 1 receptor. Circ Res. 2004;94(4):534–41.
18. Zhou W, Hashimoto K, Goleniewska K, O'Neal JF, Ji S, Blackwell TS, et al. Prostaglandin I_2 analogs inhibit proinflammatory cytokine production and T cell stimulatory function of dendritic cells. J Immunol. 2007;178:702–10.
19. Graf C, Nibbelink D. Cooperative study of intracranial aneurysms and subarachnoid hemorrhage. Stroke 1974;5:559–601.
20. Shih H, Lin C, Lee T, Lee WS, Hsu C. 17-beta-Estradiol inhibits subarachnoid hemorrhage-induced inducible nitric oxide synthase gene expression by interfering with the nuclear factor kappa B transactivation. Stroke 2006;37:3025–31.
21. Lin C, Dumont A, Su Y, Dai ZK, Cheng JT, Tsai YJ, et al. Attenuation of subarachnoid hemorrhage-induced apoptotic cell death with 17 beta-estradiol. J Neurosurg. 2009;111(5):1014–22.

Non-Aneurysm Subarachnoid Hemorrhage in Young Adults

Tianzhu Wang, John H. Zhang, and Xinyue Qin

Abstract *Objective:* The incidence of subarachnoid hemorrhage (SAH) in the young is increasing recently. Among the young patients, some of them do not have detectable aneurysms, so the cause of the disease may be non-aneurysmal. In this study, we analyzed some clinical cases of subarachnoid hemorrhage in young adults and discussed the possible causes other than present aneurysm and arteriovenous malformation (AVM).

Methods: We reviewed 11 patients with SAH below 45 years of age enrolled in our hospital from January 2007 to June 2008. Their clinical characteristics, imaging examination results were analyzed in details: nine patients were found with no obvious cause for their hemorrhage. Four of them were followed up for 1 year and the other three were followed up for half a year. We telephoned the seven patients to gain the information on their recovery by questionnaire.

Results: With an average onset age of 38 years old, all patients had similar symptoms and onset behavior according to their clinical characteristics. Based on the imaging results, two had confirmed vascular malformation; the other nine did not present detectable aneurysm or AVM, but with different morphological changes of their cerebral arteries. By 1-year or half-year follow-up, the seven patients were found to have good recovery.

Conclusion: Pathological changes of cerebral vessels due to smoking, genetic, or as an early version of formation of aneurysm, might be contributed to SAH in the young. Repeated angiogram is necessary for young patients to confirm the cause of SAH.

Keywords Cause · CTA · DSA · Subarachnoid hemorrhage · Young adults

Introduction

Subarachnoid hemorrhage, a kind of subtype of hemorrhagic stroke in subarachnoid space, accounts for 10% of stroke and 20% of hemorrhagic stroke with an incidence of 10 in 100,000 each year [1]. Compared to ischemic stroke and intracranial hemorrhage, it is commonly involved in young populations, although recent epidemiological studies showed that the incidence of SAH increase with age and the average age of onset is 49 ± 10 years old [2]. SAH is an emergency for its high fatality rate, ranging from 32 to 67% [3]. More than 2/3 of the patients cannot regain their previous occupation and lifestyle. The main reasons for patients' poor outcomes are its complications after an aneurysm ruptures are rebleeding, cerebrovascular spasm and hydrocephaly. Although the diagnosis for its etiology (aneurysms and arteriovenous malformation) becomes more specific with the development of medical imaging technology, about 20% cases are without clear causes and are classified as unknown cause SAH. Here, we report clinical cases of SAH in young adults (below 45 years of age) with unknown cause in the First Affiliated Hospital of Chongqing Medical University to discuss possible or undiscovered pathogenesis.

Methods

Subjects

Patients were admitted in our hospital from January 2007 to June 2008, with SAH diagnosed by head computed tomography (CT) and/or lumber puncture (LP). Traumatic

T. Wang and X. Qin (✉)
Department of Neurology, The First Affiliated Hospital of Chongqing Medical University, Chongqing, 400016, People's Republic of China
e-mail: Qinxinyue@yahoo.com

J.H. Zhang
Department of Physiology and Pharmacology, Loma Linda University, Loma Linda, CA, USA
Department of Neurosurgery, Loma Linda University, Loma Linda, CA, USA
Department of Anesthesiology, Loma Linda University, Loma Linda, CA, USA

SAH was excluded. Eleven adult patients below 45 years of age were selected out for study on SAH in young adults. One case was spinal subarachnoid hemorrhage; one was arteriovenous fistula in left frontal brain; the other nine patients had no clear cause but with abnormal imaging examination results. We followed these nine cases for 1 year or half a year, but two of them were lost in follow-up. Only seven patients can provide information for our investigation.

Clinical Characteristics

The clinical characteristics were retrospectively reviewed according to their medical files. We investigated the following clinical information: age, gender, onset symptoms, onset behavior, blood pressure, WFNS grade, smoking, alcohol intake, eating habits and temperament. Then we studied their imaging examination, including head CT, CTA (computed tomography angiography), DSA (digital subtraction angiography), MRI (magnetic resonance imaging), and their LP results.

Follow-Up

Eleven patients were diagnosed SAH according to their medical records. Two of them had clear cause; the other nine patients were found with no direct cause of SAH and followed up for 1 year by telephone interview, including their symptoms, lifestyle changes, activity of daily living (ADL) and modified Rankin Score (mRS).

Lawton and Brody's six-item Physical Self-maintenance Scale (PSMS) and eight-item Instrumental Activities of Daily Living (IADL) scale is used often but scored in several different ways. We gave each item four scores: one point meant independent; two, with minor assistance; three, with moderate or major assistance; four, dependent at all. Therefore, the total score was ranged from 14 to 64: 14 points meant normal; >14, with different degrees of dysfunction; ≥22 or at least two items scoring ≥3, with severe dysfunction.

Results

Clinical Characteristics

From 20 to 45, their mean onset age was 38 years old; male to female ratio was 10:1, much higher than common view (This may be biased by the small sample size). When SAH attacked, most of them had a sudden headache, and three (27.28%) lost consciousness temporarily. In addition, only one was performing heavy physical labor, and another one was playing cards excitedly. After admitted in hospital, their blood pressures were almost normal, and WFNS grades were level one except one patient with conscious disturbance who was in level four. On the aspect of lifestyle, the majority of patients did not drink wine at all; 63.64% of them are heavy

Table 1 Clinical information for 11 patients with SAH

Patients	Age, year	Gender	Symptom at onset	Behavior at onset	BP mmHg	WFNS grade	Smoking/day	Alcohol intake	Eating habits	Temperament
1	44	F	Sudden lumbocrural pain	Daily activity	120/88	1	No	No	Low-fat	Mild
2	45	M	Sudden headache	Card games	132/73	1	At least 20	No	Low-fat, spicy	Reserved
3	42	M	Sudden headache, nausea	Daily activity	125/85	1	About 40	No	Fat	Impatient
4	33	M	Sudden scruff pain, nausea	Daily activity	135/80	1	No	250 g/day	No specialty	Mild
5	33	M	Sudden conscious disturbance	Daily activity	122/77	4	About 20	No	Spicy	Mild
6	20	M	Sudden headache	Daily activity	117/78	1	About 10	No	Fat, spicy	Fidgety
7	38	M	Sudden headache, nausea	Daily activity	120/70	1	Not often	Rarely	Fat	Mild
8	41	M	Sudden dizziness, nausea	Daily activity	130/90	1	No	No	Fat	Mild
9	36	M	Headache after faint	Daily activity	124/72	1	About 40	50 g/day	No specialty	Impatient
10	41	M	Sudden headache, conscious disturbance	Heavy labor	120/80	1	About 20	No	No specialty	Mild
11	45	M	Headache, conscious disturbance	Daily activity	134/96	1	About 20	50 g/day	Spicy	Mild

This table shows the clinical information for all eleven patients with SAH. All patients had similar symptoms and onset behavior according to their clinical characteristics

smokers, ranging from 10 to 40 cigarettes per day for 5–25 years. Due to the eating habits of the living district, they usually had spicy food or greasy food. No specialty was found about individual temperament among them (Table 1).

All the imaging examination results of the patients excluded the existence of aneurysms; however, each patient had different abnormal situations on cerebral or spinal vessels. The first patient was with spinal vascular malformation, the second with vascular malformation on his Orbitofrontal lobe, the 3rd, 4th, 6th, 9th, 10th and 11th with different degrees of stenosis problems on their intracranial arteries, the fourth with suspected malformation image, and the eighth with possible venous aneurysm image. Seven among the 10 patients who underwent CTA had a further DSA to determine the exact cause for the hemorrhage. Consistently, four patients resulted in the same DSA imaging outcomes with their CTA, and the rest of them had negative results. MRI is not carried out routinely for each patient, so the clinical information on venous conditions is limited.

In our chart, only two patients took it. Only one had vascular abnormality, and the other one was negative (Table 2).

Follow-Up Results

Up to 1 year, we ended our follow-up for the nine patients (No. 3–6) with no obvious cause for SAH. Unfortunately, two patients were lost, and the remaining seven patients were included our tracing plan. Information on their prognosis was collected by telephone questionnaire, including current symptoms, lifestyle changes, ADL and mRS (Table 3).

Generally, the prognosis of the seven patients was good, although two (28.57%) of them had minor symptoms. One patient still kept smoking and playing cards almost every evening. The ADL and mRS scores were fine, consistent with their current daily functions. The one who continued

Table 2 Imaging examination and LP results for 11 patients with SAH

Patients	Head CT	CTA	DSA	MRI	LP
1	−	Spinal cord: T11-L2 vascular malformation contorted vascular image	T10 multiple vascular branches	Low thoracolumbar contorted vascular image	+
2	+	Left frontal abnormal vascular image	Orbitofrontal lobe vascular malformation	−	−
3	+	Right VB junction stenosis moderate-severe	Right VA congenital hypogenesis	−	−
4	−	Spinal cord:C1-4 vascular image enhancement, malformation possible	−	−	+
5	−	Right MCA-M1 with thin development	−	−	+
6	+ with ICH	Left ACA-A1 contorted	Left ACA with thin development	−	+
7	+	−	−	−	−
8	+	Can not exclude venous aneurysm	−	−	−
9	+	Bilateral ACA uneven	−	−	+
10	+	Left MCA uneven at Sylvius fissure	Enlargement at Right P Com A	−	−
11	+	Possible micro aneurysm at right ACA	−	−	−

This table demonstrates the imaging examination and LP results for the eleven patients with SAH. They were diagnosed with SAH by head computed tomography (CT) and/or LP. Ten of the eleven patients underwent the CTA examination
VB vertebro-basilar; *VA* vertebral artery; *MCA* middle cerebral artery; *ACA* anterior cerebral artery; *P Com A* posterior communication artery

Table 3 Follow-up results of seven patients with SAH

Patients	Current symptoms	Lifestyle changes	ADL scores	mRS scores	Others
3	−	Quit smoking Low-fat diet	14	0	
4	Sensation of chill	Quit drinking alcohol	14	0	
5	Dizziness	Continue smoking, cards	14	0	Readmitted 1 month later for dizziness
6	−	Quit smoking	14	0	
9	−	Quit smoking and drinking	14	0	
10	−	Quit smoking	14	0	
11	−	Quit smoking and drinking	14	0	

This table shows the 1-year follow-up results of seven patients with SAH. The evaluation of ADL and mRS score indicated a favorable prognosis for all of them

smoking was readmitted to the hospital, but no additional examination results turned out to be positive.

Discussion

All the 11 patients were diagnosed of SAH by head CT and/or LP. To determine the cause, particularly the source for aneurysm, they were arranged to have CTA examination. However, no evidence supported the existence of aneurysm, except that the first two patients were proved with arteriovenous problems for their SAH. Considering this result may be related to the false negative induced by vascular spasm, DSA was recommended to the other nine patients (three patients turned down the offer because of financial reasons). The final DSA results of the seven patients were either consistent with the CTA or negative. Without confirmed imaging evidence for aneurysm or vascular malformation, no surgical intervention was considered. Advice that they should repeat the CTA or DSA examination after 3 weeks was given, since the existence of microaneurysms was possible. By virtue of the expensive payment for hospitalization, no patients accepted our advice and requested only conservative medical management. They were discharged from hospital, when their clinical conditions became stable and repeated head CT showed the hemorrhage in subarachnoid space disappeared. 0.5–1 year after their first SAH, we were pleased to see the seven patients with good prognosis. Without dysfunction, they all returned to their previous workplaces. The majority of them stopped smoking or drinking alcohol, although none altered their eating habits. In our conversations, they insist that there was no need taking another imaging examination, the reason being that nothing had happened during the past year. Hitherto we have not gained the direct evidence for the cause of SAH of these patients.

Intracranial aneurysm, the most common cause of subarachnoid hemorrhage, is a local pathological expansion of the intracranial artery, ranking the first three causes of cerebrovascular accident. Approximately 75% of the cases of SAH are due to ruptured intracranial aneurysms. The incidence of intracranial aneurysm is 3.6–6% [4–5], and of ruptured aneurysm is 1–2% [5]. Other causes are craniocerebral trauma, arteriovenous malformation, dural fistulae, dural sinus thrombosis, intracranial arterial dissection, mycotic aneurysm, bleeding diseases and drugs (cocaine) [6]. Less than 10% of the patients have a perimesencephalic pattern of SAH. This type is considered to be venous in origin and have a benign course and good outcome.

Therefore, when patients were diagnosed with SAH, the first and most important step is to determine an aneurysm as soon as possible. DSA is acknowledged as a golden standard of detecting aneurysm for its high resolution. Because of its invasion, time-consuming, high expense, some severe complications, however, the clinical use of DSA has limitations. By contrast, CTA may be a good substitute for DSA as a preliminary screening technology. Teksam et al. [7] reported that the sensitivity of 4-slice CTA for aneurysms <4 mm, between 4 and 10 mm, and >10 mm was 84, 97, and 100%, respectively, on a per-aneurysm basis. Chen et al. [8] reported the sensitivity and accuracy of 16-slice CTA were 96 and 98.9% for small aneurysms (<4 mm), 98.1 and 99.2% for medium (4–10 mm), and 100 and 100% for large (>10 mm) aneurysms, respectively, on a per-aneurysm basis. The ability for 16-slice CTA to detect micro aneurysm (<2 mm) was also reported. In our study, CTA was recommended to each patient first for aneurysm screening; DSA was usually advised after CTA indicated negative or before neurosurgical operation. If possible, patients suspected to have intracranial aneurysm were recommended to undergo repeated angiogram examination after the time course of vascular spasm. In our study, the problem was that no patient wanted to spend additional money for detection for something that may be not likely present. Up to 1 year, all of them had good recoveries instead of rebleeding. In some reports, if the aneurysm is not treated, the risk of rebleeding within 1 month is estimated to be of 35–40% [9]. After the first 4 weeks, the risk decreases gradually from 1 to 2% per day to 3% per year [10]. The argument is that whether repeated angiogram examinations, particularly DSA, are necessary for patients with good outcomes after 1 year.

Excluding these causes for SAH, we speculated that their vascular pathologic changes (stenosis, buckling), due to smoking and alcohol consumption, might be contributed to SAH other than present aneurysm and arteriovenous malformation. Judged from the CT and DSA evidence, these changes were obvious in the young, which was mostly common in the old with hypertensive arteriosclerosis. However, there was no hypertension, hypercholesterolemia, or family history of stroke to be found among these patients. Thus, we focused on the relationship between smoking-induced endothelium damage and SAH. Based on epidemiological study, smoking significantly increased the risk of both aneurysm formation and SAH [11–15]; the ratio for SAH was 2.4, and 1–7 for unruptured cerebral aneurysm. Smoking especially increased the occurrence of SAH in women and in the young [16]. In China, 350,000,000 people smoke based on statistics from 2007, and the majority of this population is male. This can partly explain why the male to female ratio in our study was higher compared with other researchers'. In several studies, cigarette smoking was proven to cause damage to vascular endothelium in different organs [17–19]. The possible mechanism may be that cigarette smoking leads to endothelial dysfunction by virtue of reduced vascular responsiveness in smokers and specifically impaired both basal and stimulated nitric oxide bioactivity.

In addition, nicotine increases plasma levels of vasoconstrictors such as catecholamines, arginine vasopressin and endothelin-1, perturbs arachidonic acid metabolism and induces a thrombogenic state and smooth muscle cell proliferation [20–24]. All the effects can result in arteriosclerosis and pathological injury on vessel wall. The thickened intimal layer of the arterial wall and the increased breakdown of elastins on the wall both help to form an intracranial aneurysm. Based on these theories, our supposition that these damaged arteries were likely to be too fragile to endure the hemodynamic changes and bleeding happened before an aneurysm formed could be logical. Meanwhile, we believe smoking could make the onset of SAH to a date earlier than that of the actual occurrence. To testify our points, further endothelium function tests of cerebral artery, even biopsy from these patients are needed.

Conclusion

In summary, pathological changes of cerebral vessels, by itself or as an early version of formation of aneurysm due to smoking, might be contributed to SAH in the young. To quit smoking is necessary to stop the development of SAH. The risk of rebleeding in these patients was still high after 1 year and repeated angiogram will benefit them more than patients who have obvious cause for SAH. By the reason of small samples in our study, no statistic data could be offered for further study on young-adult subarachnoid hemorrhage. However, it is still worth of paying attention to the research on unknown-cause subarachnoid hemorrhage in the young population.

Conflict of interest statement We declare that we have no conflict of interest.

References

1. Linn FH, Rinkel GJE, van Gijn J. Incidence of subarachnoid haemorrhage: role of region, year, and rate of computed tomography: a meta-analysis. Stroke 1996;27:625–9.
2. ACROSS Group. Epidemiology of aneurismal subarachnoid haemorrhage in Australia and New Zealand. Incidence and case-fatality from the Australasian Cooperative Research on Subarachnoid Haemorrhage Study (ACROSS). Stroke 2000;31:1843–50.
3. Hop JW, Rinkel GJE, Algra A, van Gijn J. Case-fatality and functional outcome after subarachnoid hemorrhage: a systematic review. Stroke 1997;28:660–4.
4. Wardlaw JM, White PM. The detection and management of unruptured intracranial aneurysms. Brain 2000;123(2):205–21.
5. Arimura H, Li Q, Korogi Y. Computerized detection of intracranial aneurysms for three – dimensional MR angiography: feature extraction of small protrusions based on a shape – based difference image technique. Med Phys. 2006;33(2):394–401.
6. Howington JU, Kutz SC, Wilding GE, Awasthi D. Cocaine use as a predictor of outcome in aneurysmal subarachnoid haemorrhage. Neurosurgery 2003;99:271–75.
7. Teksam M, McKinney A, Casey S. Multi-section CT angiography for detection of cerebral aneurysms. AJNR Am J Neuroradiol. 2004;25:1485–92.
8. Chen W, Wang J. Accuracy of 16-row multislice computerized tomography angiography for assessment of intracranial aneurysms. Surg Neurol. 2009;71:32–42.
9. Hasan D, Lindsay KW, Wijdicks EF, Murray GD, Brouwers PJ, Bakker WH, et al. Effect of fludrocortisone acetate in patients with subarachnoid hemorrhage. Stroke 1989;20:1156–61.
10. Winn HR, Richardson AE, Jane JA. The long-term prognosis in untreated cerebral aneurysms: I The incidence of late hemorrhage in cerebral aneurysm: a 10-year evaluation of 364 patients. Ann Neurol. 1977;1:358–70.
11. Juvela S. Risk factors for multiple intracranial aneurysms. Stroke 2000;31:392–7.
12. Ellamushi HE, Grieve JP, Jager HR, Kitchen ND. Risk factors for the formation of multiple intracranial aneurysms. J Neurosurg. 2001;94:728–32.
13. Connolly ES Jr, Choudhri TF, Mack WJ, Mocco J, Spinks TJ, Slosberg J, et al. Influence of smoking, hypertension, and sex on the phenotypic expression of familial intracranial aneurysms in siblings. Neurosurgery 2001;48:64–9.
14. Feigin V, Parag V, Lawes CM, Rodgers A, Suh I, Woodward M, et al. Smoking and elevated blood pressure are the most important risk factors for subarachnoid hemorrhage in the asia-pacific region: an overview of 26 cohorts involving 306, 620 participants. Stroke 2005;36:1360–5.
15. Kurth T, Kase CS, Berger K, Gaziano JM, Cook NR, Buring JE. Smoking and risk of hemorrhagic stroke in women. Stroke 2003;34:2792–5.
16. Matsumoto K, Akagi K, Abekura M. Cigarette smoking increases the risk of developing a cerebral aneurysm and of subarachnoid hemorrhage9. Neurol Surg. 1999;27:(9): 831–5.
17. Tu YK, Ueng SWN. The effects of cigarette smoking on rabbit tibial vascular endothelium. Musculoskeletal Res. 2001;5(4):235–42.
18. Karl L, Hans JR, Paul K. Cigarette smoking and vascular pathology in renal biopsies. Kidney Int. 2002;61:648–54.
19. Butler R, Morris AD, Struthers AD. Cigarette smoking in men and vascular responsiveness. Clin Pharmacol. 2001;52:145–9.
20. Ritz E, Benck U, Franek E. Effects of smoking on renal hemodynamics in healthy volunteers and in patients with glomerular disease. J Am Soc Nephrol. 1998;9:1798–804.
21. Gambaro G, Verlato F, Budakovic A. Renal impairment in chronic cigarette smokers. J Am Soc Nephrol. 1998;9:562–7.
22. Benck U, Clorius JH, Zuna I. Renal hemodynamic changes during smoking: effects of adrenoreceptor blockade. Clin Invest. 1999;29:1010–8.
23. Hawkins RI. Smoking, platelets and thrombosis. Nature 1972;236: 450–2.
24. Barrow SE, Ward PS, Sleightholm MA. Cigarette smoking: profiles of thromboxane- and prostacyclin-derived products in human urine. Biochim Biophys Acta. 1989;993:121–7.

Cardiac Damage After Subarachnoid Hemorrhage

Bihua Wu, Xiaoming Wang, and John H. Zhang

Abstract Patients who had no heart disease had T-wave inversion and prolongation of the QT interval in electrocardiogram after Subarachnoid hemorrhage (SAH), which was reported 70 years before. Cardiac complications, including focal myocytolysis, electrocardiographic changes, arrhythmias and left ventricular wall motion abnormalities and pulmonary edema. The autonomic and cardiovascular effects of SAH, however, are modulated by concomitant factors such as pre-existent cardiac diseases, electrolyte disorders and, probably, by genetic alterations in the ionic control of myocyte repolarization. Although beta-blockers have been reported to prevent myocardial damage following SAH, adequate clinical trials are lacking, and the widespread use of these drugs in acute cerebrovascular disease is not supported by evidence. Cardiac injury occurs frequently after SAH, and the most widely investigated form of neurocardiogenic injury.

Keywords Cardiac complications · EKG · SAH

Introduction

As first reported by Wisman [1] in 1939, SAH has been recognized as being complicated by various cardiac symptoms. Cardiac complications, including focal myocytolysis, electrocardiographic changes, arrhythmias and left ventricular wall motion abnormalities, frequently occur following stroke and contribute to worsen the prognosis. Their clinical spectrum seems to be related to the type of cerebrovascular disease and its localization. Thus, the incidence of arrhythmias and pulmonary edema is significantly higher in subarachnoid hemorrhage than in ischemic stroke, and the lesions in the right insular cortex are a major risk for complex arrhythmias and sudden death. Elevated plasma norepinephrine levels are frequently associated with these events and strongly suggest an underlying sympathetically mediated mechanism. The autonomic and cardiovascular effects of stroke, however, are modulated by concomitant factors such as pre-existent cardiac diseases, electrolyte disorders and, probably, by genetic alterations in the ionic control of myocyte repolarization. Although beta-blockers have been reported to prevent myocardial damage following stroke, adequate clinical trials are lacking, and the widespread use of these drugs in acute cerebrovascular disease is not supported by evidence.

Cardiac injury occurs frequently after stroke and the mostly investigated form of neurocardiogenic injury is aneurysmal subarachnoid hemorrhage. Echocardiography and screening for elevated troponin and B-type natriuretic peptide levels may help prognosticate and guide treatment of stroke. Cardiac catheterization is not routinely recommended in subarachnoid hemorrhage patients with left ventricular dysfunction and elevated troponin. The priority should be treatment of the underlying neurologic condition, even in patients with left ventricular dysfunction. Cardiac injury that occurs after subarachnoid hemorrhage appears to be reversible. In contrast to subarachnoid hemorrhage patients, patients with ischemic stroke are more likely to have concomitant significant heart disease. For patients who develop brain death, cardiac evaluation under optimal conditions may help increase the organ donor pool.

Electrocardiogram Abnormalities

QT Prolongation

Electrocardiographic (ECG) alterations in the course of subarachnoid hemorrhage (SAH) have long been recognized.

B. Wu (✉) and X. Wang
Department of Neurology, Affiliated Hospital of North Sichuan Medical College, Nanchong, Sichuan 637007, People's Republic of China
e-mail: wubihua2008@yahoo.com

J.H. Zhang
Department of Neurosurgery, Loma Linda University School of Medicine, Loma Linda, CA 92354, USA

In particular, QT prolongation has been documented in association with SAH and may initiate severe cardiac arrhythmias [2]. Subarachnoid hemorrhage (SAH) frequently prolongs QT interval in the acute phase [3]. Several mechanisms play role in pathophysiologic basis for QTc prolongation. Sex hormones and hypokalemia lengthen the QT interval [4–6]. Female sex and hypokalemia are proven to be independent risk factors for severe QTc prolongation in patients with SAH [7]. Correlation between serum catecholamine level and QTc interval still remains unclear. The findings of a study indicated that high catecholamine levels following SAH did not play a direct role in the pathogenesis of prolonged QTc [7]. However, investigators showed that experimental serum infused-adrenaline caused prolongation of QTc interval in normal volunteers [8]. The relationship between the magnitude of intracranial bleeding and QT prolongation has also been investigated. The study demonstrated correlation between these parameters [7]. Patients with more intracranial or an intracerebral hemorrhage seen on computed tomography were more likely to have prolongation of the QT interval [9]. Significant QT interval prolongation and arrhythmias were observed after rats were given subarachnoid injections of packed red blood cells [10].

Repolarization Abnormalities

Electrocardiographic repolarization changes occur in three quarters with SAH irrespective of the presence or absence of previous cardiac disease [11]. One or more repolarization abnormalities occurred in 41% of patients [12]. Analysis revealed prolonged QTc interval >460 ms in 16%, ST segment elevation in 9%, ST depression in 3%, T wave inversion in 7%, and U wave > or = 100 microV in 15%. Electrocardiographic criteria for left ventricular hypertrophy were met in 14, and 43% of those patients had no history of hypertension. Serum cardiac troponin I was elevated in 21%, and was significantly associated with QTc interval >460 ms ($P < 0.001$). Controlling for gender, those with QTc interval >460 ms were 5.5 times more likely to have elevated serum cardiac troponin I. It is concluded that repolarization abnormalities are present in a high proportion of patients with SAH (Table 1).

Other Electrocardiogram Abnormalities

Changes in ST segment (15–51% of patients), T waves (12–92%), prominent U waves (4–47%), and sinus dysrhythmias are the most common types after SAH [13]. Prolongation of the PR interval is one of the known clinical manifestations of

Table 1 Forty-six studies reported ECG abnormalities in SAH patients

ECG changes	Number of studies	Number of patients	Abnormal patients	Incidence (%)
Abnormal ECG	37	2,727	1,554	57.4
Abnormal ST-segment	40	2,781	1,268	45.6
Long QTs	34	2,739	859	31.5
Bradycardia	37	2,845	346	12.2
Cardiac arrest	40	2,114	19	0.8
Ventricular tachycardia	44	3,096	32	1.0
Ventricular fibrillation	44	3,095	5	0.2

hypomagnesemia [14], but it has also been described with the existence of hypermagnesemia. Moreover, there is convincing evidence that magnesium infusion is slowing conduction through the atrioventricular node and thus prolongs the PR interval [15]. The duration of the QRS complex in our study population was longer than could be expected in a normal population. Widening of the QRS complex has been described with even modest magnesium loss [14] but also with hypermagnesemia. The effect of magnesium therapy on the QRS complex is not consistent, but mostly a widening of the QRS complex has been reported [15].

Implication of Electrocardiogram Abnormalities

In earlier studies [16] of the prognostic importance of ECG changes, sample sizes were small and the results were equivocal. In a more recent retrospective study, Zaroff et al. [17] examined mortality due to cardiac abnormalities and to all causes in 58 patients with SAH who had ECG changes consistent with myocardial ischemia or infarction. The results indicated that ECG abnormalities were not a significant predictor of mortality. However, 20% of patients in the source SAH database were excluded from the study because their medical records did not include ECG findings, perhaps leading to selection bias. This study was further limited by its small sample size and inclusion of only three "snapshot" ECG recordings per subject. To date, patients' outcomes have not been studied in a prospective investigation that included a large sample size.

Left Ventricular Dysfunction

Ventricular wall motion abnormalities is one of characteristic of early myocardial damage, many studies reported that patients have wall motion abnormalities after SAH. Kuroiwa reported [18] 23 patients had ventricular wall motion abnormalities with ST elevation after SAH, eight patients had no abnormality by coronarography. Zaroff [19] identified 589 patients with SAH, 147 had ultrasonic cardiogram findings indicative whom had Left ventricular dysfunction are up to 28%. Regional or focal wall-motion abnormalities on echocardiogram have been observed in some patients with SAH, as have increased levels of creatine kinase, MB fraction (CK-MB) [20]. These findings often raise concern about ongoing cardiac ischemia from coronary artery disease and may cause treatment to be delayed. There is a common misperception among trainees at our institution that patients who have coronary artery disease with neurologic causes do not have elevations in cardiac enzymes. This turns out not to be the case. Cardiac troponin I (cTnI) has been shown to be a more sensitive and specific marker for cardiac dysfunction in patients with SAH than is CK-MB. Parekh [21] found 32 patients with SAH, eight of whom had cTnI elevated; these patients are more likely to manifest echocardiographic and clinical evidence of left ventricular dysfunction.

Pathology

Over 50% of patients had cardiac muscle contraction band necrosis; these findings were in autopsy specimens from patients with SAH [22]. Transient low ejection fraction is the physiologic parameter that correlates with this pathologic finding. A model has been proposed for how SAH can cause cardiac damage. Brain injury can damage the insular cortex of the cerebral hemisphere or cause hypothalamic pressure, either of which causes catecholamine release at the nerve terminal at the cardiac myocyte. As the heart muscles contract, adenosine triphosphate (ATP) is depleted, mitochondria malfunction, and there is ensuing myocardial cell death. However, some studies have reported no correlation between concentrations of plasma catecholamine and ECG abnormalities, which suggests a more complicated pathophysiology [23, 24].

Directions for Future Research

SAH is a serious neurological disorder that is often complicated by the occurrence of ECG abnormalities unexplained by preexisting cardiac conditions. ECG changes that occur during cardiac repolarization, such as abnormalities in the ST segment and the T wave, must be interpreted in the context of the patient's neurological abnormalities. Most researchers considered this damage of cardio-pulmonary function after SAH temporary and reversible, which couldn't increase mortality rate. But, we also need do EEG, CK, cTnI, ultrasonic cardiogram and X-ray as routine examination, so we can discover cardiac damage early and give electrocardiographic monitoring to patients of SAH. At the same time, in order to clarify the mechanism of cardiac damage and effects of prognosis of patients with SAH, a large study scale will be needed.

Conflict of interest statement We declare that we have no conflict of interest.

References

1. Weisman SJ. Edemaa and congeestion of lungs resulting from intracranial hemorrhage. Surgery 1939;6:722–9.
2. Andreoli A, di Pasquale G, Pinelli G, Grazi P, Tognetti F, Testa C. Subarachnoid hemorrhage: frequency and severity of cardiac arrhythmias. A survey of 70 cases studied in the acute phase. Stroke 1987;18:558–64.
3. Colkesen AY, Sen O, Giray S, Acil T, Ozin B, Muderrisoglu H. Correlation between QTc interval and clinical severity of subarachnoid hemorrhage depends on the QTc formula used. Pacing Clin Electrophysiol. 2007;30(12):1482–6.
4. Machado C, Baga JJ, Kawasaki R, Reinoehl J, Steinman RT, Lehmann MH. Torsade de pointes as a complication of subarachnoid hemorrhage: A critical reappraisal. J Electrocardiol. 1997;30: 31–7.
5. Drici MD, Burklow TR, Haridasse V, Glazer RI, Woosley RL. Sex hormones prolong the QT interval and downregulate potassium channel expression in the rabbit heart. Circulation 1996;94:1471–4.
6. Akita M, Kuwahara M, Tsubone H, Sugano S. ECG changes during furosemide-induced hypokalemia in the rat. J Electrocardiol. 1998; 31:45–9.
7. Fukui S, Katoh H, Tsuzuki N, Ishihara S, Otani N, Ooigawa H, et al. Multivariate analysis of risk factors for QT prolongation following subarachnoid hemorrhage. Crit Care. 2003;7:R7–12.
8. Reid JL, Whyte KF, Struthers AD. Epinephrine-induced hypokalemia: the role of beta adrenoceptors. Am J Cardiol. 1986;57:23F–7F.
9. Lanzino G, Kongable GL, Kassell NF. Electrocardiographic abnormalities after nontraumatic subarachnoid hemorrhage. J Neurosurg Anesthesiol. 1994;6:156–62.
10. Randell T, Tanskanen P, Scheinin M, Kytta J, Ohman J, Lindgren L. QT dispersion after subarachnoid hemorrhage. J Neurosurg Anesthesiol. 1999;11:163–6.
11. Schuiling WJ, Algra A, de Weerd AW, Leemans P, Rinkel GJ. ECG abnormalities in predicting secondary cerebral ischemia after subarachnoid haemorrhage. Acta Neurochir (Wien). 2006;148 (8):853–8; discussion 858.
12. Sommargren CE, Zaroff JG, Banki N, Drew BJ. Electrocardiographic repolarization abnormalities in subarachnoid hemorrhage. J Electrocardiol. 2002;35(Suppl):257–62.
13. van den Bergh WM, Algra A, Rinkel GJ. Electrocardiographic abnormalities and serum magnesium in patients with subarachnoid hemorrhage. Stroke 2004;35(3):644–8.
14. Dyckner T. Serum magnesium in acute myocardial infarction: relation to arrhythmias. Acta Med Scand. 1980;207:59–66.
15. Akazawa S, Shimizu R, Nakaigawa Y, Ishii R, Ikeno S, Yamato R. Effects of magnesium sulphate on atrioventricular conduction

times and surface electrocardiogram in dogs anaesthetized with sevoflurane. Br J Anaesth. 1997;78:75–80.
16. Carruth JE, Silverman ME. Torsade de pointe atypical ventricular tachycardia complicating subarachnoid hemorrhage. Chest 1980;78: 886–8.
17. Zaroff JG, Rordorf GA, Newell BA, Ogilvy CS, Levinson JR. Cardiac outcome in patients with subarachnoid hemorrhage and electrocardiographic abnormalities. Neurosurgery 1999;44: 34–40.
18. Kuroiwa T, Morita H, Tanabe H, Ohta T. Siganificance of ST segment elevation in electrocardiodrams in patients with euptured cerebral aneurysms. Acta Neu rochir (Wien). 1995;133:141–6.
19. Zaroff JG, Rordorf GA, Ogilvy CS, Picard MH. Regional patterns OF LEFT ventricular systolic dysfunction after subarachnoid hemorrhage: evidence for neurally mediated cardiac injury. J Am Soc Echocardiogr. 2000;13:774–9.
20. Mashaly HA, Provencio JJ. Inflammation as a link between brain injury and heart damage: the model of subarachnoid hemorrhage. Cleve Clin J Med. 2008;75(2):26–30.
21. Parekh N, Venkatesh B, Cross D, Leditschke A, Atherton J, Miles W, et al. Cardiac troponin-1 predicts meyocardial dysfunction in aneurismal subarachnoid hemorrhage. J Am Coll Cardiol. 2000;36:1328–35.
22. Bergh WM, Algra A, Rinkel GJ. Electrocardiographic abnormalities and serum magnesium in patients with subarachnoid hemorrhage. Stroke 2004;35:644–8.
23. Kawahara E, Ikeda S, Miyahara Y, Kohno S. Role of autonomic nervous dysfunction in electrocardiographic abnormalities and cardiac injury in patients with acute subarachnoid hemorrhage. Circ J. 2003;67:753–6.
24. Mashaly HA, Provencio JJ. Inflammation as a link between brain injury and heart damage: the model of subarachnoid hemorrhage. Cleve Clin J Med. 2008;75:2:S26–30.

Analysis on Death-Associated Factors of Patients with Subarachnoid Hemorrhage During Hospitalization

Tianzhu Wang, John H. Zhang, and Xinyue Qin

Abstract *Objective*: The prognosis of patients with high-clinical-score subarachnoid hemorrhage remains poor, with early high mortality rate. Therefore, to predict the early outcome of patients after subarachnoid hemorrhage, several clinical factors were hypothesized to be related to death during hospitalization.

Methods: Eighty-nine cases after subarachnoid hemorrhage, divided into two groups (① death group; ② survival group) according to their clinical situations during hospitalization, were studied. Twelve factors, including gender, hypertension, intracranial aneurysm, cerebral vascular spasm, hydrocephalus and conscious disturbance during hospitalization, smoking, age, WFNS (World Federation of Neurological Surgeons) scale, Fisher grade, white blood cell count and blood glucose level at admission, were analyzed by using Chi-square test, *t* test, and Logistic multiple regression analysis.

Results: The results of single-factor analysis indicated that ruptured intracranial aneurysm, conscious disturbance, increasing age, high WFNS scale, high Fisher grade, increasing white blood cell count and blood glucose level were statistically significant different between the two groups. The logistic analysis results showed that ruptured intracranial aneurysm (odds ratio [OR], 9.253; 95% confidence interval [CI], 0.617–98.263), high WFNS score (OR, 2.105; 95% CI, 1.275–5.204) and increasing white blood cell count (OR, 1.397; 95% CI 1.062–2.013) were the independent risk factors associated with death during hospitalization for patients with subarachnoid hemorrhage.

Conclusions: Increased white blood cell count may indicate poor outcomes for patients during hospitalization, even early death.

Keywords Death · Factors · Logistic regression analysis · Subarachnoid hemorrhage

Introduction

Although less frequent than ischemic stroke and intracranial hemorrhage, subarachnoid hemorrhage is a devastating condition: global mortality ranges from 32 to 67% [1]. One quarter of the patients who reach a hospital will die from complications of subarachnoid hemorrhage within 2 weeks. In addition, it can affect young and middle-aged adults and cause disabilities among 20–30% of the survivors. In the recent two decades, advancements in medical imaging technology and endovascular interventions have led to significant decrease in the mortality of subarachnoid hemorrhage and improvements in long-term outcomes. However, some patients will still die during hospitalization, even on the first day after admission. Risk factors for subarachnoid hemorrhage have been studied in a number of settings in the United States [2, 3], Japan [4], the Netherlands [5, 6], Finland [7, 8], and Portugal [9]. In China, the differences in individual financial conditions, personal educational level and medical care may be additional risk factors. Therefore, we reviewed 89 cases with subarachnoid hemorrhage and tried to analyze the death-associated factors.

T. Wang (✉) and X. Qin
Department of Neurology, The First Affiliated Hospital of Chongqing Medical University, Chongqing, 400016, People's Republic of China
e-mail: Qinxinyue@yahoo.com

J.H. Zhang
Department of Physiology and Pharmacology, Loma Linda University, Loma Linda, CA, USA
Department of Neurosurgery, Loma Linda University, Loma Linda, CA, USA
Department of Anesthesiology, Loma Linda University, Loma Linda, CA, USA

Methods

Subjects and Clinical Information

The data of 89 patients with subarachnoid hemorrhage, admitted to the department of neurology in our hospital from January 2006 to December 2008, was collected from the medical records department. The diagnosis of subarachnoid hemorrhage was established by clinical manifestations, computed tomographic scan or lumber puncture. Traumatic subarachnoid hemorrhage and spinal subarachnoid hemorrhage were excluded. Of the 89 patients, 53 were male and 36 female, with an average age of (57.10 ± 1.55) years and a mean length of hospital stay of (12.58 ± 1.31) days. Conventional medical and surgical treatments were carried out to all patients to prevent the incidence of complications and deal with other symptoms. A majority of patients took angiography to determine etiology. No difference was found among drugs or other medical management among them.

Groups, Variables and Scales

All patients were divided into two groups: Death group; Survival group. Outcome was assessed during hospitalization after subarachnoid hemorrhage. The following variables are used for data analysis.

Discrete variables: gender, hypertension history, intracranial aneurysm, cerebral vascular spasm, hydrocephalus and conscious disturbance during hospitalization, smoking history.

Continuous variables: age, admission WFNS scale, Fisher grade, white blood cell count and blood glucose level.

Symptomatic vasospasm was defined a ≥2 point decrease in Glasgow coma score. Confirmation with transcranial Doppler ultrasound or cerebral angiography was recommended but not mandatory. WFNS scale [10] (Table 1), based on Glasgow Coma Score (GCS), was used to assess the clinical conditions of the patients with subarachnoid hemorrhage; Fisher Grade [11] (Table 2) classifies the appearance of subarachnoid hemorrhage on CT scan. Both scores were determined immediately after hospitalization.

Statistical Analysis

Single-factor analysis of discrete variables was by using Chi-square test, continuous variables by using t test; multifactor Logistic regression analysis with stepwise backward selection was used to determine death-associated factors of subarachnoid hemorrhage during hospitalization. All statistics were finished by SPSS 13.0 for Windows software, $\alpha = 0.05$. OR and 95% CI were calculated.

Results

Missing Data

In the death group, some data was missing because 22 patients died during a short stay in the hospital (Fig. 1). In these cases, information about the existence of intracranial

Table 1 World federation of neurological surgeons (WFNS) grading scale

WFNS grade	Glasgow coma score	Motor deficit
I	15	Absent
II	14-13	Absent
III	14-13	Present
IV	12-7	Present or absent
V	6-3	Present or absent

Table 2 Fisher grade on SAH CT scan

Points	Description
1	No blood detected
2	Diffuse or vertical layer <1 mm thick
3	Clot and/or vertical layer >1 mm thick
4	Intracerebral or intraventricular clot

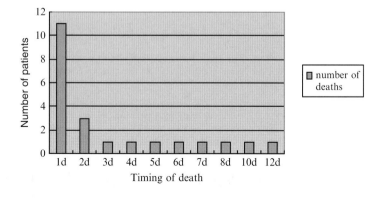

Fig. 1 Early death of 22 patients in death group. These patients died during a short stay in hospital which led to a data gap for etiological investigation. The number of deaths within 72 h accounted for 42.86% of the total number of deaths

aneurysm was incomplete, and then data was modified appropriately to accomplish multi-factor logistic regression analysis.

Single-Factor Analysis

Table 3 shows the results of single-factor analysis of discrete dates that intracranial aneurysm and conscious disturbance were statistically significant between the two groups, indicating both factors were potentially concerned with death after subarachnoid hemorrhage during hospitalization. Although some data about intracranial aneurysm and cerebral vascular spasm was incomplete, the results could still partly reflect the relationship between death and intracranial aneurysm.

The results of single-factor analysis of continuous data in Table 4 indicate that age, WFNS scale, Fisher grade, white blood cell count and blood glucose level were statistically significant different between the two groups. They were very likely to be the candidate risk factors of death after subarachnoid hemorrhage during hospitalization.

Multi-Factor Logistic Regression Analysis

The results of multi-factor stepwise logistic regression (Backward: Wald) analysis suggested that WFNS scale and white blood cell count were high risk death-associated factors after subarachnoid hemorrhage during hospitalization (Table 5).

Discussion

Subarachnoid hemorrhage is a major clinical problem worldwide. Of 22 patients in the death group, who did not get the chance to have computed tomographic angiography examination, 50% died within 24 h after admission and 63.6% within 48 h and 68.2% within 72 h. Of 89 patients, the early case fatality (within 1 month) is 39.3%, which is higher than the fatality (30%) in high-income countries but lower than that (43.9%) in low to middle income countries in 2000–2008 [12]. To decrease the mortality of patients after bleeding during hospitalization and help patients to gain a long-term favorable outcome, predictors of death in hospital should be recognized by neurologists and aggressive measures are supposed to be carried out in particular to patients with high risk factors of death.

In our single-factor analysis of factors associated with death in 89 patients after subarachnoid hemorrhage, six factors (decreased consciousness, age, high WFNS scale, increased Fisher grade, increased leukocyte count and blood glucose) were proved to be relevant to the unfavorable outcome, and the other five factors (gender, hypertension history, vasospasm, hydrocephalus, smoking history) seemed much more related to the incidence of subarachnoid hemorrhage than to the fatality. However, univariate statistical analysis is deficient to evaluate the influence between variables and unlikely to tell the relations between potential predictors and unfavorable outcome. Therefore, multivariate Logistic regression analysis was used to estimate how the independent variables affect the dependent variable in our study.

The results showed that only three factors (intracranial aneurysm, high WFNS scale and increased leukocyte count) were finally believed to be the high risk factors related to death after subarachnoid hemorrhage during hospitalization. The reason that decreased consciousness, age, increased Fisher grade and blood glucose were excluded from the regression equation is that these factors can be partially replaced by intracranial aneurysm, high WFNS scale and increased leukocyte count. Simply, patients with older age, decreased consciousness and increased blood glucose can

Table 3 Single-factor analysis of discrete data

Variables	Death group	Survival group	χ2	P value
Cases	35	54		
Gender M/F	19/16	34/20	0.664	>0.05
HBP history Y/N	16/19	16/38	2.386	>0.05
Aneurysm Y/N	8/5	14/38	5.566	<0.05
CVS Y/N	3/10	17/37	0.173	>0.05
Hydrocephalus Y/N	4/31	8/46	0.209	>0.05
Conscious dis Y/N	31/4	16/38	29.604	<0.01
Smoking history Y/N	7/28	17/37	1.421	>0.05

Table 4 Single-factor analysis of continuous data ($\bar{x} \pm s$)

Variables	Death group	Survival group	t	P value
Cases	35	54		
Age year	61.54 ± 14.80	54.22 ± 13.87	2.369	<0.05
WFNS scale	4.46 ± 1.20	1.35 ± 0.87	14.148	<0.01
Fisher grade	3.23 ± 0.91	2.37 ± 0.92	4.324	<0.01
WBC counts (×10E9/L)	17.87 ± 5.38	9.10 ± 3.24	9.603	<0.01
Blood glucose (mmol/L)	10 ± 5.25	6.86 ± 1.63	4.100	<0.01

Table 5 Multi-factor logistic regression analysis

Variables	B coefficient	OR	95% CI	P value
Aneurysm	2.225	9.253	0.617–98.263	<0.05
WFNS scale	0.744	2.105	1.275–5.204	<0.01
WBC counts (×10E9/L)	0.334	1.397	1.062–2.013	<0.05

make their WFNS scales higher than young and conscious patients do; patients with intracranial aneurysm are more likely to have higher Fisher grades than non-aneurysmal patients. Although the rupture of intracranial aneurysm may cause thick blood in the subarachnoid space, which can lead to decreased consciousness and worsen WFNS grade of patients, it cannot explain the effects of other factors on high WFNS grade, such as older age and high blood glucose. Increased blood leukocyte count is another independent predictor of poor prognosis [13–15]. It is strongly associated with poor clinical grade on admission and with a mortality of 50% when exceeding 20,000. In this study, ten patients with a white blood cell count greater than 20,000 died and the mortality was up to 100%. In addition, a blood leukocyte count >15,000 is concerned with an increased likelihood of cerebral vasospasm (OR, 3.33) [14]. It suggests that high blood leukocyte count is not only a risk factor of death after subarachnoid hemorrhage, but also an early warning to delayed ischemia caused by vasospasm.

In China, it is difficult to control these medical risk factors to reduce the occurrence of subarachnoid hemorrhage because of the different educational levels and financial states among people who are high risk group of the bleeding. Instead, to treat the death-associated factors during hospitalization is more feasible and effective to decrease the mortality and morbidity of patients with subarachnoid hemorrhage. Intracranial aneurysm is the factor which strongly influences the outcome after subarachnoid hemorrhage. For one reason, the volume of blood when aneurysms burst for the first time is much more than non-aneurysm hemorrhage dose; for another reason, the incidence of rebleeding of an aneurysm is also much higher than non-aneurysm SAH. Therefore, it is crucial to determine the presence of intracranial aneurysm or not. With advanced imaging technology, its size, location in the circle of Willis and possibly morphology can be detected by digital subtraction angiography. Once the presence of aneurysm is confirmed, surgery should be recommended to patients with low risk of surgical complications. However, the problem we meet is that when patients with decreased consciousness and high WFNS score come to the hospital, digital subtraction angiography is not accepted by majority of the families for it is invasive, expensive and has a high risk of complications. So these patients, treated only by medical therapies first, waiting for computed tomographic angiography available, usually die before the confirmation of the etiology of subarachnoid hemorrhage. Based on our analysis, we believe that poor WFNS score can predict a poor clinical outcome and imply the presence of intracranial aneurysm. Further, early diagnosis and treatment of intracranial aneurysm can change the prognosis from unfavorable to favorable. Therefore, emergency computed tomography angiography should be recommended to patients with poor clinical grades, since it has a reported sensitivity for aneurysm between 77 and 100% and specificity between 79 and 100% [16–19], and is a less invasive alternative to catheter angiography. In addition, endovascular intervention should be taken into consideration preferentially than surgery, for the latter will be less beneficial to patients in bad condition [20–22].

Conclusion

In conclusion, intracranial aneurysm, high clinical grade and increased white blood cell count are highly related to death after subarachnoid hemorrhage in hospital. Neurologists are supposed to assess the overall condition of patients with subarachnoid hemorrhage and the WFNS grade accurately. According to the evaluation, emergency computed tomographic angiography should be arranged as soon as possible to determine the etiological factors of subarachnoid hemorrhage. Once the intracranial aneurysm is diagnosed, endovascular obliteration of the aneurysm should be recommended immediately to those with high score of WFNS grade who cannot tolerate surgery. In addition, increased white blood cell count may allow for poor outcomes for patients during hospitalization, even early death.

Conflict of interest statement We declare that we have no conflict of interest.

References

1. Hop JW, Rinkel GJE, Algra A, van Gijn J. Case-fatality and functional outcome after subarachnoid hemorrhage. A systematic review. Stroke 1997;28:660–4.
2. Qureshi AI, Suri MF, Yahia AM, Suarez JI, Guterman LR, Hopkins LN et al. Risk factors for subarachnoid hemorrhage. Neurosurgery 2001;49:607–12.
3. Taylor CL, Yuan Z, Selman WR, Ratcheson RA, Rimm AA. Cerebral arterial aneurysm formation and rupture in 20,767 elderly patients: hypertension and other risk factors. J Neurosurg. 1995;83:812–9.
4. Kubota M, Yamaura A, Ono J. Prevalence of risk factors for aneurysmal subarachnoid haemorrhage: results of a Japanese multicentre case control study for stroke. Br J Neurosurg. 2001;15:474–8.
5. van der Schaaf IC, Ruigrok YM, Rinkel GJ, Algra A, van Gijn J. Study design and outcome measures in studies on aneurysmal subarachnoid hemorrhage. Stroke 2002;33:2043–6.
6. Teunissen LL, Rinkel GJ, Algra A, van Gijn J. Risk factors for subarachnoid hemorrhage: a systematic review. Stroke 1996;27:544–9.
7. Knekt P, Reunanen A, Aho K, Heliovaara M, Rissanen A, Aromaa A, et al. Risk factors for subarachnoid hemorrhage in a longitudinal population study. J Clin Epidemiol. 1991;44:933–9.
8. Juvela S, Hillbom M, Numminen M, Koskinen P. Cigarette smoking and alcohol consumption as risk factors for aneurysmal subarachnoid hemorrhage. Stroke 1993;24:639–46.

9. Pinto AN, Canhao P, Ferro JM. Seizures at the onset of subarachnoid haemorrhage. J Neurol. 1996;243:161–4.
10. Teasdale GM, Drake CG, Hunt W, Kassell N, Sano K, Pertuiset B, et al. A universal subarachnoid hemorrhage scale: report of a committee of the World Federation of Neurosurgical Societies. J Neurol Neurosurg Psychiatry. 1988;11:1457.
11. Fisher C, Kistler J, Davis J. Relation of cerebral vasospasm to subarachnoid hemorrhage visualized by computerized tomographic scanning. Neurosurgery 1980;1:1–9.
12. Feigin VL, Lawes CMM, Bennett DA, Barker-Collo SL, Parag V. Worldwide stroke incidence and early case fatality reported in 56 population-based studies: a systematic review. Lancet Neurol. 2009;8:355–69.
13. Maiuri F, Gallicchio B, Donati P, Carandente M. The blood leukocyte count and its prognostic significance in subarachnoid hemorrhage. J Neurosurg Sci. 1987;31:45–8.
14. McGirt MJ, Mavropoulos JC, McGirt LY, Alexander MJ, Friedman AH, Laskowitz DT, et al. Leukocytosis as an independent risk factor for cerebral vasospasm following aneurysmal subarachnoid hemorrhage. J Neurosurg. 2003;98:1222–6.
15. Parkinson D, Stephensen S. Leukocytosis and subarachnoid hemorrhage. Surg Neurol. 1984;21:132–4.
16. Dehdashti AR, Rufenacht DA, Delavelle J, Reverdin A, de Tribolet N. Therapeutic decision and management of aneurysmal subarachnoid haemorrhage based on computed tomographic angiography. Br J Neurosurg. 2003;17:46–53.
17. Siablis D, Kagadis GC, Karamessini MT. Intracranial aneurysms: reproduction of the surgical view using 3D-CT angiography. Eur J Radiol. 2005;55:92–5.
18. Boet R, Poon WS, Lam JM, Yu SC. The surgical treatment of intracranial aneurysms based on computer tomographic angiography alone – streamlining the acute management of symptomatic aneurysms. Acta Neurochir. 2003;145:101–5.
19. Hoh BL, Cheung AC, Rabinov JD. Results of a prospective protocol of computed tomographic angiography in place of catheter angiography as the only diagnostic and pretreatment planning study for cerebral aneurysms by a combined neurovascular team. Neurosurgery 2004;54:1329–40.
20. Britz GW. ISAT trial: coiling or clipping for intracranial aneurysms? Lancet 2005;366:783–5.
21. Johnston SC, Higashida RT, Barrow DL. Recommendations for the endovascular treatment of intracranial aneurysms: a statement for healthcare professionals from the Committee on Cerebrovascular Imaging of the American Heart Association Council on Cardiovascular Radiology. Stroke 2002;33:2536–44.
22. Lozier AP, Connolly ES Jr, Lavine SD, Solomon RA. Guglielmi detachable coil embolization of posterior circulation aneurysms: a systematic review of the literature. Stroke 2002;33:2509–18.

Clinical Study of Changes of Cerebral Microcirculation in Cerebral Vasospasm After SAH

Wei-na Chai, Xiao-chuan Sun, Fa-jin Lv, Bin Wan, and Li Jiang

Abstract Aim to investigate the changes of cerebral microcirculation after subarachnoid hemorrhage (SAH) and its association with cerebral vasospasm (CVS) after SAH. CTP was performed in 85 patients with SAH and 35 controls. Cerebral blood flow (CBF), cerebral blood volume (CBV) and mean transit time (MTT) were recorded for final analysis. CTP parameters were compared between (1) SAH group and control group, (2) CVS group and non-CVS group (nCVS), (3) symptomatic CVS (sCVS) group and asymptomatic CVS (asCVS) group. Compared to control group, there were significant differences in CBF and MTT of SAH patients ($P < 0.05$). Among SAH patients, the CBF and MTT (a decreased CBF and a prolonged MTT) of CVS patients were significantly different from those of non-CVS patients ($P < 0.05$). In 46 CVS patients, sCVS group presented significantly lower CBF and more prolonged MTT than asCVS patients ($P < 0.05$). Seven cases with MTT between 6.31 and 12.72 s showed delayed ischemic neurological deficit (DIND), two of whom had hemiplegia, and one died. Our findings suggest that CTP examination contributes to uncover the changes of cerebral microcirculation after SAH, and the changes of cerebral microcirculation are associated with CVS post SAH.

Keywords Cerebral microcirculation · Cerebral vasospasm · CT perfusion · Subarachnoid hemorrhage

Introduction

Cerebral vasospasm (CVS) is a common complication of subarachnoid hemorrhage (SAH) and an important reason for poor prognosis. Until now, the diagnosis of CVS mainly depends on clinical symptoms and signs, DSA, CTA and TCD images. However, the major accessory examinations can only identify the changes of large intracranial blood vessels which are not entirely consistent with clinical symptoms and signs. This phenomenon could be explained by the changes of microcirculation [3] which cannot be revealed on DSA, CTA and TCD images.

Have microcirculation remarkably changed when large intracranial vasospasm happened? Can changes in microcirculation predict and be more representative of the occurrence of CVS? Are changes in microcirculation more consistent with clinical manifestations? CTP is a new method to identify the microcirculation homodynamic which has been applied to the study of cerebral ischemic diseases and brain tumor. CTP parameters are used to investigate the changes of microcirculation after SAH as follows.

Methods

General Information

A total of 85 SAH cases and 35 normal subjects were enrolled in this prospective study. If SAH was established on a non-contrast CT scan, we immediately proceeded to CTP and CT angiography (CTA). Patients were brought into the current study if CTP was performed within 14 days after SAH. Patients with SAH from causes other than ruptured aneurysms, patients had cerebrovascular disease, brain tumor, brain injury or functional encephalopathy in the past, and patients had severe blood system diseases were excluded from the current study. All patients' clinical status on admission was assessed by means of Hunt–Hess scale.

CVS Criteria

If there's only arterial segments demonstrating vasospasm by DSA and/or CTA, and/or peak blood flow velocity (BFV) of middle cerebral artery (MCA) greater than 200 cm/s or average BFV greater than 120 cm/s on TCD [1], while patients do not have neurological deficit observed, it can be called asymptomatic CVS (asCVS) [7]. Otherwise, it could be called symptomatic CVS (sCVS) [7].

Sub-Group Study

Patients were divided into CVS group and nCVS group, and CVS group was further divided into sCVS group and asCVS group according to the criteria above. We divided SAH group into I–II group and III–V group by Hunt–Hess scale according to the studies which indicated high association between Hunt–Hess grades and CVS [2]. In addition, 35 normal persons were enrolled as control group, which referred to people who had no cerebrovascular diseases in the past, and there were no abnormalities on head CT scan, and agreed with CTP check (Table 1).

Imaging Technique

All images studies were performed on a 64-slice spiral CT scanner (GE Lightspeed). CTP source data were derived from sequential scans covering a slab of 0.5 cm thickness selected the sella turcica and angulated parallel to the meato-orbital line to contain the upper parts of the lateral ventricles and the basal ganglia. Thirty milliliter of nonionic contrast agent (iopromide, Ultravist 370 mg iodine per milliliter) was injected into the cubital vein at a rate of 4 ml/s followed by a 15 ml saline flush at a rate of 4 ml/s with high-pressure syringe. The following parameters were used: 80 kVp, 200 mAs, 280 layers.

Table 1 Sub-group of objects

Data	Men	Women	Mean age (years ± SD)
Control	18	17	55.12 ± 10.53
CVS-group	20	26	52.78 ± 13.52
nCVS-group	19	20	43.56 ± 18.24
sCVS-group	12	10	55.52 ± 10.78
asCVS-group	11	13	47.57 ± 8.31
Hunt–Hess I–II group	26	22	44.38 ± 19.06
Hunt–Hess III–V group	17	20	52.43 ± 13.87

The original images were transmitted to adw4.2 workstation after scanning to be post-processed using GE perfusion-3-software package. Anterior cerebral artery (ACA), MCA, or internal carotid artery siphon (CS) was selected as an input artery, superior sagittal sinus as the venous output.

One side and the contralateral mirror area of the frontal lobe, temporal lobe, occipital lobe, parietal lobe, thalamus, basal ganglia was selected as region of interest (ROI) to measure the perfusion parameters.

The perfusion parameters used in this study including CBF, CBV and MTT. CBF (ml/min • 100g) refers to a certain amount of blood through the vascular of brain tissue per minute. CBV (ml/g) refers to the blood volume exists in the vascular of brain tissue. MTT (s) refers to the mean time of blood flows through the cerebral vascular structures including arteries, capillaries, venous sinus and vein, for the time is different when the blood flow different path.

Statistical Methods

The differences of parameters between groups were analyzed with one-way ANOVA (F test) using SPSS 13.0 software. The correlation between clinical factors and parameters was analyzed by Logistic single and multi-factor regression.

Results

CTP Parameters of Sub-Groups

The age and sex constitute among CVS group, nCVS group, and control group are of no remarkable difference ($P > 0.05$). The nCVS group's, CVS group's and CVS group's MTT are greater than the normal group, the normal group and nCVS group ($P < 0.05$) and CBF are smaller ($P < 0.05$), respectively. The differences in CBV are not remarkable ($P > 0.05$).

Homogeneously, the age and sex constitute among sCVS group, asCVS group, and control group are also of no remarkable difference ($P > 0.05$). The asCVS group's, sCVS group's and sCVS group's MTT are greater than the normal group, the normal group and asCVS group ($P < 0.05$) and CBF are smaller ($P < 0.05$), respectively, too. The differences in CBV are not remarkable either ($P > 0.05$).

It was shown in Table 2 that the Hunt–Hess III–V patients' MTT are remarkably greater than I–II scale, the former's CBF statistically are lower than the latter ($F = 6.77$, $P < 0.005$; $F = 1.31$, $P < 0.005$), CBV between the two

Table 2 Parameters of sub-groups

	n	MTT(s)	CBF(ml/min·ml)	CBV(ml/g)
CVS	46	4.72 ± 1.67^a	29.87 ± 26.53^a	1.76 ± 1.47
nCVS	39	$3.49 \pm 0.7^{a,b}$	$37.23 \pm 14.59^{a,b}$	1.78 ± 1.46
sCVS	22	5.53 ± 0.83^a	23.14 ± 9.32^a	1.85 ± 0.75
asCVS	24	$4.37 \pm 0.92^{a,c}$	$35.55 \pm 10.03^{a,c}$	1.77 ± 0.96
Control	35	3.13 ± 1.08	47.41 ± 27.23	2.26 ± 1.52
I–II	48	3.92 ± 0.85	30.02 ± 24.59	1.80 ± 1.61
III–V	37	6.29 ± 1.52^d	22.97 ± 19.07^d	1.73 ± 1.29

$^a P < 0.05$ compared with control group
$^b P < 0.05$ compared with CVS group
$^c P < 0.05$ compared with sCVS group
$^d P < 0.05$ compared with Hunt–Hess I–II group

Table 3 The degree of association between related clinical information and MTT↑ and CBF↓

Related factors		MTT↑	P-value	CBF↓	P-value
Age(year)	<45	23	0.0082	22	0.0053
	45–60	37		26	
	>60	25		15	
Sex	Male	44	0.0965	26	0.0023
	Female	41		41	
Hypertension history	Yes	28	0.0658	33	0.0851
	No	57		32	
Hunt–Hess grade	I–II	48	0.2847	37	0.1512
	III–V	37		30	

groups have no significant difference ($F = 0.06$, $P = 0.7987$). The results of perfusion parameters compared are as shown in Table 2.

The Correlation Analysis Between CTP Parameters and the Clinical Data

Single-factor Logistic regression analysis about age, gender, history of hypertension, Hunt–Hess grade with the increase of MTT and CBF reduction (as shown in Table 3) found that gender, high blood pressure have no significant correlation with MTT increase; high blood pressure has no significant correlation with CBF; age and Hunt–Hess grade have good relevance with CBF and MTT; gender also has a better correlation with the CBF. Results of multi-factor Logistic regression analysis after adjusting the clinical data showed Hunt–Hess level is a risk factor for MTT increase.

CTP Parameters and Prognosis

Seven cases with MTT between 6.31 and 12.72 s had delayed neurological deficit (DIND), two of whom were hemiplegic and one died.

Conclusion

CVS is the continuous contraction of affected intracranial arterial with remote reduced supply of cerebral perfusion at the same time. There are "false negative" (severe vasospasm on images but no symptoms and signs) and "false positive" (severe symptoms and signs but no vasospasm on images) results in DSA, CTA and TCD when diagnosing CVS. These phenomena may due to changes in peripheral circulation.

The great basicranial vessels may ensure their diameters after SAH by self-regulatory mechanism but microcirculation's changes may lead to functional changes which result corresponding clinical symptoms, signs, and etc. So studying the changes in microcirculation may help for further understanding CVS.

The viewpoint was supported by latest research. Orthogonal polarization spectral imaging (OPS) is a qualitative and quantitative imaging method which can identify blood flow of cerebral microcirculation. In 2003, Uhl et al. [5] found that more than 50% of patients after SAH (before clipping) have microvascular segmental spasm by OPS, and the reduction of vessel diameter can be up to 75%, which caused a series of clinical symptoms, and affected the clinical outcome ultimately. The study showed that, CVS can not only happen to the great intracranial arteries but also to the brain microcirculation. But angiography couldn't identify spasm of small blood vessels up to now.

CBF and MTT of CVS group have significant differences from nCVS group prompts that, there may be some connection between brain microcirculation's homodynamic and CVS; While SAH group's MTT and CBF remarkably vary with normal group suggests there are changes in microcirculation even in the absence of CVS, and large vessels' spasm makes intracranial cerebral microcirculation more obviously changed.

During the further study, it was found that MTT and CBF of asCVS group and sCVS group both remarkably changed based on the normal group, MTT in sCVS group remarkably extended than asCVS group, CBF decreased remarkably, which suggests that there're still some changes in cerebral microcirculation even no clinical symptoms and signs can be observed, more apparent changes in cerebral microcirculation make clinical symptoms and signs occur.

MTT of patients with higher Hunt–Hess scales remarkably prolonged compared with lower grades, while the former's CBF decreased remarkably, and results of single-factor logistic regression analysis showed that the Hunt–Hess grades had a good correlation with MTT extension and CBF reduction meanwhile, indicated that changes in cerebral microcirculation are associated with clinical symptoms and/or signs, so parameters MTT and CBF may be of important research and clinical application value for cerebral microcirculation.

Turowski et al. [4] found in his study that patients with MTT in 3.2–4 s had loss of nervous system symptoms and signs, and cases with MT $\geq$ 4 s had poor prognosis, and patients with MTT at 3.2 s were compatible for DSA. Our study also found seven cases with MTT in 6.31–12.72 s appeared DIND and had poor prognosis. Wintermark et al. [6] performed CTP and DSA examination in 33 cases of SAH patients in acute stage to evaluate vasospasm and found that, CBF and DSA also have a high relevance in addition to MTT, and their sensitivity and specificity were 92 and 86% (MTT), 75 and 95% (CBF), respectively. He held that MTT map can be used to screen vasospasm and CBF confirm vasospasm. In our study, there were significant differences in MTT and CBF between groups such as CVS group and nCVS Group, sCVS group and as CVS. These may indicate that CTP parameters can be used to help diagnose CVS.

The study found cerebral microcirculation after SAH and clinical manifestations have close correlation through research on CTP of post-SAH, which may help for further understanding CVS. But there may still be some impact on the evaluation of CVS because of the different locations of CTP, DSA, and TCD equipment though the time intervals between inspections were shortened as far as possible. During the next period of research, patients with SAH will be detected dynamically to identify cerebral homodynamic changes before and after CVS. It may help diagnose CVS and improve the prognosis. With relatively less sample, the above conclusions need to be further confirmed with more cases.

Conflict of interest statement We declare that we have no conflict of interest.

References

1. Gonzalez NR, Boscardin WJ, Glenn T, Vinuela F, Martin NA. Vasospasm probability index: a combination of transcranial doppler velocities, cerebral blood flow, and clinical risk factors to predict cerebral vasospasm after aneurysmal subarachnoid hemorrhage. Neurosurgery 2007;107(6):1101–12.
2. Greenberg MS, Arredondo N. Handbook of Neurosurgery (M) 6th ed. New York: Thieme Medical Publishers; 2006;1: p. 785.
3. Macdonald RL, Pluta RM, Zhang JH. Cerebral vasospasm after subarachnoid hemorrhage: the emerging revolution. Nat Clin Pract Neurol. 2007;3:256–63.
4. Turowski B, Haenggi D, Wittsack J, Beck A, Moedder U. Cerebral perfusion computerized tomography in vasospasm after subarachnoid hemorrhage: diagnostic value of MTT. Rofo 2007;179(8): 847–54.
5. Uhl E, Lehmberg J, Steiger HJ, Messmer K. Intraoperative detection of early microvasospasm in patients with subarachnoid hemorrhage by using orthogonal polarization spectral imaging. Neurosurgery 2003;52(6):1307–17.
6. Wintermark M, Dillon WP, Smith WS, Lau BC, Chaudhary S, Liu S, et al. Visual grading system for vasospasm based on perfusion CT imaging: comparisons with conventional angiography and quantitative perfusion CT. Cerebrovasc Dis. 2008;26(2):163–70.
7. Wu J. Cerebral vasospasm after spontaneous subarachnoid hemorrhage. Chinese medical digest. 2004;25(4):538–40.

Effect of Weekend Admission on in-Hospital Mortality After Subarachnoid Hemorrhage in Chongqing China

Guanghui Zhang, John H. Zhang, and Xinyue Qin

Abstract *Background*: Medical resources are usually not the same throughout the week. It is reported that the mortality rate of some disease was higher in patients admitted on weekends than on weekdays. Our study will try to evaluate whether this "weekend effect" acts on in-hospital mortality rate after SAH.

Methods: We performed a retrospective study of patients with SAH admitted to our hospital from January 2006–2009. Patients were classified according to their admission days. The following information, including patient demographics, living habits, systemic complications and Charlson comorbidity index, were documented. Descriptive statistics were used to assess the characteristics between patients admitted on weekends and weekdays. The comparison of mortality between the two groups was carried out by chi-square test. Multivariable regression model was used to analyze the influence of weekend admission on in-hospital mortality and adjust for potential confounders.

Results: Weekend admission accounted for about 29% of the 183 patients with SAH. There were no differences in general characteristics between patients admitted on weekends and those on weekdays. The chi-square test showed the mortality between two groups was not significantly different (0.082). In logistic regression model, weekend admission was not an independent predictor of higher in-hospital mortality (OR 1.77, 95% CI 0.83–3.77) after SAH.

Conclusion: Weekend admission was not closely related to higher in-hospital mortality. There was no weekend effect observed in our hospital in Chongqing, China.

Keywords In-hospital mortality · Subarachnoid hemorrhage · Weekend admission

Introduction

Subarachnoid hemorrhage (SAH) is an acute and intensely life-threating neurologic disease with extremely high rates of morbidity and mortality. SAH occupies about 5–10% of total strokes, and contributes to 10–20% long-term disability and 32–67% case fatality rate [1]. Hydrocephalus, rebleeding and cerebral vascular spasm are the main complications in the acute phase of SAH. Besides neurological complications, there are many severe systemic compilations that might also cause death, such as systemic inflammatory response syndrome (SIRS), myocardial damage, and neurogenic pulmonary edema [2–4]. The treatment of SAH requires immediate examination (skull CT scan or lumbar puncture), diagnosis and relative emergent therapy, which needs a great deal of medical resources. But medical resources may not be uniformly available throughout the week. There is usually a decreased level of staffing on weekends than on weekdays [5].

Weekend admission is associated with increased mortality in different illness or conditions such as cancer, duodenal ulcer, gastrointestinal hemorrhage and cardiovascular symptoms [6, 7]. This weekend effect also occurs in stroke. In a study including 26,676 patients, weekend admission for ischemia stroke was associated with higher short-term mortality when compared with admission during the remainder of the week [8]. Webster et al. found that patients with intracerebral hemorrhage admitted on weekends had increased mortality than did patients admitted on weekdays [9]. But there were few studies involving the effect of week-

G. Zhang and X. Qin (✉)
Department of Neurology, The First Affiliated Hospital, Chongqing Medical University, Chongqing 400016, People's Republic of China
e-mail: Qinxinyue@yahoo.com

J.H. Zhang
Department of Physiology and Pharmacology, Loma Linda University, Loma Linda, CA, USA
Department of Neurosurgery, Loma Linda University, Loma Linda, CA, USA
Department of Anesthesiology, Loma Linda University, Loma Linda, CA, USA

end admission on SAH. The aims of our study were to calculate mortality rates of patients admitted on weekends and those admitted on weekdays, to investigate whether there were any differences of in-hospital mortality between two groups, and to test whether weekend admission was a predictor of increased in-hospital mortality in SAH.

Patients and Methods

This study included 183 patients with SAH admitted to our hospital, the First Affiliated Hospital of Chongqing Medical University in China, between January 2006 and 2009. Detailed clinical data regarding all patients during the period were obtained from medical record library in our hospital. Our study was authorized by the department of scientific research, which administrates scientific research activities in our hospital. The diagnosis of patients was according to the International Classification of Diseases, ninth revision, Clinical Modification (ICD-9-CM) diagnostic code for SAH (ICD-9-CM diagnostic code 430).

Patient demographics, including sex, age and past history of alcohol abuse, were traced. Systemic complications such as pneumonia, urinary tract infections (UTI) and electrolyte disorder were also documented. Pneumonia was defined as symptoms of lower respiratory tract infection as well as an infiltration lesion on chest radiograph or CT scan. Urinary tract infection was defined by patients' reported symptoms plus laboratory tests such as bacterial culture or urine sample with pyuria. Any abnormalities in the levels of sodium iron or potassium iron in fasting plasma during hospital stays were presumed to be electrolyte disorder. Charlson comorbidity index [10] (CCI), which reflects the number and seriousness of comorbid diseases, was reckoned. CCI is widely used in adjusting for the severity of illness.

Patients were classified according to the day of the week that they were admitted. The period from midnight on Friday to midnight on Sunday was defined as weekend, and the remainder of times in the week were considered to be weekdays. This way of defining weekend was also used in other studies involving the weekend effect [11].

Statistical Analysis

SPSS 10.0 software tools were used for data processing. Differences in demographic characteristics, systemic complication, CCI and in-hospital mortality between patients admitted on weekends and on weekdays were compared using the chi-square test or the t-test. Logistic regression model was used to test for predictors of increased in-hospital mortality rates after adjusting for age, sex, alcohol abuse, systemic complication and score on the CCI. Only variables with P value of less than 0.10 on univariate analysis were adopted to multivariate logistic regression model. A statistically significant probability value was defined as $P < 0.05$.

Results

From January 2006 to 2009, there were 198 patients diagnosed with SAH in our hospital. Fifteen patients were excluded from this study because of incomplete clinical information. Of the 183 patients included in our study, the median age was 54.63 ± 11.48 years for males and 57.13 ± 13.61 years for females. There were 53 patients admitted to our hospital on weekends, accounting for about 29% of the total group. One hundred and thirty patients were admitted on weekdays. There were no significant differences in baseline characteristics between patients admitted on weekends and those admitted on weekdays (Table 1).

A total of 62 (33.9%) patients died in hospital; 23 (12.6%) of them were weekend admissions, and 39 (21.3%) were weekday admissions. The in-hospital mortality of weekend admission (43.4%) was higher than that of weekday admission (30%), but Chi test showed there was no significant difference between two groups (p = 0.082). Univariate analysis identified five factors that closely related to in-hospital mortality: CCI (p = 0.03), electrolyte disorder (p < 0.001), pneumonia (p = 0.002), UTI (p = 0.068) and older age (p < 0.001). Two variates were excluded from logistic

Table 1 Characteristics of the patients admitted on weekdays and weekends

Variables	Weekday admissions (n = 130)	Weekend admissions (n = 53)	p value
Age, year (mean ± SD)	55.28 ± 12.42	57.06 ± 12.89	0.386
Sex, male (%)	71(55)	27(51)	0.651
History of alcohol abuse (%)	11(8)	5(9)	0.83
CCI (%)			0.983
0	80(62)	31(59)	
1	19(15)	8(15)	
2	20(15)	9(17)	
≥3	11(7)	5(9)	
Pneumonia (%)	24(18)	12(23)	0.519
UTI (%)	13(10)	6(11)	0.790
Electrolyte disorder (%)	51(39)	17(32)	0.364
Death (%)	39(30)	23(43)	0.082

CCI Charlson comorbidity index; *UTI* urinary tract infections

Table 2 Univariate analysis of predictive factors for in-hospital mortality

Variable	Survivor	Death	p value
Age, year, mean ± SD	53.45 ± 11.83	60.29 ± 12.78	<0.001
Sex, male (%)	66(55)	32(52)	0.707
History of alcohol abuse (%)	11(9)	5(8)	0.816
CCI (%)			0.030
0	80(66)	31(50)	
1	19(16)	8(13)	
2	15(12)	14(22)	
≥3	7(6)	9(15)	
Pneumonia (%)	16(13)	20(32)	0.002
UTI (%)	9(7)	10(16)	0.068
Electrolyte disorder (%)	34(28)	34(55)	<0.001
Weekend admission (%)	30(25)	23(37)	0.082

CCI Charlson comorbidity index; *UTI* urinary tract infections

Table 3 Multivariate analysis of predictive factors for in-hospital mortality

Variable	OR	95% CI	p value
Weekend admission	1.77	0.83–3.77	0.137
Age	1.04	1.01–1.07	0.009
Pneumonia	3.11	1.30–7.40	0.011
UTI	2.16	0.72–6.46	0.169
Electrolyte disorder	2.55	1.24–5.22	0.011

OR odds ratio; *UTI* urinary tract infections

regression model because of unsuitable p value: alcohol abuse (p = 0.816) and sex (p = 0.707) (Table 2).

After adjusting for CCI, electrolyte disorder, pneumonia, UTI and age, logistic regression illustrated that weekend admission was not an independent predictor of higher in-hospital mortality (OR 1.77, 95% CI 0.83–3.77; Table 3).

Discussion

In recent years, the weekend effect is receiving great concern from clinical researchers. In the present study, in-hospital mortality of weekend admission was slightly higher than that of weekday admission, but chi-square test demonstrated there was no significant difference between two groups, and logistic regression analysis showed that weekend admission was not an independent predictor of higher in-hospital mortality, which meant that weekend admission was not closely related to increased in-hospital mortality in SAH.

A number of research reported that weekend admission was associated with higher mortality. Barnett and his colleagues [12] performed a study including 1,56,136 patients admitted to intensive care units. They found that patients admitted to ICU on weekends experienced higher mortality and longer stay in ICU. However, they also found there was similar higher risk for death in patients admitted on Monday and Friday. A study involving 6,41,860 patients with 50 common diagnoses illustrated that patients admitted to hospital on the weekend had higher in-hospital mortality than those admitted on weekdays, and interestingly, this phenomenon was more evident in major teaching hospitals [13]. Later, Ensminger et al. [14] conducted another study regarding weekend effect on in-hospital mortality, and a total of 29,084 patients were included. They reported that there was no difference of the total mortality between patients admitted to ICU on weekends and those on weekdays, but in surgical ICU, weekend admission possessed higher in-hospital mortality than weekday admission.

Hasegawa et al. [15] reported weekend effect on stroke. They illustrated that weekday admission was associated with decreased case fatality and positive outcome at discharge in the acute stroke unit, and a reduction in the weekday ratio caused worse outcome in patients with rehabilitative therapy. But in a retrospective study conducted by Webster [16], weekend admission was not closely related to short-term mortality in patient with SAH.

There are some possible reasons for the weekend effect. Fewer doctors and nurses on weekends is the most popular. Inexperienced staff, lessened interventions and operations, unavailable facilities and tests on weekends are also taken into account. The disparity between patients admitted on weekends and weekdays may be another explanation for the weekend effect. LaBounty et al. [17] found that patients admitted on weekends were more likely to appear the condition of AMI than those admitted on weekdays.

But in our study, there were no significant differences in general characteristics between patients admitted on weekends and weekdays, including patient demographics, CCI, and systemic complications. Here may be some reasons for our negative weekend effect. As we know, being the most acute and life-threating illness in neurology, SAH attracts great attention from clinical staff. A relatively standard procedure has been constructed, including treatment in acute stage and intervention on intracranial aneurysm. There is no delay in the entire hospital stay. All necessary equipment is open to patients with SAH. Special staff for treatment of intracranial aneurysm are ready all week. Furthermore, in our study, a large part of patients with SAH were in severe conditions at early stage of illness, and there was little chance of them surviving even under the help of the best experienced medical staff, which also contribute to the negative weekend effect.

Some limitations of this study should be mentioned. As a retrospective study, we could not pursue the survival state of discharged patients, and the effect of weekend admission on long-term mortality was not accomplished. We also failed to detect the relation between weekend admission and neurofunctional rehabilitation, cognitive, and behavioral outcome, while weekend admission may have influence on outcome irrespective of mortality. In addition, we did not take long holidays into account, such as National Day or New Year's Day, which might exert more impact on mortality than weekend admission in China. Further research is needed to investigate the weekend effect on SAH.

Conflict of interest statement We declare that we have no conflict of interest.

References

1. Hop JW, Rinkel GJ, Algra A, van Gijn J. Case-fatality rates and functional outcome after subarachnoid hemorrhage: a systematic review. Stroke 1997;28(3):660–4.
2. Wartenberg KE, Mayer SA. Medical complications after subarachnoid hemorrhage: new strategies for prevention and management. Curr Opin Crit Care. 2006;12(2):78–84.
3. Wartenberg KE, Schmidt JM, Claassen J, Temes RE, Frontera JA, Ostapkovich N, et al. Impact of medical complications on outcome after subarachnoid hemorrhage. Crit Care Med. 2006;34(3):617–23.
4. Stevens RD, Nyquist PA. The systemic implications of aneurysmal subarachnoid hemorrhage. Neurol Sci. 2007;261(1–2):143–56.
5. Bell CM, Redelmeier DA. Mortality among patients admitted to hospitals on weekends as compared with weekdays. N Engl J Med. 2001;345(9):663–8.
6. Cram P, Hillis SL, Barnett M, Rosenthal GE. Effects of weekend admission and hospital teaching status on in-hospital mortality. Am J Med. 2004;117(3):151–7.
7. Shaheen AA, Kaplan GG, Myers RP. Weekend versus weekday admission and mortality from gastrointestinal hemorrhage caused by peptic ulcer disease. Clin Gastroenterol Hepatol. 2009;7(3):303–10.
8. Saposnik G, Baibergenova A, Bayer N, Hachinski V. Weekends: a dangerous time for having a stroke? Stroke 2007;38(4):1211–5.
9. Crowley RW, Yeoh HK, Stukenborg GJ, Medel R, Kassell NF, Dumont AS. Influence of weekend hospital admission on short-term mortality after intracerebral hemorrhage. Stroke 2009;40(7):2387–92.
10. Charlson ME, Pompei P, Ales KL, MacKenzie CR. A new method of classifying prognostic comorbidity in longitudinal studies: development and validation. J Chronic Dis. 1987;40(5):373–83.
11. Bell CM, Redelmeier DA. Mortality among patients admitted to hospitals on weekends as compared with weekdays. N Engl J Med. 2001;345(9):663–8.
12. Barnett MJ, Kaboli PJ, Sirio CA, Rosenthal GE. Day of the week of intensive care admission and patient outcomes: a multisite regional evaluation. Med Care. 2002;40(6):530–9.
13. Cram P, Hillis SL, Barnett M, Rosenthal GE. Effects of weekend admission and hospital teaching status on in-hospital mortality. Am J Med. 2004;117(3):151–7.
14. Ensminger SA, Morales IJ, Peters SG, Keegan MT, Finkielman JD, Lymp JF, et al. The hospital mortality of patients admitted to the ICU on weekends. Chest 2004;126(4):1292–8.
15. Hasegawa Y, Yoneda Y, Okuda S, Hamada R, Toyota A, Gotoh J, et al. The effect of weekends and holidays on stroke outcome in acute stroke units. Cerebrovasc Dis. 2005;20(5):325–31.
16. Crowley RW, Yeoh HK, Stukenborg GJ, Ionescu AA, Kassell NF, Dumont AS. Influence of weekend versus weekday hospital admission on mortality following subarachnoid hemorrhage. J Neurosurg. 2009;111(1):60–6.
17. LaBounty T, Eagle KA, Manfredini R, Fang J, Tsai T, Smith D, et al. The impact of time and day on the presentation of acute coronary syndromes. Clin Cardiol. 2006;29(12):542–6.

The Correlation Between COMT Gene Polymorphism and Early Cerebral Vasospasm After Subarachnoid Hemorrhage

Zhaohui He, Xiaochuan Sun, Zongduo Guo, and John H. Zhang

Abstract *Background*: The individual difference of cerebral vasospasm (CVS) degree after subarachnoid hemorrhage (SAH) is common in clinic observation. Numerous studies have found that early CVS after SAH is associated with derangements in catecholamine(CA) metabolism. Catechol-O-methyltransferase (COMT) is a key rate-limiting enzyme in the degradation of CA. In this study, we investigate the correlation between COMT gene polymorphism of patients and early CVS after SAH.

Methods: One hundred and sixty-seven patients with spontaneous SAH in early stage were selected in this study. COMT genotyping was performed by means of polymerase chain reaction-restriction fragment length polymorphism (PCR-RFLP). The degree of CVS was identified by TCD. Hunt–Hess classification was used to evaluate the severity of the patients' condition. The bleeding amount was evaluated by means of Fisher classification of head CT. $\chi 2$ test (SPSS13.0 software) and logistic regression were adopted to analyze the correlation of COMT gene polymorphism and other clinical data of patients with early CVS after SAH.

Results: The distribution of each allele matched Hardy–Weinberg law and research samples were heredity equilibrium population. Early CVS incidence of patients with COMT-A allele was much higher than those with COMT-G allele ($P < 0.01$). Early CVS incidence of patients with COMT A/A genotype was obviously higher than those with COMT G/G genotype ($P < 0.05$). Univariate logistic regression demonstrated that COMT-A allele, A/A genotype and Grade 3–5 of Hunt–Hess classification were all associated with early CVS. After adjustment of general information, further multivariate logistic regression demonstrated that COMT-A allele, A/A genotype were risk factors of early CVS after SAH.

Conclusion: COMT-A allele, A/A genotype were risk factors of early CVS after SAH.

Keywords Cerebral vasospasm · COMT · Gene polymorphism · Subarachnoid hemorrhage

Introduction

CVS after SAH frequently results in severe cerebral ischemia and other brain injuries and is the main cause of aneurysm-related death or disability [1–3]. "Dual-phase phenomenon" has been observed in CVS after SAH: early (acute) CVS and delayed (chronic) CVS. Early CVS affects the occurrence and development of delayed CVS [4]. It has been observed that early brain injury (EBI) after SAH is the main cause of death induced by SAH [5].

The individual difference of CVS degree after SAH is common in clinical observation. It was discovered that polymorphism of some gene is associated with the individual difference of CVS degree after SAH [6–7]. Numerous studies have found that early CVS after SAH is associated with derangements in CA metabolism. COMT is a key rate-limiting enzyme in CA degradation [1–2]. So we hypothesize that the individual difference of early CVS degree after SAH is related to the individual difference of COMT activity which was produced by gene polymorphism.

The recent discovery that COMT gene polymorphism is associated with the hereditary susceptibility of PD, schizophrenia and attention deficit hyperactivity disorder support our hypothesis [8–10]. Up to now, there is no report on the correlation between COMT gene polymorphism and individual difference of early CVS degree after SAH. The present

Z. He, X. Sun (✉), and Z. Guo
Department of Neurosurgery, First Affiliated Hospital of Chongqing Medical University, Chongqing 400016, People's Republic of China
e-mail: sunxch1445@gmail.com

J.H. Zhang
Department of Neurosurgery, Loma Linda University, Loma Linda, CA, USA

study aims to analyze this correlation and explore the cause of the individual difference of early CVS degree after SAH.

Materials and Methods

Inclusion Criteria and Exclusion Criteria of Patients Selection

Patients with sSAH (sSAH onsetting time is shorter than 3 days) which were confirmed by CT scanning and lumbar puncture were selected. Patients with doubtful head injury history and brain herniation within 3 days, who could not survive beyond 3 days after SAH, were excluded.

Record of Clinical Information

The clinical data of the patients included were recorded, such as age, sex, having hypertension or not, having hyperlipemia or not, Hunt–Hess grade and Fisher grade on admission, traunscranial doppler sonography (TCD) examination and treatment as well. According to patients' individual condition, blood pressure (BP) was controlled to 90–140/50–90 mmHg. Besides that, patients received spasmolytic therapy, hemostatic treatment, as well as symptomatic treatment.

This study was approved by the ethics committee of the Department of Medical Research. An informed consent was obtained from the patient himself/herself directly or their family members if the status of patients' consciousness restricted such procedure.

Judgment of CVS

Before operation or interventional therapy, the blood flow rate of middle cerebral artery (MCA) and anterior cerebral artery (ACA) were measured by TCD every day from first to third days after hemorrhage. The peak flow rate of MCA (Vm) in each patients were regarded as judgment evidence, Vm $\geq$ 120 cm/s were deemed to present CVS, while Vm < 120 cm/s were ruled out [11].

Genotyping of COMT

Venous blood was collected from patients on admission, and then frozen and stored for extraction of DNA by standard techniques. The primer was designed and synthesized by Shanghai Sangon Biological Engineering Technology& Service Limited Company, gene order of the 158th amino acids in forth exon in COMT gene was amplified. The sequence is P_1: 5'TCGTGGACGCCGTGATTCAGG3', P_2: 5'AGGTCTGACAACGGGTCAGGC3'. PCR amplification was carried out under reaction system with DNA, 2 μl; P_1, 0.5 μl; P_2, 0.5 μl; Taq enzyme, 10 μl; H_2O, 7 μl and reaction condition of 94°C–5 min→ (94°C–30 s→57°C–30 s→72°C–30 s) × 30→72°C–10 min. The PCR products were digested by NIaIII and the fragments were separated by agarose gel electrophoresis (5V/1 cm) for genotype determination. DNA fragments were visualized by ultraviolet illumination.

The total length of PCR product is 217 bp. G allele contains two enzyme reaction site on 83 bp and 197 bp which should present three strap of 83, 114, and 20 bp after N1aIII enzyme reaction. A allele contains three enzyme reaction site on 83, 179, and 197 bp which should present four strap of 83, 96, 18, and 20 bp after N1aIII enzyme reaction.

The results were interpreted according to the simplified Richard method.

Statistic Analysis

The SPSS 13.0 software was used. The constituent ratio of each correlation factor in clinical data of SAH patients was analyzed using χ^2 test, the statistical difference of incidence of each COMT genotype and allele was analyzed by χ^2 test. Univariate logistic regression was performed to analyze the association of each clinical correlation factor, COMT genotype and allele with CVS, after adjustment of clinical data, further multivariate logistic regression was used to analyze the association of COMT genotype and allele with CVS.

Results

Clinical Information of SAH Suffers

According to the inclusion and exclusion criteria, a total of 167 SAH sufferers admitted to Dept. Neurosurgery, the First Affiliated Hospital of Chongqing Medical University from January 1, 2008 to December 30, 2008, were involved in the current research.

The clinical data such as age, sex, having hypertension or not, having hyperlipemia or not, Hunt–Hess grade and Fisher grade of CT scanning were available (Table 1). TCD

Table 1 The distribution of related clinical data of patients with spontaneous SAH

		CVS(−)	CVS(+)	X^2	P value
Age	<60	48	32	0.2316	0.6306
	≥60	49	38		
Sex	Male	43	28	0.3119	0.5765
	Female	54	42		
Hypertension or not	Yes	36	29	0.3185	0.5725
	No	61	41		
Hyperlipemia or not	Yes	40	31	0.1546	0.6942
	No	57	39		
Hunt & Hess grade	1–2	84	51	4.9559	0.0226
	3–5	13	19		
Fisher grade	1–2	66	38	3.2747	0.0704
	3–4	31	32		

Table 2 The distribution of COMT genotypes and allele frequency

Genotype			Allele	
G/G	G/A	A/A	G	A
92 (55.1%)	63 (37.7%)	12 (7.2%)	247 (74.0%)	87 (26.0%)

Table 3 The association of COMT genetype and allele frequency with CVS

	Genotype						Allele	
	G/G	G/A	G/G	A/A	G/A	A/A	G	A
CVS(+)	64	34	64	4	34	4	162	42
CVS(−)	28	29	28	8	29	8	85	45
X^2	3.2754		6.1571		1.7171		8.1104	
P value	0.0873		0.0131		0.1901		0.0044	

showed that 70 patients presented with CVS and 97 patients presented with no CVS, which divided patients into CVS(+) group and CVS(−) group. χ2 test demonstrated no statistical difference in constituent ratio of age, sex, hypertension, hyperlipemia and Fisher grade in two groups (P > 0.05), but the constituent ratio of Hunt–Hess 3–5 grade in CVS(+) group is significantly higher than that of CVS(−) group (P = 0.0226).

The Distributions of COMT Genotypes and Allele Frequency

The distributions of COMT genotypes and allele frequency of 167 patients were given in Table 2. Genotypic distribution was consistent with Hardy–Weinberg equilibrium (P > 0.05), the research sample are genetic equilibrium population.

COMT Gene Polymorphism and CVS

COMT Genotype and CVS

The incidence of CVS in patients with A/A genotype (66.7%) is significantly higher than that in patients with G/G genotype (30.4%) (X^2 = 6.1571, P = 0.0131) and showed statistical difference. The incidence of CVS in patients with A/A genotype (66.7%) is higher than that in patients with G/A genotype (46.0%) (X^2 = 1.7171, P = 0.1901), but no significant difference was found between the two groups. The incidence of CVS in patients with G/A genotype (46.0%) is higher than that in patients with G/G genotype (30.4%) (X^2 = 3.2754, P = 0.0873), but significant difference was not noted in these two groups.

COMT Allele and CVS

The incidence of CVS in patients carrying A allele (51.7%) is significantly higher than that of patients with G allele (34.4%) (X^2 = 8.1104, P = 0.0044) (Table 3).

Univariate and Multiple Logistic Regression on Each Related Clinical Factor

Univariate logistic regression revealed the association of CVS with COMT-A allele, A/A genotype and Grade 3–5 of Hunt–Hess. After adjustment for general information, including age, sex, having hypertension or not, having hyperlipemia or not, Hunt–Hess grade and Fisher grade, the further multiple logistic regression showed that COMT-A allele, A/A genotype were still risk factors to predispose to SAH induced CVS. (OR = 2.798, OR95%CI = (0.575, 9.112), P = 0.0397; OR = 3.875, OR 95%CI = (1.991, 7.351), P = 0.0310) (Table 4).

Conclusion

Although DSA angiograph is always regarded as the gold standard of diagnosis to cerebrovascular disease and cerebralvasospasm, the limit of invasion and inability of repeated measurement confine its continuous monitoring on occurrence, development and turnover of CVS. After its application in clinic in 1982, TCD makes it possible to measure, atraumatically and repeatedly, the changes in blood flow velocity that occur with vasospasm after SAH. Up to now, TCD is still the most frequently used approach to assess CVS which can continuously monitor the cerebral haemodynamics changes [12].

Table 4 The logistic regression analysis of each single factor and CVS

correlation factor	P	OR	OR95%CI
Sex	0.5202	0.792	(0.389, 1.611)
Age	0.0569	2.248	(1.011, 4.997)
Blood fat	0.2933	1.470	(0.717, 3.014)
Blood pressure	0.5403	0.768	(0.577, 2.366)
Fisher grade	0.0587	4.540	(2.040, 19.840)
H-H grade	0.0432	5.110	(1.600, 24.060)
G/G	0.1974	1.013	(0.532, 4.565)
G/A	0.0736	1.580	(0.770, 6.570)
A/A	0.0224	3.105	(1.174, 8.208)
G	0.1356	1.204	(0.662, 4.505)
A	0.0217	4.422	(1.243, 15.735)

A great number of studies proved the clear correlation between increasing of blood flow velocity reflected by TCD and CVS presented in angiograph, especially in middle cerebral artery [13–14]. Aäslid et al. carried out the clinical scale of CVS induced by SAH according to the clinical follow-up observation by TCD. Blood flow velocity of 120–140 cm/s were deemed to mild CVS, 140–200 cm/s were regarded as moderate CVS, exceed to 200 cm/s were defined as serious CVS, while slower than 120 cm/s were ruled out of CVS [15].

Angiographic middle and anterior cerebral artery diameter and transcranial ultrasound flow velocity measurements were performed by Grosset et al. in 102 patients with recent aneurysmal subarachnoid haemorrhage [16]. There was a significant inverse correlation between middle cerebral artery diameter and flow velocity. No such correlation was seen for anterior cerebral arteries. This discovery was consistent with the hemodynamic principle that the velocity of blood flow is inversely related to the lumen area. But this principle is not suitable to ACA because of its sufficient collateral circulation. Therefore, when CVS degree of MCA was measured, TCD displayed an accuracy of 85–90%, which was much higher than that of ACA or PCA [17]. Based on the hemodynamic principle, we adopt TCD to detect the blood flow velocity of SAH patients in early stage (1–3 days) and choose MCA as the observation spot to evaluate CVS degree.

It is common in clinical observation that some patients with large amount of bleeding displayed less severe CVS, while some patients with mild hemorrhage showed severe CVS; some patients with severe CVS in TCD, CTA, DSA displayed mild condition, while some patients with mild CVS in TCD, CTA, DSA presented severe condition. The conflicting phenomena above implies significant individual difference in CVS degree and prognosis of sufferers with SAH, which has been believed be associated with gene polymorphisms.

Accumulating evidence indicated that several gene may influence CVS degree and outcome of SAH victims [6–7].

It was mentioned above that early CVS after SAH is associated with increased CA [1–2]. COMT is a chief rate-limiting enzyme in degradation of CA, widespread in forebrain, striatum, neurogliocyte limbic system and displayed higher activity in synaptic cleft, especially in postsynaptic membrane. Under the catalysis of magnesium, the enzyme introduces a methyl group to CA, which is donated by S-adenosyl methionine (SAM) to produce 3-methoxy-4-hydroxy derivatives resulting in the activation of CA or inactivation of toxic effects of CA [18]. Therefore, COMT should be an important factor impacting CA content and CVS degree. Based on the deduction, we hypothesize that the COMT activity of some patients is relatively lower with homologous weaker inactivation on CA, as a result, the CVS is more severe with a longer duration and the patients' condition is more serious with a worse prognosis. On the other hand, the COMT activity of some patients is relatively higher with homologous stronger inactivation on CA, consequently, the CVS is milder with a shorter duration and the patients' condition is milder with a better prognosis.

It was proven that the individual difference of COMT activity is great with three phenotype as mild, moderate, high activity. A functional G to A polymorphism in the fourth exon of COMT gene results in a valine to methionine amino acid transition at codon 158 (COMT Val158Met polymorphism) leading to thermolability and lower activity of the enzyme [19–20].

The three phenotype of COMT is determined by the two alleles of Val-COMT and Met-COMT and inherit by means of codominance style. The former enhanced the enzyme activity for 3–4 times, the activity of enzyme with Val/Val genotype is high, the activity of enzyme with Val/Met is moderate, while the activity of enzyme with Met/Met is low [21–22].

The phenomenon above imply the polymorphism of COMT gene. The association of COMT gene polymorphism with hereditary susceptibility of Parkinson's disease, schizophrenia and attention deficit hyperactivity disorder proven in previous studies hinted potentiality of our hypothesis [8–10].

But up to now, the report on association between COMT gene polymorphism and CVS degree in early stage after SAH is not available.

In this study, univariate logistic regression demonstrated that, in the Chinese Han population, the CVS incidence of patients with A/A genotype is significantly higher than that of patients with G/G genotype (P = 0.013) and the CVS incidence of A allele carrier is obviously higher that of G allele carrier (P = 0.0044). Furthermore, after the adjustment of general information, including age, sex, having hypertension or not, having hyperlipemia or not, Hunt–Hess grade and Fisher grade, the further multiple logistic regression showed that the A allele and A/A genotype are still risk factors to predispose to SAH induced CVS. From the current study results, it could be presumed that high activity COMT can more effectively decompose, inactivate CA and CVS is milder, while low activity COMT cannot sufficiently deactivate increased CA and induce more severe CVS consequently.

It was presumed in previous reports that the association of blood volume in Fisher's classification with latent risk of CVS is helpful to estimate the potentiality of CVS after SAH [23]. Moreover, it was reported that blood volume of SAH presented in CT is a chief risk factor of CVS [24]. In our study, although the CVS incidence of patients with 3–4 Fisher's grade is obviously higher than those with 1–2 Fishers grade, no statistic difference can be found, furthermore, univariate logistic regression showed no correlation between the Fisher's classification and CVS incidence, which is not consistent with previous studies. The results above confirmed the clinical phenomenon that the CVS degree of patients with larger size of hemorrhage is not severe correspondingly, implied the possibility of individual difference induced by gene polymorphism, if the statistical discrepancy due to small sample size can be excluded.

It was reported that CVS degree can be predicted by Hunt & Hess score, that means if the Hunt & Hess score of patients is higher, the incidence of the CVS is higher [25]. In our study, the CVS incidence of patients with 3–5 Hunt & Hess score is significantly higher than that of patients with 1–2 Hunt & Hess score (P = 0.0226), and univariate logistic regression demonstrated that 3–5 Hunt & Hess score is a risk factor, which was consistent with previous study. The above results indicated that CVS is one of the chief causes of grave condition of patients, that is to say, the more severe condition of patients implied larger opportunity of CVS.

COMT is just one of the rate-limiting enzymes in the CA metabolic pathway and plays a role in the mechanism of CA increasing. The association of COMT gene polymorphism with CVS is one of the important factors of individual difference of CVS and cooperates with other enzymes in CA metabolic pathway to exert its effect on polymorphism. Individual difference of CVS should be related to the gene polymorphism of other enzymes in CA metabolic pathway, which is the target of our next research.

As an important complication of SAH, numerous studies were carried out to treat CVS through the gene engineering approach. However, the treatments adopted in present clinical work aimed at the external factor of CVS, instead of the most principal cause of the individual difference – genetics. As the development of mechanism on CVS and gene technology, gene polymorphism analysis could be undertaken in a short time and the risk of SAH patients can be evaluated and predicted individually. According to the specific gene type, homologous gene intervention could be selected to achieve the purpose of individual treatment.

Acknowledgements Financial support from the Nature Science Funds of Chongqing Science and Technology Committee (CSTC, 2008BB5219) is gratefully acknowledged.

Conflict of interest statement We declare that we have no conflict of interest.

References

1. Dilraj A, Botha JH, Rambiritch V, Miller R, van Dellen JR. Levels of catecholamine in plasma and cerebrospinal fluid in aneurysmal subarachnoid hemorrhage. Neurosurgery 1992;31(1):42–50.
2. Naredi S, Lambert G, Edén E, Zäll S, Runnerstam M, Rydenhag B, et al. Increased sympathetic nervous activity in patients with nontraumatic subarachnoid hemorrhage. Stroke 2000;31:901–6.
3. Condette-Auliac S, Bracard S, Anxionnat R, Schmitt E, Lacour JC, Braun M, et al. Vasospasm after SAH: interest in diffusion-weighted MR imaging. Stroke 2001;32:1818–24.
4. Shen JK. The pathogenesis of cerebral vasospasm and its prevention and treatment. Int J Cerebrovasc Dis. 2006;14(7):481–93.
5. Ostrowski RP, Colohan AR, Zhang JH. Molecular mechanisms of early brain injury after subarachnoid hemorrhage. Neurolog Res. 2006;28:399–414.
6. Khurana VG, Sohni YR, Mangrum WI, McClelland RL, O'Kane DJ, Meyer FB, et al. Section on cerebrovascular surgery: Galbraith award: endothelial nitric oxide synthase (eNOS) and heme oxygenase-1 (HO-1) gene polymorphisms predict susceptibility to aneurysmal subarachnoid hemorrhage (SAH) and post-SAH cerebral vasospasm. Clin Neurosurg. 2004;51:343–50.
7. Ko NU, Rajendran P, Kim H, Rutkowski M, Pawlikowska L, Kwok PY, et al. Endothelial nitric oxide synthase polymorphism (-786T- > C) and increased risk of angiographic vasospasm after aneurysmal subarachnoid hemorrhage. Stroke 2008;39(4):1103–8.
8. Kunugi H, Nanko S, Ueki A, Otsuka E, Hattori M, Hoda F, et al. High and low activity alleles of catechol-O-methyltransferase gene: ethnic difference and possible association with Parkinson's disease. Neurosci Lett. 1997;221:202–4.
9. Goldberg TE, Egan MF, Gscheidle T, Coppola R, Weickert T, Kolachana BS. Executive subprocesses in working memory: relationship to catechol-O-methyltransferase Val158Met genotype and schizophrenia. Arch Gen Psychiatry. 2003;60:889–96.
10. Eisenberg J, Mei-Tal G, Steinberg A, Tartakovsky E, Zohar A, Gritsenko I, et al. Haplotype relative risk study of catechol-o-methyltransferase (COMT) and attention deficit hyperactivity disorder (ADHD): association of the high-enzyme activity Valallele with ADHD impulsive-hyperactive phenotype. Am J Med Gene. 1999;88:497–502.
11. Kochanowicz J, Krejza J, Mariak Z, Ustymowicz A, Lewko J. Diagnosis of middle cerebral artery spasm by determination of flow velocity and the Lindegaard index with transcranial color Doppler sonography. Neurol Neurochir Pol. 2005;39:11–6.
12. Lindegaard KF. The role of transcranial Doppler in the management of patients with subarachnoid haemorrhage: a review. Acta Neurochir (Wien). 1999;72:59–71.
13. Aaslid R, Huber R, Nomes H. Evaluation of cerebrovascular spasm with transcranial Doppler ultrasound. J Neurosurg. 1984;60:37–42.
14. Harders AG, Gilsbach JM. Time course of blood velocity changes related to vasospasm in the circle of Willis measured by transcranial Doppler ultrasound. J Neurosurg. 1987;66:718–22.
15. Aäslid R et al. Transcranial doppler sonography. New York: Springer; 1986.

16. Grosset DG, Straiton J, McDonald I, Bullock R. Angiographic and Doppler diagnosis of cerebral artery vasospasm following subarachnoid Hemorrhage. Br J Neurosurg. 1993;7(3):291–8.
17. Aaslid R. Transcranial Doppler assessment of cerebral vasospasm. Eur J Ultrasound. 2002;16:3–10.
18. Männistö PT, Kaakkola S. Catechol-O-methyltransferase (COMT): biochemistry molecular biology, pharmacology, and clinical efficacy of the new selective COMT inhibitors. Pharmacol Rev. 1999;51(4):594–622.
19. Chen X, Wang X, O'Neill AF, Walsh D, Kendler KS. Variants in the catechol-o-methyltransferase (COMT) gene are associated with schizophrenia in Irish high – density families. Mol Psychiatry. 2004;9:(10):962–7.
20. Spielman RS, Weinshilboum RM. Genetics of red cell COMT activity: analysis of thermal stability and family data. Am J Med Genet. 1981;10:279–90.
21. Lotta T, Vidgren J, Tilgmann C, Ulmanen I, Melén K, Julkunen I, et al. Kinetics of human soluble and membrane-bound catechol-O-methyltransferase: a revised mechanism and description of the thermolabile variant of the enzyme. Biochemisty 1995;34:4202–10.
22. Palmatier MA, Kang AM, Kidd KK. Global variation in the frequencies of functional different catechol-O-methyltransferase alleles. Biol Psychiatry. 1999;46:557–67.
23. Janjua N, Mayer SA. Cerebral vasospasm after subaracnoid hemorrhage. Curr Opin Crit Care. 2003;9(2):113–9.
24. Hirashima Y, Kurimoto M, Hori E, Origasa H, Endo S. Lower incidence of symptomatic vasospasm after subarachnoid hemorrhage owing to ruptured vertebrobasilar aneurysms. Neurosurgery 2005;57(6):1110–6.
25. Dietrich HH, Dacey RG Jr. Molecular keys to the problems of cerebral vasospasm. Neurosurgery 2000;46:517–30.

Fever Increased In-Hospital Mortality After Subarachnoid Hemorrhage

Guanghui Zhang, John H. Zhang, and Xinyue Qin

Abstract *Objective*: Fever is a common clinical complication in patients with subarachnoid hemorrhage (SAH), and is usually related to prognosis in early stage of diseases. In our study, we try to help improve the outcome of SAH by assessing possible risk factors for fever and investigating the influence of fever on in-hospital mortality.

Methods: Fever was defined as axillary temperature above 38.3°C appearing at least two times (not in the same day). One hundred and fifty-five patients with SAH were divided into febrile group and afebrile group. The following data were documented: patient demographics, clinical grade on admission Glasgow Coma Scale score, Hunt–Hess grade), conscious state on admission, presence of seizure, imaging assessment, admission glucose levels and plasma electrolytes levels. Univariate analysis and multivariate logistic regression analysis were used to determine factors associated with fever or in-hospital mortality.

Results: Forty-one percent of patients with SAH developed fever. As determined by univariate analysis, older age, history of hypertension, Glasgow Coma Scale score, Hunt–Hess grade, Fisher CT grade, conscious state on admission, presence of intraventricular hemorrhage (IVH), admission glucose levels and plasma electrolytes levels were factors for fever. Multivariate analysis indicated that three factors independently predicted the occurrence of fever: poor Hunt–Hess grade (OR 5.37, 95% CI 1.56–18.44), presence of IVH (OR 5.18, 95% CI 1.43–18.85) and older age (OR 1.06, 95% CI 1.02–1.09). In-hospital mortality after SAH was associated with fever (OR 17.36, 95% CI 4.47–67.35), consciousness disorders on admission (OR 5.89, 95% CI 1.16–29.89) and older age (OR 1.07, 95% CI 1.00–1.13).

Conclusions: Poor Hunt–Hess grade, presence of IVH and older age are independent predictors of fever in SAH. Fever is closely related to increased in-hospital mortality after SAH.

Keywords Fever · In-hospital mortality · Subarachnoid hemorrhage

Introduction

In ischemic stroke, fever usually aggravates ischemic damage, enlarges infarct area, worsens cerebral edema, suppresses neural recovery [1–3], and is related to bad outcomes [4–6]. Similarly, fever often presents in subarachnoid hemorrhage (SAH), especially in patients with complications such as severe infection, consciousness disorders [7], hydrocephalus, and symptomatic vasospasm [8]. A number of factors contribute to fever in SAH. Except for infection, there are many other nonseptic factors associated with fever, such as systemic inflammatory response syndrome (SIRS), blood in CSF [9], vasospasm [10] and hydrocephalus.

A prospective study showed that intraventricular hemorrhage (IVH), symptomatic cerebral vasospasm, and older age were independent predictors of fever, and fever was related to poor outcome after SAH [11]. Another research found that treatment-refractory fever was predicted by poor Hunt–Hess grade and IVH, and was in relation to more functional disability and cognitive impairment [12]. But these studies were different in the definition of fever, including concrete body temperature and the phase of fever. The inclusion criteria for patient enrollment were also various. Data in patients' clinical conditions and severity of illness were not overall in these studies. Until now, there has been no study exclusively deals with the relation between fever

G. Zhang and X. Qin (✉)
Department of Neurology, The First Affiliated Hospital, Chongqing Medical University, Chongqing 400016, People's Republic of China
e-mail: Qinxinyue@yahoo.com

J.H. Zhang
Department of Physiology and Pharmacology, Loma Linda University, Loma Linda, CA, USA
Department of Neurosurgery, Loma Linda University, Loma Linda, CA, USA
Department of Anesthesiology, Loma Linda University, Loma Linda, CA, USA

and in hospital mortality. Here we reviewed patients suffered from SAH in our hospital, examined various factors relative to fever and detected the possible effect of fever on in-hospital mortality.

Patients and Methods

We retrospectively studied 183 medical records of patients suffering from SAH who were admitted to the First Affiliated Hospital of ChongQing Medical University between January 2006 and 2009. Our study was authorized by the department of scientific research which administrates scientific research activities in our hospital. SAH was diagnosed by computed tomographic (CT) scan or by lumbar puncture if the CT scan was negative while the symptoms implied SAH. Patients with an age of more than 18, spontaneous SAH, an admission to hospital within 7 days after onset were included. Exclusion criteria included insufficient clinical information) no available CT image information and uncompleted records of temperature. Patients were divided into febrile group and afebrile group according to their temperature records and the definition of fever.

We traced every patient's axillary temperature from their medical records. Patients' temperatures were measured at least three times a day. Fever was defined as temperature exceeding 38.3° at least two times (not in the same day). Besides temperature, the following data were also collected: patient demographics including sex, age, past medical history of hypertension and alcohol abuse, admission conditions including conscious state, Glasgow Coma Scale (GCS) score and Hunt–Hess grade. Other messages such as admission glucose levels, electrolytes levels in plasma, presence of seizure and imaging assessment were also reviewed.

Admission glucose levels were assayed on the next morning of the first day after admission, with a fast of at least 8 h. Admission glucose level more than 7.0 mmol/l was considered to be hyperglycemia. Any abnormalities in the levels of sodium ion or potassium ion in fasting plasma during hospital days were defined to be electrolyte disorder. Imaging assessment was based on the manifestations of CT scans of the brain on admission. The amount of hemorrhage was described by Fisher CT Grade Scale. In addition, we recorded the presence of IVH and intracerebral hemorrhage (ICH).

Analysis

Statistical analysis was processed by SPSS for Windows. Descriptive analysis was performed to detect possible factors related to fever or in-hospital mortality. Categorical variables were analyzed by chi-square test. We used Student t-test for normally distributed continuous variables and the Mann–Whitney U test for nonnormally distributed ones. Logistic regression model was performed to analyses the adjusted risk of fever or in-hospital mortality. Only variables with P value of less than 0.10 on univariate analysis were adopted to multivariate logistic regression model. A significant probability value was defined as $P < 0.05$.

Results

From January 2006 to 2009, there were 198 patients diagnosed with SAH. One hundred and fifty-five of these patients corresponded to our requirement and were included in subsequent study. Patient demographic and clinical characteristics of the entire study group are shown in Table 1. Of the 155 patients, 76 were males and 79 were females, and their mean age was 54.12 ± 12.12 years for males and 58.46 ± 13.08 years for females. There were 63 (41%) patients who experienced fever, and they were classified into febrile group. The other 92 patients were the afebrile group. In the total study group, there were 56 (36%) patients who died in hospital.

Univariate analysis revealed nine factors related to fever: age, history of hypertension, consciousness disorders on admission, GCS score, Hunt–Hess grade, Fisher

Table 1 Characteristics of 155 patients with SAH

Clinical factors	n (%)
Age	56.36 ± 12.76
Sex, M/F	76/79
History of hypertension	55(35.5)
History of alcohol abuse	15(10)
Conscious disorder on admission	57(36.7)
GCS score	
<8	31(20)
8–12	17(11)
12–15	107(69)
Hunt–Hess grade	
1, 2, or 3	110(71)
4 or 5	45(29)
Fisher CT grade	
1, 2, or 3	90(58)
4	65(42)
Seizure	17(11)
IVH	50(32)
ICH	30(19)
Admission hyperglycemia	58(37)
Electrolytes disturbance	68(44)
Fever	63(41)
Death	56(36)

GCS glasgow coma scale, *IVH* intraventricular hemorrhage, *ICH* intracerebral hemorrhage

CT grade, presence of IVH, admission glucose levels, electrolytes levels in plasma (Table 2). After exclusion of the least significant predictive factors, multivariate regression model showed three significant predictors closely related to fever: poor Hunt–Hess grade (OR 5.37, 95% CI 1.56–18.44), presence of IVH (OR 5.18, 95% CI 1.43–18.85) and older age (OR 1.06, 95% CI 1.02–1.09) (Table 3). Fever was not in relation to sex and the presence of seizure or ICH.

Univariate analysis primarily identified ten factors that were associated with in-hospital mortality: fever, age, history of hypertension, consciousness disorders on admission, GCS score, Hunt–Hess grade, Fisher CT grade, presence of IVH, admission glucose levels and electrolytes levels in plasma (Table 4). In the multivariate model, only three variables were predictive factor of higher mortality (Table 5): fever (OR 17.36, 95% CI 4.47–67.35), consciousness disorders on admission (OR 5.89, 95% CI 1.16–29.89) and older age (OR 1.07, 95% CI 1.00–1.13).

Discussion

Fever is a common symptom of stroke, especially in SAH [7]. Although fever possesses high incidence rate and potential hazards to patients with SAH [13], there are relatively

Table 2 Univariate analysis of related factors for fever

Variable	Afebrile group	Febrile group	p value
Age (x ± s)	52.40 ± 11.77	62.14 ± 11.99	<0.001
Sex			0.11
Male (%)	50(54)	26(41)	
Female (%)	42(46)	37(59)	
History of hypertension (%)	25(27)	31(49)	0.005
History of Alcohol abuse (%)	9(10)	6(10)	0.96
Seizure (%)	8(9)	9(14)	0.274
GCS score, median	10	15	<0.001
Hunt–Hess grade (%)			<0.001
1, 2 or 3	80(87)	28(44)	
4 or 5	12(13)	35(56)	
Conscious disorder (%)	17(18)	40(63)	<0.001
Fisher CT grade (%)			<0.001
1, 2, or 3	64(70)	26(41)	
4	28(30)	37(59)	
Admission hyperglycemia (%)	24(26)	34(54)	<0.001
Electrolytes disturbance (%)	29(32)	39(62)	<0.001
ICH (%)	15(16)	15(24)	0.245
IVH (%)	15(16)	36(58)	<0.001

GCS glasgow coma scale, IVH intraventricular hemorrhage, ICH intracerebral hemorrhage

Table 3 Multivariate analysis of related factors for fever

Variable	OR	95% CI	P Value
Hunt–Hess grade	5.37	1.56–18.44	0.008
Fisher CT grade	0.96	0.41–2.26	0.921
Conscious disorder	2.51	0.75–8.39	0.136
ICH	1.37	0.42–4.44	0.600
IVH	5.18	1.43–18.85	0.012
GCS score	1.08	0.89–1.30	0.433
Admission hyperglycemia	1.62	0.61–4.34	0.334
History hypertension	2.04	0.81–5.15	0.130
Electrolytes disturbance	0.67	0.24–1.87	0.449
Older age	1.06	1.02–1.09	0.007

OR odds ratio, GCS glasgow coma scale, IVH intraventricular hemorrhage, ICH intracerebral hemorrhage

Table 4 Univariate analysis of related factors for in-hospital mortality

Variable	Survivor group	Death group	p value
Age (x ± s)	52.31 ± 11.38	63.33 ± 12.03	<0.001
Sex			0.752
Male (%)	49(50)	27(47)	
Female (%)	49(50)	30(53)	
Hypertension (%)	28(29)	27(47)	0.018
Alcohol abuse (%)	11(11)	5(9)	0.628
Seizure (%)	11(11)	6(11)	0.893
GCS score (median)	15	7	<0.001
Hunt–Hess grade (%)			<0.001
1, 2, or 3	88(90)	20(35)	
4 or 5	10(10)	37(65)	
Conscious disorder (%)	13(13)	44(77)	<0.001
Fisher CT grade (%)			<0.001
1, 2, or 3	71(72)	19(33)	
4	27(28)	38(67)	
Admission hyperglycemia (%)	21(21)	37(65)	<0.001
Electrolytes disturbance (%)	26(26)	42(74)	<0.001
ICH (%)	17(17)	13(23)	0.407
IVH (%)	15(15)	36(63)	<0.001
Fever (%)	15(15)	48(84)	<0.001

GCS glasgow coma scale, IVH intraventricular hemorrhage, ICH intracerebral hemorrhage

Table 5 Multivariate analysis of related factors for in-hospital mortality

Variable	OR	95% CI	p Value
GCS score	1.07	1.00–1.30	0.736
Hunt–Hess grade	2.81	0.42–18.89	0.289
Fisher CT Grade	3.83	0.47–31.45	0.211
Conscious disorders	5.89	1.16–29.89	0.032
ICH	0.25	0.03–1.88	0.180
IVH	0.89	0.12–6.92	0.915
Admission hyperglycemia	3.43	0.77–15.17	0.105
Hypertension	1.10	0.28–4.36	0.895
Electrolytes disturbance	0.673	1.55–0.35	0.565
Older age	1.07	1.00–1.13	0.038
Fever	17.36	4.47–67.35	<0.001

OR odds ratio, GCS glasgow coma scale, IVH intraventricular hemorrhage, ICH intracerebral hemorrhage

sparse studies demonstrating predictive factors that might allow clinicians to recognize the presence of fever promptly and help patients get better outcomes. There are many reasons for elevated temperature in SAH, such as infection, SIRS, losing control of regulation to temperature, but the mechanism has not been fully discovered. Compared with afebrile groups, patients with fever usually are accompanied with serious systematic complications and worse outcomes. We analyzed different factors that might be predictive of fever in SAH, and investigated the relation between fever and in-hospital mortality.

In our study, we found that 63 of the 155 patients experienced fever, with a ratio of 41%, which were basically in accord with previous research [11]. This ratio may be slightly down-regulated because of the application of antipyretic drugs and physical cooling therapy to heightened temperature. Univariate analysis implied nine factors that were predictive of fever. Of these factors, five were indicative of illness severity: consciousness disorders on admission, presence of IVH, worse GCS score, higher Hunt–Hess grade and Fisher CT grade, which means that serious SAH were more sensitive to fever. In this study, admission hyperglycemia as well as electrolytes disturbance were also in relation to fever. A similar phenomenon was found by Fernandez and his colleagues [12], they detected that anemia and hyperglycemia were also associated with fever, and these physiologic disturbance may be caused by lose of the brain's ability to sustain physiological homeostasis in severe impairment [14].

Multivariate analysis also showed that temperature elevation was more common in older patients. The predisposition to infection because of worse constitution may partly contribute to high incidence rate of fever in older patients. Interestingly, we also found that, of the 51 patients with IVH, there were 32 patients at an age of more than 56 years, whereas IVH might have an effect on thermoregulatory centre in hypothalamus, which also contributed to higher temperature in older patients. But why IVH was inclined to appear in older patients deserves deeper research. In our study, poor Hunt–Hess grade and presence of IVH were also independent risk factors for fever, which the same results were found in another research [12]. Hunt–Hess grade is most frequently used in assessing the severity of neurological injury after SAH. Higher Hunt–Hess grade commonly means worse state of an illness and more serious neurological injury. Logistic regression verified the view that fever was inclined to appear in patients with severe SAH. IVH is linked to central hyperthermia [7], and it also increases the risk of hydrocephalus [15] and predicts poor outcome in acute stroke [16–18]. Its impact on hypothalamus and brain stem may cause elevated temperature [19].

In the present study, fever intensely predicted higher in-hospital mortality after SAH (OR 17.36, 95% CI 4.47–67.35). It has been reported that patients with fever had worse outcomes in stroke, and in a meta-analysis including 14,431 patients with various kinds of strokes and other brain injuries, fever was consistently linked to worse outcomes and higher mortality. As known to all, fever significantly exacerbates neurological injury and inhibits restoration after stroke, which partly explains our result that fever independently predicted higher in-hospital mortality [20]. Besides fever, there were two other variables in relation to higher in-hospital mortality: older age and consciousness disorders on admission. In a study of 629 consecutive patients with ICH, age was an independent predictor of Glasgow Outcome Score ≥ 4 [21]. A prospective study also found that older age was related to poor outcome after SAH [11]. Worse constitution, more severe complications or comorbidities, lessened ability to recovery from injury may contribute to the connection between older age and mortality. Consciousness disorders mean worse GCS score and higher Hunt–Hess grade, which indicates severe illness and thus contributes to higher mortality.

There were some limitations in our research. As a retrospective study, we could not follow the survival state of outpatients, so only in-hospital mortality was traced. Our study did not differentiate between infective fever and noninfective fever, whereas it was possible that the predictor may be distinct between two kinds of fever. In spite of some limitations, our study has prominent advantages. For all we know, this is the first study especially on the effect of fever on in-hospital mortality. Compared with other relative researches, we collected clinical data as far as possible and analyzed factors involved in patients' conditions.

Conflict of interest statement We declare that we have no conflict of interest.

References

1. Barone FC, Feuerstein GZ, White RF. Brain cooling during transient focal ischemia provides complete neuroprotection. Neurosci Biobehav Rev. 1997;21(1):31–44.
2. Kim Y, Busto R, Dietrich WD, Kraydich S, Ginsberg MD. Delayed postischemic hyperthermia in awake rats worsens the histopathologic outcome of transient forebrain ischemia. Stroke 1996;27(12):2274–81.
3. Ginsberg MD, Busto R. Combating hyperthermia in acute stroke: a significant clinical concern. Stroke 1998;29(2):529–34.
4. Todd MM, Hindman BJ, Clarke WR, Torner JC, Weeks JB, Bayman EO, et al. Perioperative fever and outcome in surgical patients with aneurysmal subarachnoid hemorrhage. Neurosurgery, 2009; 64:897–908
5. Azzimondi G, Bassein L, Nonino F, Fiorani L, Vignatelli L, Re Get al., Fever in acute stroke worsens prognosis: a prospective study. Stroke 1995;26(11):2040–3.

6. Georgilis K, Plomaritoglou A, Dafni U, Bassiakos Y, Vemmos K. Aetiology of fever in patients with acute stroke. J Intern Med. 1999;246(2):203–9.
7. Commichau C, Mayer SA, Scarmeas N. Risk factors for fever in the neurological intensive care unit. Neurology 2003;60(5):837–41.
8. Albrecht RFI, Wass CT, Lanier WL. Occurrence of potentially detrimental temperature alterations in hospitalized patients at risk for brain injury. Mayo Clin Proc. 1998;73(7):629–35.
9. Frosini M, Sesti C, Valoti M, Palmi M, Fusi F, Parente L, Sgaragli G. Rectal temperature and prostaglandin E2 increase in cerebrospinal fluid of conscious rabbits after intracerebroventricular injection of hemoglobin. Exp Brain Res. 1999;126:252–8
10. Weir B, Disney L, Grace M, Roberts P. Daily trends in white blood cell count and temperature after subarachnoid hemorrhage from aneurysm. Neruosurgery. 1989;25:161–5
11. Oliveira-Filho J, Ezzeddine MA, Segal AZ, Buonanno FS, Chang Y, Ogilvy CS, et al. Fever in subarachnoid hemorrhage: relationship to vasospasm and outcome. Neurology. 2001;56:1299–1304
12. Fernandez A, Schmidt JM, Claassen J, Pavlicova M, Huddleston D, Kreiter KT, et al. Fever after subarachnoid hemorrhage: risk factors and impact on outcome. Neurology. 2007;68:1013–19.
13. Ling GSF. More heat to treat fever in subarachnoid hemorrhage? Neurology 2007;68(13):973–4.
14. Menon DK. Cerebral protection in severe brain injury: physiological determinants of outcome and their optimisation. Br Med Bull. 1999;55(1):226–58.
15. Kazan S, Gura A, Ucar T, Korkmaz E, Ongun H, Akyuz M. Hydrocephalus after intraventricular hemorrhage in preterm and low-birth weight infants: analysis of associated risk factors for ventriculoperitoneal shunting. Surg Neurol. 2005;64:(suppl 2):S77–81.
16. Mayfrank L, Hütter BO, Kohorst Y, Kreitschmann-Andermahr I, Rohde V, Thron A, et al. Influence of intraventricular hemorrhage on outcome after rupture of intracranial aneurysm. Neurosurgical review. 2001;24:185–191.
17. Wildrick D. Intraventricular hemorrhage and long-term outcome in the premature infant. J Neurosci Nurs. 1997;29(5):281–9.
18. Ment LR, Allan WC, Makuch RW, Vohr B. Grade 3 to 4 intraventricular hemorrhage and Bayley scores predict outcome. Pediatrics 2005;116(6):1597–8.
19. Sung CY, Lee TH, Chu NS. Central hyperthermia in acute stroke. Eur Neurol. 2009;62(2):86–92.
20. Greer DM, Funk SE, Reaven NL, Ouzounelli M, Uman GC. Impact of fever on outcome in patients with stroke and neurologic injury: a comprehensive meta-analysis. Stroke 2008;39(11):3029–35.
21. Rost NS, Smith EE, Chang Y, Snider SW. Prediction of functional outcome in patients with primary intracerebral hemorrhage: the FUNC score. Stroke 2008;39(8):2304–9.

Subarachnoid Hemorrhage in Old Patients in Chongqing China

Yan Zhang, Tianzhu Wang, John H. Zhang, Jiayu Zhang, and Xinyue Qin

Abstract *Background*: Subarachnoid hemorrhage (SAH) is a disorder with high mortality in central nervous system, especially in old population. Misdiagnosis and poor outcome frequently occur in old patients with SAH. This research is to investigate the demographic characteristics, clinical features, neuroimaging data, and the outcome of the old patients (≥ 60 of age) with SAH.

Methods: The data was from both neurosurgical and neurology departments of two hospitals in Chongqing, China, from October 2007 to March 2009. One hundred and seventy eight patients were enrolled and divided into two groups: the elderly group (≥ 60 of age) and the non-elderly group (≥ 18 but <60 of age). The condition on admission was assessed by Hunt–Hess grade (H–H) and the Glasgow scales of coma (GCS). Findings on computerized tomography (CT) were measured by Fisher grades. The outcome after 3 months was evaluated by the modified Rankin Scale (mRS). Statistic analysis was managed by Chi-square test and *t*-test.

Findings: Compared to the non-elderly group, the clinical conditions on admission in the elderly group was worse, with lower average scores of GCS, higher Fisher grades, systolic blood pressure, and percentage of the H-H IV and V. Some preexisting medical conditions with the old such as arterial hypertension, pulmonary diseases, and diabetes mellitus were worsening. During the clinical course, the elderly group had the following characteristics: the incidence of rebleeding, asymptomatic vasospasm, hydrocephalus, and other severe medical complications were all higher, while the percentage of early surgery was lower. The outcome after 3 months was poorer in the elderly.

Conclusions: It is indicated that the elderly patients with SAH have poorer clinical conditions, much lower ratio of early surgery and higher incidence of rebleeding. Together, these factors contribute to a poorer short-term outcome after SAH.

Keywords Clinical features · Old patients · Outcome · Subarachnoid hemorrhage

Y. Zhang, T. Wang, and X. Qin (✉)
Department of Neurology, The First Affiliated Hospital of Chongqing Medical University of Chongqing 400016, People's Republic of China
e-mail: Qinxinyue@yahoo.com

J.H. Zhang
Department of Physiology and Pharmacology, Loma Linda University, Loma Linda, CA, USA
Department of Neurosurgery, Loma Linda University, Loma Linda, CA, USA
Department of Anesthesiology, Loma Linda University, Loma Linda, CA, USA

J. Zhang
Department of Neurology, Xinqiao Hospital Third Military Medical University, Chongqing, China

Introduction

As a hemorrhagic stroke, a high rate of mortality is observed in SAH [1, 2]. It has been reported that in China 33.3% of the first-ever SAH patients die within 28 days [3]. Up to now, with the increase of the elderly population, the number of elderly patients with SAH is rising [4]. In despite of the advancement of neuroimaging technology, misdiagnosis and poor outcome frequently occur in old patients with SAH [5–7]. Additionally, it is common that elderly patients with SAH have various complications. Thus, the mortality in the old was up to 50% [8]. In this sense, more complete and systematic data are required for the further study on SAH in the old so as to reduce the mortality and improve the prognosis. Therefore, we studied retrospectively the demographics, clinical data (previous and on admission clinical conditions, clinical course, and outcome of the elderly patients with SAH in Chongqing China.

Clinical Materials and Methods

The patients were selected from all the patients admitted to both neurosurgical and neurology departments of two hospitals in Chongqing, China, from October 2007 to March 2009. One hundred and seventy eight patients (aged 18–89) with SAH, which were not attributed to trauma, tumor, or vascular malformation, within 14 days, were enrolled in this retrospective consecutive study. The diagnosis of SAH was on the basis of clinical presentation and confirmed by head CT (computed tomography) scan or lumbar puncture. Patients with severe medical illnesses, usage of calcium antagonist drugs at the prior time of hemorrhage, history of other neurological or psychiatric illnesses, allergy to calcium antagonist drugs, pregnancy or the suspicion of pregnancy, and inability to obtain informed consent were excluded. Patients with clinical Grade IV to V based on the H–H (Hunt and Hess grading system) [9] were included. Then they were divided into two groups: the elderly group ($\geq$60 of age) and the non-elderly group ($\geq$18 but <60 of age).

The preexisting illnesses (such as hypertension, cardiac disease, and the pulmonary disease, diabetes, nephropathy, hepatopathy, gastroenteropathy) were all noted. H-H and GCS (Glasgow Coma Scale) [10] were used to evaluate the clinical conditions of patients on admission. The findings on CT scan were assessed by Fisher grade [11]. The information of daily neurological examinations, the medical and surgical complications such as vasospasm and the treatment during the hospitalization were checked. Severe complications are defined as those medical complications threatening lives. The outcome after 3 months was measured by mRS at last.

The Chi-square test and t-test were used to compare variables between the two groups. The student's t test was used to compare the scores of GCS, Fisher grades, blood pressure, and mRS. The Chi-square test was used to compare the percentage of H-H IV to V, ratio of hydrocephalus on CT, preexisting medical conditions, and clinical course.

Results

Clinical Characteristics

With the mean age of 55.8 (18–89)-years-old, one hundred and seventy eight patients were enrolled. Forty four percent of the patients were over 60-years-old. In the elderly group the number of female ($n = 47$) exceeded male ($n = 30$), while in the non-elderly group the male ($n = 59$) was over the female ($n = 42$).

The clinical characteristics of the elderly patients compared with the non-elderly patients are summarized in Table 1. The average score of GCS was lower in the elderly (9.95 $\pm$ 0.56, p = 0.042), suggesting the elderly patients were more likely to have severe consciousness disturbance on admission. The percentage of the HH IV and V was higher in the elderly, respectively 30% (p = 0.016) and 21% (p = 0.002). The mean systolic blood pressure on admission was significantly higher in the elderly (147.63 $\pm$ 3.37, p = 0.001). On CT scan, the elderly patients got a higher Fisher scale (3 $\pm$ 0.11, p = 0.042), and the incidence of hydrocephalus was higher (15.4%, p = 0.045), compared to the non-elderly group.

Associated Health Status

The main preexisting illnesses are shown in Table 2. Higher rates in the elderly patients with arterial hypertension (39%, p = 0.001), pulmonary diseases (21%, p = 0.013), diabetes mellitus (9%, p = 0.022) and hepatic diseases (13%, p = 0.005) were significant. While the incidence of other illnesses such as cardiac diseases (9%, p = 0.058), renal diseases (6%, p = 0.295) or cerebrovascular diseases (10%, p = 0.131) had no significant difference between the two groups.

Table 1 Clinical characteristics of patients with SAH on admission

Clinical characteristics	Elderly group	Non-elderly group	P value
Average score of GCS	9.95 $\pm$ 0.56	11.47 $\pm$ .49	0.042
HH grade I	5%	4%	0.277
HH grade II	21%	57%	<0.01
HH grade III	22%	19%	0.591
HH grade IV	30%	15%	0.016
HH grade V	21%	5%	0.002
HH grade VI	1%	0%	0.433
MSBP (mmHg)	147.63 $\pm$ 3.37	136.06 $\pm$ 2.26	0.001
Average scale of Fisher grades	3.00 $\pm$ 0.11	2.68 $\pm$ 0.12	0.004
Percentage of hydrocephalus on CT	15%	5%	0.045

Table 2 Preexisting illnesses of patients with SAH

Preexisting illnesses	Elderly group No. of patients (%)	Non-elderly group No. of patients (%)	P value
Arterial hypertension	30(39)	2(16)	0.001
Cardiac diseases	8(11)	3(3)	0.058
Pulmonary diseases	16(21)	8(8)	0.013
Diabetes mellitus	7(9)	1(1)	0.022
Renal diseases	5(6)	3(3)	0.295
Hepatic diseases	10(13)	2(2)	0.005
Cerebrovascular diseases	8(10)	4(4.0)	0.131

Clinical Course

The elderly patients with SAH had less chance of undergoing early surgery. During hospitalization, their incidence of rebleeding and asymptomatic vasospasm were higher than that in the non-elderly group, respectively 16%, p = 0.035; 16%, p = 0.045. Besides, they were vulnerable to other severe complications (p = 0.037). While the incidence of symptomatic vasospasm and surgical complication was found no statistic difference. (Table 3)

Outcome at 3 Months After SAH

The average score of mRS at 3 months after SAH was 2.86 ± 0.25 in the elderly group and 2.01 ± 0.20 in the non-elderly group, whose difference was statistic significant (p = 0.008). The mortality was also compared between the two groups, but no difference was found.

Discussion

In the demographic analysis in this study, the average age of the 178 patients was very close to other studies [6]. But males with SAH were more prevalent than females in the elderly group, which was not similar to the results in another research [12], in which the female had a higher incidence of SAH than the male no matter in the elderly population or not. The cause of the difference may lie in the fact that the population with smoking, hypertension and hyperlipidemia are all higher in males in China. And we all know these events are risk factors for SAH.

Most previous studies [5, 6, 13, 14] indicated that the elderly patients had worse medical conditions on admission. Our results are consistent with the majority. The elderly patients showed poorer performance when evaluated by H-H grades. In particular, patients with H-H grade IV or V were more prevalent in the elderly group than in the non-elderly group. However, John et al. [15] suggested that no difference was found when H-H grade on admission was compared between the elderly and the non-elderly.

It was found that the incidence of symptomatic vasospasm had no associations with age, H-H grade and Fisher grade on admission [16]. Michael et al. [17] also showed that the development of symptomatic vasospasm was associated with the admission Fisher grade only in the half of the patients. In our research it seemed that the elderly patients had poorer H-H and Fisher grades, but their incidence of symptomatic vasospasm was not higher than that of the non-elderly. Instead, the incidence of asymptomatic vasospasm was higher in the elderly. This may explained by the decreased sensitivity of cerebral vessels to the initial bleed, and the diseases in other systems.

It has been shown that poor conditions on admission and the development of rebleeding can prompt a worse outcome [18, 19]. Otherwise, a better outcome was seen in the operated patients with SAH and those without incidence of rebleeding [20]. It is well known that rebleeding is the most common cause resulting in worse outcome (death and disability) [21, 22]. Therefore, in elderly patients with SAH, a vicious cascade exists and prevents them from favorable prognosis: the old are more likely to be accompanied by other systematic diseases when hit by SAH, which may aggravate the clinical manifestations; poor clinical performances lead to the delay of early surgical treatment, so the patients are highly exposed to the danger of rebleeding; once rebleeding happens, they may die or have permanent disability. It turned out in our study that the elderly patients with SAH had higher mRS scores and poorer outcomes at 3 months after the hemorrhage.

Conclusion

To sum up, this study provides an overall description of SAH in the elderly patients in Chongqing, China. Since the elderly patients with SAH may have higher risk of rebleeding and severe complication, lower chance of early surgery, and unfavorable outcomes, it is critical to diagnose the old patients in an early stage of SAH, take the comprehensive management, and strive for the possibility of surgery for the sake of the improved outcomes.

Conflict of interest statement We declare that we have no conflict of interest.

Table 3 Clinical course of patients with SAH

Clinical Course	Elderly No. of patients (%)	Non-elderly No. of patients (%)	P value
undergoing early surgery	17(22)	38(38)	0.025
Asymptomatic vasospasm	12(16)	6(6)	0.035
Symptomatic vasospasm	9(12)	19(19)	0.19
Rebleeding	12(16)	6(6)	0.045
Severe complications	11(14)	4(5)	0.037
Surgical complications	2(3)	0(0)	0.214

References

1. de Rooij NK, Linn FHH, van der Plas JA, Algra A, Rinkel GJE. Incidence of subarachnoid haemorrhage: a systematic review with emphasis on region, age, gender and time trends. J Neurol Neurosurg Psychiatry. 2007;78:1365–72.

2. Bonita R, Thomson S. Subarachnoid hemorrhage: epidemiology, diagnosis, management, and outcome. Stroke 1985;16;591–4.
3. Zhao YNH, Chen J, Yang-Feng W, Zhang LF, Yang J, Hong Z, et al. Proportion of different subtypes of stroke in China; Stroke 2003;34;2091–6.
4. Pobereskin LH. Incidence and outcome of subarachnoid haemorrhage: a retrospective population based study. J Neurol Neurosurg Psychiatry. 2001;70:340–3.
5. Lanzino G, Kassell NF, Germanson TP, et al. Age and outcome after aneurysmal subarachnoid hemorrhage: why do older patients fare worse? J Neurosurg. 1996;85:410–8.
6. Arboix A, García-Eroles L, Massons J, Oliveres M, Targa C. Acute stroke in very old people: clinical features and predictors of in-hospital mortality. J Am Geriatr Soc. 2000;48(1):36–41.
7. Taylor CL, Yuan Z, Selman WR, Ratcheson RA, Rimm AA. Mortality rates, hospital length of stay, and the cost of treating subarachnoid hemorrhage in older patients: institutional and geographical differences. J neurosurg. 1997;86:4.
8. Broderick JP, Brott TG, Duldner JE, Tomsick T, Leach A. Initial and recurrent bleeding are themajor causes of death following subarachnoid hemorrhage. Stroke 1994;25:1342–7.
9. Hunt WE, Hess RM. Surgical risk as related to time of intervention in the repair of intracranial aneurysm. J Neurosurg. 1968; 28:14–20.
10. Teasdale GM, Jennett B. Assessment of coma and impaired consciousness. A practical scale. Lancet 1974;2:81–4.
11. Fisher CM, Kistler JP, Davis JM. Relation of cerebral vasospasm to subarachnoid hemorrhage visualized by computerized tomographic scanning. Neurosurgery 1980;6:1–9.
12. Lindvall P, Runnerstam M, Birgander R, Koskinen LO. The Fisher grading correlated to outcome in patients with subarachnoid haemorrhage. Br J Neurosurg. 2009;23(2):188–92.
13. Asano S, Hara T, Haisa T, Okamoto K, Kato T, Ohno H, et al. Outcomes of 24 patients with subarachnoid hemorrhage aged 80 years or older in a single center. Clin Neurol Neurosurg. 2007;109: 853–7.
14. Ogilvy CS, Cheung AC, Mitha AP, Hoh BL, Carter BS. Outcomes for surgical and endovascular management of intracranial aneurysms using a comprehensive grading system. Neurosurgery 2006; 59:1037–42.
15. Laidlaw JD, Siu KH. Aggressive surgical treatment of elderly patients following subarachnoid haemorrhage: management outcome results, J Clin Neurosci. 2002;9(4):404–10.
16. Miranda P, Lagares A, Alen J, Perez-Nuñez A, Arrese I, Lobato RD. Early transcranial Doppler after subarachnoid hemorrhage: clinical and radiological correlations. Surg Neurol. 2006;65(3): 247–52.
17. Smith ML, Abrahams JM, Chandela S, Smith MJ, Hurst RW, Le Roux PD. Subarachnoid hemorrhage on computed tomography scanning and the development of cerebral vasospasm: the Fisher grade revisited. Surg Neurol. 2005;63(3):229–34.
18. Starke RM, Komotar RJ, Kim GH, Kellner CP, Otten ML, Hahn DK, et al. Evaluation of a revised glasgow coma score scale in predicting long-term outcome of poor grade aneurismal subarachnoid hemorrhage patients, J Clin Neurosci. 2009;16(7):894–9.
19. Locksley HB. Natural history of subarachnoid hemorrhage, intracranial aneurysms and arteriovenous malformations, based on 6368 cases in the cooperative study. J Neurosurg. 1966;25:321–68.
20. Nieuwkamp DJ, Rinkel GJE, Silva R, Greebe P, Schokking DA, Ferro JM. Subarachnoid haemorrhage in patients > 75 years: clinical course, treatment and outcome. J Neurol Neurosurg Psychiatry. 2006;77:933–7.
21. Rosenørn J, Eskesen V, Schmidt K, Espersen JO, Haase J, Harmsen A, et al. Clinical features and outcome in 1076 patients with ruptured intracranial saccular aneurysms: a prospective consecutive study. Br J Neurosurg. 1987;1(1):33–45.
22. Kassell NF, Torner JC. The International cooperative study on timing of aneurysm surgery – an update. Stroke 1984;15:566–70.

Author Index

A
Ai, J., 105
Altay, O., 43
Ayer, R., 75

B
Bakhtian, K.D., 93
Bederson, J.B., 99
Bellut, D., 191
Biehle, S.J., 157
Brayden, J.E., 145

C
Chai, W.-n., 225
Chen, K., 151
Chen, W., 75
Chen, Y., 167
Chen, Z., 151, 167
Chi, L., 151
Clark, J.F., 157

D
Dan, W., 39
Dorsch, N., 5
Dreier, J.P., 111, 119
Duris, K., 67

F
Fandino, J., 163, 173, 191
Fan, W., 151
Fathi, A.R., 93
Feng, H., 151, 167
Friedrich, V., 49
Fuhr, S., 119

G
Gui, L., 151
Guo, Z., 181
Guo, Z.-d., 63, 71, 81
Gu, Y.X., 203

H
Hansen-Schwartz, J., 23
Harm, A., 157
Hasegawa, Y., 43, 57, 67, 75, 133
Haux, D., 125
Hegewald, A.A., 35

H
Hertle, D.N., 125
He, Z., 181, 233
Hu, R., 167

J
Jadhav, V., 57
Jakob, S., 163
Jiang, L., 39, 225
Jiang, Y., 141
Jorks, D., 111
Jung, C.S., 87

K
Kanamaru, K., 75, 133
Keller, E., 191
Kiening, K.L., 125
Kitchen, N., 173
Kleeberg, J., 111
Koide, M., 145
Konczalla, J., 177
Kong, Y., 197
Krajewski, K.L., 125

L
Leng, B., 203
Li, L., 151
Lin, B., 39, 81
Li, P.L., 203
Liu, Z., 167
Lu, A., 157
Luo, C., 151, 167
Lv, F.-j., 225

M
Macdonald, R.L., 105
Major, S., 111
Manville, J., 35
Mao, Y., 203
Marbacher, S., 163, 173
Martin, R.D., 15
Mink, S., 191
Muroi, C., 191

N
Neuschmelting, V., 163
Nishizawa, S., 57
Nishziawa, S., 27

Ni, W., 203
Nystoriak, M., 145

O
Offenhauser, N., 119
Oliveira-Ferreira, A.I., 111
Orakcioglu, B., 125

P
Pluta, R.M., 7, 93
Pyne, G., 157

Q
Qin, X., 197, 209, 229, 245

S
Sabri, M., 105
Saffire, A., 157
Sakowitz, O.W., 125
Santos, E., 125
Schläppi, J.-A., 163
Schubert, G.A., 35
Sehba, F.A., 49, 99
Seifert, V., 177
Seiz, M., 35
Seule, M., 191
Sherchan, P., 67
Sherif, C., 163
Song, D.L, 203
Sozen, T., 43, 57, 75
Strong, A.J., 119
Sugawara, T., 75
Su, H., 141
Sun, X., 181
Sun, X.-c., 39, 63, 71, 81, 141, 225
Suzuki, H., 43, 57, 67, 75, 133

T
Takala, J., 163
Tang, W., 167
Thomé, C., 35
Tsuchiyama, R., 57

U
Unterberg, A.W., 125

V
Vatter, H., 177

W
Wan, B., 225
Wang, T., 209, 219, 245
Wang, X., 215
Wellman, G.C., 145
Windmüller, O., 119
Wu, B., 215
Wu, H.-t., 39, 71, 81, 141

Y
Yi, B., 151, 167
Yin, X.-h., 39

Z
Zhang, G., 229, 239
Zhang, J., 245
Zhang, J.H., 15, 43, 57, 63, 67, 71, 75, 81, 133, 167, 181, 197, 209, 215, 229, 245
Zhang, X.-d., 71, 81, 141
Zhang, Y., 245
Zhan, Y., 67
Zhou, S., 141
Zhou, Y., 15

Subject Index

A
Akt (protein kinase B), 44–45
Angiogenesis
    ecdysterone (EDS)
        astrocyte activation, 152–153
        microvessel density, 152
        neurological recovery, 152, 153
    grouping and drug administration, 152
    immunohistostaining and image analysis, 152, 153
    materials, 151
    microvessel density detection, 152
    neurological scores, 152
    statistical analysis, 152
Angiographic spasm, 5
Anti-proinflammatory cytokine treatment, 58–59
APOE. *See* Apolipoprotein E (APOE)
Apolipoprotein E (APOE)
    CVS
        assessment, 142
        pathological nature, 143
    genotyping, 142
    neuropsychological outcomes, 143
    patient population, 141–142
    polymorphism and EBI in SAH
        distribution of, 40
        EEG detection and interpretation, 40
        EEG deterioration *vs.* stabilization, 40–41
        genome-wide linkage analyses, 41
        genotyping, 40
        Glasgow outcome scale (GOS), 41
        pathogenesis of, 39
        patient study, 40
        statistical analysis, 40
    SAH, acute phase, 143
    statistical analysis, 142
Apoptosis
    CVS/EBI and, 18
    EBI and, 63–64
    extrinsic pathway of, 46
    neuronal, 46
    SAH and mechanism of
        caspase-dependent pathway, 44–45
        caspase-independent pathway, 45
Arginase, 8
Arterial smooth muscle contraction, 133
Astrocyte activation, 151–154
Asymmetric methylated L-arginine (ADMA), 8, 88–89

B
Basal lamina degradation, 51
Bilirubin oxidation products (BOXes)
    heat shock protein expression, 159–160
    HO-1, 159–160
    HSP-25, 159
    immunohistochemistry, 159–160
    SAH, 157–158
    toxicity effects analysis
        bilirubin peroxidation, 158
        cranial window, 158–159
        immunohistochemistry, 159
        male sprague dawley rats, 158
        spectrophotometric analysis, 158
        surgical methods, 158
        time dependence, 159
Biochemical potentials, 95–96
Biological activity, NO
    nitrite/nitrate recycling, 10–11
    nitrite, on-demand NO donor, 9–10
Blood-brain barrier, 15, 17, 18, 57, 59, 63–65, 76, 78
BOX. *See* Bilirubin oxidation products (BOXes)

C
Calcium antagonists, 6, 23–24
Calcium signaling
    cerebral artery myocytes
        Ca^{2+} sparks measurement, 146, 147
        cytosolic Ca^{2+} arterial diameter measurement, 146–147
        membrane potential, 149
        SAH model, 146
    cerebral circulation, 148
    fluorescent images, 148
    K^+ channels, 149
    voltage-dependent calcium^{2+} channel (VDCC), 149
CAMSC. *See* Cerebral arterial smooth muscle cell (CAMSC)
Cardiac complications
    electrocardiogram abnormalities
        implication, 216
        magnesium loss, 216
        QT prolongation, 215–216
        repolarization abnormalities, 216
    left ventricular dysfunction, 216–217
    magnesium loss, 216
Caspase-dependent pathway, 44–45
Caspase-independent pathway, 45
Catechol-O-methyl-transferase (COMT)

Catechol-O-methyl-transferase (COMT) (cont.)
   animals and experimental groups, 181–182
   basilar artery, morphology and measurements, 183–185
   catecholamine (CA)
      detection, 183
      metabolic pathway, 186
   CVS, 185
   gene polymorphism
      allele and CVS, 235
      allele frequency, 235
      cerebral artery, 234
      clinical information, 234
      CVS, 233
      genotype and CVS, 235
      genotyping, 234
      inclusion and exclusion, patients, 234–235
      logistic regression analysis, 235, 236
      patients selection, 234
      phenotype, 236
      statistic analysis, 234
   high performance liquid chromatography (HPLC), 182, 183
   mRNA expression, 183
   plasma CA, 184
   protein expression, 183–184
   reverse transcription polymerase chain reaction, 182
   SAH Induction, 182
   samples collection and HE staining, 182
   statistical analysis, 183
   western blot analysis, 182–183
Cerebral arterial smooth muscle cell (CAMSC)
   culturing and grouping, 168
   pathogenesis, CVS, 170
Cerebral blood flow
   animal recordings, 120
   cortical spreading ischemia, 119–120, 123
   data analysis, 120
   human recordings, 120
   magnitudes of non-physiological, 123
   spectrum of, 121–122
Cerebral ischemia
   ecdysterone (EDS) treatment, 151–154
   minocycline, 71
   NO biosynthetic pathways, 100
   SOV, 67
Cerebral microcirculation
   clinical data, 225
   CTP parameters, 226–227
   CVS, 227
   imaging technique, 226
   logistic regression analysis, 227
   mean transit time (MTT), 227
   statistical methods, 226
   sub-group, 226
Cerebral microvasculature
   anatomical architecture, 49–50
   injury
      basal lamina degradation, 51
      endothelium, 50
      platelet aggregation, 51–52
   occlusive cerebral ischemia, 50
cGMP regulation, 9
COMT. See Catechol-O-methyl-transferase (COMT)
Cortical spreading depolarizations. See Spreading depolarization
Cortical spreading ischemia (CSI), 119–123

D
DDAH, 89
Delayed cerebral vasospasm (DCVS)
   animal models
      canine, 174
      methods, 173
      murine, 173–174
      primate, 174
      rabbit, 174
      rat, 174
   ICP-controlled subarachnoid hemorrhage, 163
Delayed ischemic neurological deficits (DIND), 5–6, 106–107
Diazeniumdiolates. See NONOates
DID. See Delayed ischemic neurological deficits

E
Ecdysterone (EDS)
   astrocyte activation, 152–153
   microvessel density, 152
   neurological recovery, 152, 153
Electrocardiogram (ECG)
   implication, 216
   magnesium loss, 216
   QT prolongation, 215–216
   repolarization abnormalities, 216
Electrocortigraphy (ECoG), 125–126
Electroencephalogram (EEG)
   correlation of APOE with, 41
   detection and interpretation, 40
   deterioration vs. stabilization groups, 41
Endogenous NOS inhibitor, 88
Endothelial NOS
   gene transfer therapy, 96
   mRNA, 100
   pathogenesis of CVS, 106
   phosphorylation, 8
   single nucleotide polymorphism (SNP), 7–8
Endothelin-1$_{(1-31)}$
   biological activity of, 115
   induced SD, 115
   materials and methods
      animals, 112–113
      data analysis, 113
      experimental protocols, 113
      physiological variables, 113
      SD, 114
   pathophysiological role, 115
   peptides and receptors, 112
   role in chronic vasospasm, 111–112
   in vasospasm after aSAH, 115
Endothelin (ET)
   alteration of (B)-receptor, 179
   cerebrovasculature vessel wall, 178
   CVS, 177
   expression and function, receptor, 178–179
   metabolism, 178
   receptors changes, 178
   smooth muscle cells (SMC), 177
   synthesis, 178
Endothelium injury, 50
ERK1/2, 29, 134–136
ET. See Endothelin (ET)
ET(B)-receptor, 179
Evans blue dye extravasation, 58

Subject Index

F
Fasudil hydrochloride, 25

G
Gelatinase-B. *See* Matrix metalloproteinase-9
Gelatin zymogram, 72
Glucose and lactate, 129
Glutamate, 129
GTN. *See* Nitroglycerin

H
Heat shock protein 27 (HSP27), 133, 137
Hemodynamic response, 120–122
High performance liquid chromatography (HPLC), 182, 183
HO-1, 159–160
Hospital mortality
　factor analysis, 231
　fever
　　Hunt–Hess grade, 242
　　intraventricular hemorrhage (IVH), 242
　　patients and methods, 240
　　risk factors, 240–241
　　statistical analysis, 240
　patients and methods, 230
　statistical analysis, 230, 231
　systemic complications, 230
　weekday effect, 231
　weekend admission, 229
Hunt-Hess scale, 226
Hypoxia inducible factor-1 (HIF-1), 16–17

I
Inflammatory response monitoring
　acute stage, 192
　central nervous system (CNS), 191
　cytokines, 192
　ET-1, 192
　factors, 192
　IL-6, 194
　leukocytes, 192
　modalities, 194
Interleukin-6 (IL-6)
　clinical material and methods
　　admission condition, 203–204
　　patients, 203
　　test methods, 204
　　therapeutic methods, 204
　CSF, 205
　ET-1, 207
　Fisher scale, 205
　transcranial Doppler (TCD), 205, 207
　vasospasm, 204
Interleukin-1β, 57–58

L
Laminin, 64
L-Arginine, 89
Logistic regression analysis, 221

M
Magnesium sulphate, 24–25
Mann–Whitney test, 36
MAPKs. *See* Mitogen-activated protein kinases
Matrix metalloproteinase-9 (MMP-9)
　antibodies and reagents, 82
　basal lamina degradation, 51
　early brain injury and apoptosis, 63–64
　histology, 82
　hypothesis, 64–65
　IL-1β and, 57–58
　and laminin, 64
　laminin and TUNEL staining, 82–83
　minocycline, 64
　preparation of tissue extracts, 82
　SAH Rat model, 81–82
　statistical analysis, 82
　western blot analysis, 82, 83
Microdialysis, 125, 128–129
Microthrombosis, 107
Minocycline
　EBI, protection of
　　antibodies and reagents, 71
　　behavior scores assessment, 72–73
　　clinical assessment, 72
　　experimental groups, 71
　　gelatin zymogram, 72
　　MMP-9 protein, 73
　　SAH rat model, 71–72
　　statistics, 72
　　tissue extracts, preparation of, 72
　　western blot analysis, 72
　with MMP-9, 64
Mitogen-activated protein (MAP), 29
Mitogen-activated protein kinases (MAPKs)
　arterial smooth muscle contraction, 133
　HSP27, 133
　IL-1β and, 58
　intracellular signal transduction, 29
　pathways to induce vasospasm, 136–137
　role in EBI, 45
　in vitro studies, 134–135
　in vivo studies, 135–136
Mono methylated L-arginine (L-NMMA), 88–89
Myosin light chain phosphorylation, 28

N
Neuronal apoptosis, 44, 46
Nitric oxide (NO)
　biological activity
　　nitrate as source of NO, 10–11
　　nitrite, on-demand NO donor, 9–10
　cerebral vasospasm, pathogenesis of, 106
　DIND, 106–107
　donors
　　biochemical potentials, 95–96
　　classic, 93–94
　　new generation of, 94–95
　　pathway of, 95
　early brain injury
　　cerebral ischemia, 100
　　phase I (0–60 min After SAH), 100
　　phase II (1–6 h After SAH), 100–101
　　phase III (6–72 h After SAH), 101
　microthrombosis, 107
　nitrite/nitrate recycling, 10–11
　pathophysiological changes, SAH, 105–107
　radicals and oxidative stress, 107
　signaling pathways, new regulatory
　　eNOS phosphorylation, 8
　　single nucleotide polymorphism (SNP), 7–8
　synthesis of
　　arginase, 8

asymmetric dimethylarginine (ADMA), 8
erythropoietin, 9
soluble guanylyl cyclase and cGMP regulation, 9
substrate and coenzyme deficiency, 8–9
therapeutic application of, 107
and vasoconstriction, 105–106
Nitric oxide synthase (NOS)
CVS and, 16
inhibitors
ADMA and L-NMMA, 88–89
endogenous, production and hydrolysis, 88
NO and NOS-pathway, 87–88
therapeutic approach, 89
structure, 9
synthesis and regulation
eNOS SNP, 7–8
phosphorylation, 8
Nitroglycerin, 94
NONOates, 94

O
OPN. *See* Osteopontin
Osteopontin (OPN)
brain water content and BBB permeability, 76
described, 75
effects of endogenous, 77
effects of r-OPN, 77
experimental model of SAH and study protocol, 76
expression levels in brain after SAH, 76–77
intracerebroventricular infusion of siRNA or r-OPN, 76
neurological scoring and SAH grading, 76
neuroprotection against NF-κB-dependent MMP-9, 78
statistics, 76
western blot analyses, 76
Oxidative stress
CVS/EBI and, 17–18
early brain injury, 45
NO-related pathophysiological changes, 107
Oxyhemoglobin (Oxyhb), 167

P
Pathophysiological pathways and treatment strategies
apoptosis, 18
endothelin pathway, 16
HIF-1, 16–17
inflammation, 17
NOS-NO pathway, 16
oxidative stress, 17–18
statin, 18
thrombin, 18
Perimesencephalic nonaneurysmal subarachnoid hemorrhage (PNSH)
angiography, 200–201
clinical presentations, 199
computed tomography (CT), 197
etiological factor, 199
patients and procedure, 198
risk factor, 198–199
vs. SAH, 199–200
statistic analysis, 198
Phosphorylation
Akt, 45
eNOS, 8
of HSP27, 133
myosin light chain, 28
PKG. *See* Protein kinase G (PKG)

Platelet aggregation, 51–52
Protein arginine methyltransferases, 89
Protein kinase C (PKC), 27–28
Protein kinase G (PKG)
CASMC, culturing and grouping, 168
^{3}H-TdR incorporation test, 168, 169
MTT assay, 168, 169
PKG mRNA examination and protein expression, 168, 169
reagents and instruments, 167–168
statistical analysis, 168–169
types, 167
Protein tyrosine kinase (PTK), 28

R
Rho A, 28
Rho-kinase, 28

S
S-adenosylmethionine, 89
SAH. *See* Subarachnoid hemorrhage (SAH)
SD. *See* Spreading depolarization
Signal transduction mechanisms
MAPK/MAP, 29
myosin light chain phosphorylation, 28
protein kinase C (PKC), 27–28
protein tyrosine kinase (PTK), 28
Rho-kinase and Rho A, 28
vascular smooth muscle cells, phenotypic change of, 28–29
SIRS. *See* Systemic inflammatory response syndrome (SIRS)
S-Nitrosothiols, 94
Sodium nitrite, 94–95
Sodium nitroprusside, 93–94
Sodium orthovanadate (SOV)
brain water content, 68, 69
DNA fragmentation, 69
experiment by rat, 67–68
Induction of SAH, 68
neurological scoring and mortality, 68, 69
SAH severity, 68
Soluble guanylyl cyclase (sGC), 9
Spreading depolarization (SD)
animal recordings, 120
data analysis, 120
DIND, 111
electrocortigraphy (ECoG), 125–126
ET-1
biological activity of, 115
induced SD, 114–115
pathophysiological role, 115
peptides and receptors, 112
in vasospasm after aSAH, 115
glucose and lactate, 129
glutamate, 129
human recordings, 120
materials and methods, 112–114
methods
data reduction and statistics, 127
monitoring, 126–127
operative procedures, 126
patients, 126
postoperative care, 126
microdialysis, 125, 128–129
partial correlation, 128
pathological monitoring values, 127–128
rCBF response, 122–123
spectrum of hemodynamic responses, 120–122

Subject Index

Statins, 18, 24, 89
Subarachnoid haemorrhage (SAH)
    APOE polymorphism and EBI
        distribution of, 40
        EEG detection and interpretation, 40
        EEG deterioration *vs.* stabilization, 40–41
        genome-wide linkage analyses, 41
        genotyping, 40
        Glasgow outcome scale (GOS), 41
        pathogenesis of, 39
        patient study, 40
        statistical analysis, 40
    arterial narrowing, 15
    cerebral vasospasm, 15
    cytokine activity after, 57–58
    early brain injury, 15
    early micro vascular changes
        animal studies, 49
        cerebral microvasculature, anatomical architecture, 49–50
        microvascular injury, 50–52
    EBI
        Ac-YVAD-CMK treatment, 59
        anti-proinflammatory cytokine treatment, 58–59
            cytokine activity, 57–58
            DNA damage, 45–46
            extrinsic pathway of apoptosis, 46
            intrinsic apoptosis mechanisms, 44–45
            neuronal apoptosis in, 46
            oxidative stress and, 45
            pathophysiology of, 43–44
            tyrosine phosphatase inhibitor, 67–70
            western blotting analysis, 59–60
    hypoperfusion
        cerebral blood flow, 36
        CPP-dependent, 37
        cumulative morbidity and mortality, 35
        Mann-Whitney and t-test, 36
        methods, 36
        results, 36–37
        xenon-CT scanning, 37
    incidence of vasospasm
        angiographic spasm, 5
        delayed ischaemic deficits, 5–6
    matrix metalloproteinase-9
        antibodies and reagents, 82
        apoptosis, 63–64
        histology, 82
        hypothesis, implication of, 64–65
        laminin, 64, 82–83
        minocycline, 64
        SAH rat model, 81–82
        TUNEL staining, 82–83
        western blot of, 83
    minocycline
        antibodies and reagents, 71
        behavior scores assessment, 72–73
        clinical assessment, 72
        experimental groups, 71
        gelatin zymogram, 72
        MMP-9 protein evaluation, 73
        rat model, 71–72
        western blot analysis, 72
    nitric oxide donors, role of
        biochemical potentials, 95–96
        classic, 93–94
        new generation, 94–95
    NO/NOS pathway, 100
    NO-related pathophysiological changes
        cerebral vasospasm, pathogenesis of, 106
        DIND, 106–107
        microthrombosis, 107
        pathophysiological changes, SAH, 105–107
        radicals and oxidative stress, 107
        therapeutic application of, 107
        and vasoconstriction, 105–106
    osteopontin in EBI, role of, 75–78
    outcome of, 6
    pathophysiological pathways and treatment strategies
        CVS and endothelin pathway, 16
        CVS and HIF-1, 16–17
        CVS and inflammation, 17
        CVS and NOS-NO pathway, 16
        CVS/EBI and apoptosis, 18
        CVS/EBI and oxidative stress, 17–18
        statin and CVS/EBI, 18
        thrombin and CVS/EBI, 18
    phase I (0–60 min After SAH), 100
    phase II (1–6 h After SAH), 100–101
    phase III (6–72 h After SAH), 101
    sodium orthovanadate (SOV)
        animal experiment, 67–68
        brain water content, 68, 69
        DNA fragmentation, 69
        induction of SAH, 68
        neurological scoring and mortality, 68
        SAH grading, 68, 69
        statistical analysis, 68
Subarachnoid hemorrhage (SAH)
    BOXes, 157–158
    calcium signaling, cerebral artery myocytes, 145–149
    cardiac complications
        electrocardiogram abnormalities, 215–217
        pathology, 217
    COMT expression, 186
    COMT gene polymorphism, 233–237
    DCVS, 163
    death factor analysis, patients
        clinical information, 220
        groups, 220
        increased white blood cell, 222
        intracranial aneurysm, 220–221
        multi-factor logistic regression analysis, 221
        single-factor analysis, 221
        statistical analysis, 220
        variables and scales, 220
    hospital mortality, fever 239–242
    hospital mortality, weekend admission
        factor analysis, 231
        patients and methods, 230
    inflammatory response monitoring, 191–194
    intracranial pressure (ICP), 164
    old patients
        clinical characteristics, 246
        demographic analysis, 247
        illnesses, 246
        materials and methods, 246
        rebleeding and asymptomatic vasospasm, 247
    rabbit model
        anaesthesia and clinical observation, 163
        angiography, 164
        brain, gross examination, 164, 165
        induction and monitoring, 164

statistical methods, 164
young adults, non-aneurysm
  clinical characteristics, 210
  CTA examination, 212
  digital subtraction angiography (DSA), 212
  imaging examination, 211
  medical records, 210
  patients, 209–210
  prognosis, 211
  vascular pathologic changes, 212
Systemic inflammatory response syndrome (SIRS), 194

T

Terminal deoxynucleotidyl transferase-mediated uridine 5′-triphosphate-biotin nick end-labeling (TUNEL) staining, 68
Thrombin, 18
Treatment, CVS
  calcium antagonists, 23–24
  fasudil hydrochloride, 25
  magnesium sulphate, 24–25
  statins, 24

Tyrosine phosphatase inhibition
  brain water content measurement, 68
  cell death evaluation, 69
  DNA fragmentation, 69
  experimental animals, 67–68
  induction of SAH, 68
  neurological scoring and mortality, 68, 69
  SAH severity, 68
  statistical analysis, 68
  TUNEL staining, 68

V

Vascular endothelial growth factor (VEGF), 17, 45, 51, 69–70
Vascular smooth muscle cells, 28–29
Vasoconstriction, 105–106
Voltage-dependent calcium^{2+} channel (VDCC), 145, 148–149

W

Western blotting analysis, 59–60
World federation of neurological surgeons (WFNS) scale, 220–221

Table of Contents for Vol. 1

Part I: Advances in Subarachnoid Hemorrhage and Cerebral Vasospasm

Section I: Honored Guest & Honored Speaker Speeches

A Clinical Review of Cerebral Vasospasm and Delayed Ischaemia
Following Aneurysm Rupture 5
Dorsch, N.

New Regulatory, Signaling Pathways, and Sources of Nitric Oxide 7
Pluta, R.M.

Section II: Advances in Subarachnoid Hemorrhage Research

Advances in Experimental Subarachnoid Hemorrhage 15
Zhou, Y., Martin, R.D., and Zhang, J.H.

Advances in Treatment of Cerebral Vasospasm: an Update 23
Hansen-Schwartz, J.

Roles of Signal Transduction Mechanisms in Cerebral Vasospasm
Following Subarachnoid Hemorrhge: Overview 27
Nishziawa, S.

Part II: Mechanistic Studies

Section III: Early Brain Injury After Subarachnoid Hemorrhage

Hypoperfusion in the Acute Phase of Subarachnoid Hemorrhage 35
Schubert, G.A., Seiz, M., Hegewald, A.A., Manville, J., and Thomé, C.

Association of APOE Polymorphism with the Change of Brain Function
in the Early Stage of Aneurysmal Subarachnoid Hemorrhage 39
Lin, B., Dan, W., Jiang, L., Yin, X.-h., Wu, H.-t., and Sun, X.-c.

Apoptotic Mechanisms for Neuronal Cells in Early Brain Injury
After Subarachnoid Hemorrhage 43
Hasegawa, Y., Suzuki, H., Sozen, T., Altay O., and Zhang, J.H.

Early Micro Vascular Changes After Subarachnoid Hemorrhage 49
Sehba, F.A. and Friedrich, V.

Immunological Response in Early Brain Injury After SAH 57
Sozen, T., Tsuchiyama, R., Hasegawa, Y., Suzuki, H., Jadhav, V.,
Nishizawa, S., and Zhang, J.H.

Mechanisms of Early Brain Injury After SAH: Matrixmetalloproteinase 9 63
Guo, Z.-d., Sun, X.-c., and Zhang, J.H.

**Tyrosine Phosphatase Inhibition Attenuates Early Brain Injury
After Subarachnoid Hemorrhage in Rats** 67
Hasegawa, Y., Suzuki, H., Sherchan, P., Zhan, Y., Duris, K., and Zhang, J.H.

**Protection of Minocycline on Early Brain Injury After Subarachnoid
Hemorrhage in Rats** 71
Guo, Z.-d., Wu, H.-t., Sun, X.-c., Zhang, X.-d., and Zhang, J.H.

**Role of Osteopontin in Early Brain Injury After Subarachnoid
Hemorrhage in Rats** 75
Suzuki, H., Ayer, R., Sugawara, T., Chen, W., Sozen, T., Hasegawa, Y.,
Kanamaru, K., and Zhang, J.H.

**Matrix Metalloproteinase 9 Inhibition Reduces Early Brain Injury
in Cortex After Subarachnoid Hemorrhage** 81
Guo, Z.-d., Zhang, X.-d., Wu, H.-t., Lin, B., Sun, X.-c., and Zhang, J.H.

**Section IV: Nitric Oxide & Cortical Spreading Depolarization After
Subarachnoid Hemorrhage**

Nitric Oxide Synthase Inhibitors and Cerebral Vasospasm 87
Jung, C.S.

**The Role of Nitric Oxide Donors in Treating Cerebral Vasospasm
After Subarachnoid Hemorrhage** 93
Fathi, A.R., Bakhtian, K.D., and Pluta, R.M.

Nitric Oxide in Early Brain Injury After Subarachnoid Hemorrhage 99
Sehba, F.A., and Bederson, J.B.

**Nitric Oxide Related Pathophysiological Changes Following
Subarachnoid Haemorrhage** 105
Sabri, M., Ai, J., and Macdonald, R.L.

Endothelin-1$_{(1-31)}$ Induces Spreading Depolarization in Rats 111
Jorks, D., Major, S., Oliveira-Ferreira, A.I., Kleeberg, J., and Dreier, J.P.

**The Gamut of Blood Flow Responses Coupled to Spreading Depolarization
in Rat and Human Brain: from Hyperemia to Prolonged Ischemia** 119
Offenhauser, N., Windmüller, O., Strong, A.J., Fuhr, S., and Dreier, J.P.

**Cerebral Microdialysis in Acutely Brain-Injured Patients
with Spreading Depolarizations** 125
Krajewski, K.L., Orakcioglu, B., Haux, D., Hertle, D.N., Santos, E.,
Kiening, K.L., Unterberg, A.W., and Sakowitz, O.W.

Section V: Pathophysiology of Cerebral Vasospasm

Mitogen-Activated Protein Kinases in Cerebral Vasospasm After Subarachnoid Hemorrhage: A Review 133
Suzuki, H., Hasegawa, Y., Kanamaru, K., and Zhang, J.H.

Association of Apolipoprotein E Polymorphisms with Cerebral Vasospasm After Spontaneous Subarachnoid Hemorrhage 141
Wu, H.-t., Zhang, X.-d., Su, H., Jiang, Y., Zhou, S., and Sun, X.-c.

Impact of Subarachnoid Hemorrhage on Local and Global Calcium Signaling in Cerebral Artery Myocytes 145
Koide, M., Nystoriak, M.A., Brayden, J.E., and Wellman, G.C.

Enhanced Angiogenesis and Astrocyte Activation by Ecdysterone Treatment in a Focal Cerebral Ischemia Rat Model 151
Luo, C., Yi, B., Fan, W., Chen, K., Gui, L., Chen, Z., Li, L., Feng, H., and Chi, L.

Bilirubin Oxidation Products Seen Post Subarachnoid Hemorrhage Have Greater Effects on Aged Rat Brain Compared to Young 157
Clark, J.F., Harm, A., Saffire, A., Biehle, S.J., Lu, A., and Pyne-Geithman, G.J.

Preliminary Results of an ICP-Controlled Subarachnoid Hemorrhage Rabbit Model for the Study of Delayed Cerebral Vasospasm 163
Marbacher, S., Sherif, C., Neuschmelting, V., Schläppi, J.-A., Takala, J., Jakob, S., and Fandino, J.

PKGIα Inhibits the Proliferation of Cerebral Arterial Smooth Muscle Cell Induced by Oxyhemoglobin After Subarachnoid Hemorrhage 167
Luo, C., Yi, B., Chen, Z., Tang, W., Chen, Y., Hu, R., Liu, Z., Feng, H., and Zhang, J.H.

Characteristics of In Vivo Animal Models of Delayed Cerebral Vasospasm 173
Marbacher, S., Fandino, J., and Kitchen, N.

Endothelin Related Pathophysiology in Cerebral Vasospasm: What Happens to the Cerebral Vessels? 177
Vatter, H., Konczalla, J., and Seifert, V.

Expression and Role of COMT in a Rat Subarachnoid Hemorrhage Model 181
He, Z., Sun, X., Guo, Z., and Zhang, J.H.

Section VI: Clinical Manifestations of Subarachnoid Hemorrhage

Monitoring of the Inflammatory Response After Aneurysmal Subarachnoid Haemorrhage in the Clinical Setting: Review of Literature and Report of Preliminary Clinical Experience 191
Muroi, C., Mink, S., Seule, M., Bellut, D., Fandino, J., and Keller, E.

Perimesencephalic Subarachnoid Hemorrhage: Risk Factors, Clinical Presentations, and Outcome 197
Kong, Y., Zhang, J.H., and Qin, X.

The Relationship Between IL-6 in CSF and Occurrence of Vasospasm After Subarachnoid Hemorrhage 203
Ni, W., Gu, Y.X., Song, D.L., Leng, B., Li, P.L., and Mao, Y.

Non-Aneurysm Subarachnoid Hemorrhage in Young Adults 209
Wang, T., Zhang, J.H., and Qin, X.

Cardiac Damage After Subarachnoid Hemorrhage 215
Wu, B., Wang, X., and Zhang, J.H.

Analysis on Death-Associated Factors of Patients with Subarachnoid Hemorrhage During Hospitalization 219
Wang, T., Zhang, J.H., and Qin, X.

Clinical Study of Changes of Cerebral Microcirculation in Cerebral Vasospasm After SAH 225
Chai, W.-n., Sun, X.-c., Lv, F.-j., Wan, B., and Jiang, L.

Effect of Weekend Admission on in-Hospital Mortality After Subarachnoid Hemorrhage in Chongqing China 229
Zhang, G., Zhang, J.H., and Qin, X.

The Correlation Between COMT Gene Polymorphism and Early Cerebral Vasospasm After Subarachnoid Hemorrhage 233
He, Z., Sun, X., Guo, Z., and Zhang, J.H.

Fever Increased In-Hospital Mortality After Subarachnoid Hemorrhage 239
Zhang, G., Zhang, J.H., and Qin, X.

Subarachnoid Hemorrhage in Old Patients in Chongqing China 245
Zhang, Y., Wang, T., Zhang, J.H., Zhang, J., and Qin, X.

Author Index 249

Subject Index 251

Table of Contents (Vols. 1 and 2) 257

Table of Contents for Vol. 2

Part III: Therapeutical Studies

Section VII: Experimental Treatment for Cerebral Vasospasm

The Role of Apolipoprotein E in the Pathological Events Following
Subarachnoid Hemorrhage: A Review 5
Guo, Z.-d., Sun, X.-c., and Zhang, J.H.

Mechanisms of Statin Treatment in Cerebral Vasospasm 9
Sugawara, T., Ayer, R., Jadhav, V., Chen, W.,
Tsubokawa, T., and Zhang, J.H.

The Effect of Phosphodiesterase Inhibitor Tadalafil on Vasospasm Following
Subarachnoid Hemorrhage in an Experimental Rabbit Model 13
Narin, F., Bilginer, B., Isikay, A.I., Onal, M.B.,
Soylemezoglu, F., and Akalan, N.

Effect of a Free Radical Scavenger, Edaravone, on Free Radical Reactions:
Related Signal Transduction and Cerebral Vasospasm in the Rabbit
Subarachnoid Hemorrhage Model 17
Munakata, A., Ohkuma, H., and Shimamura, N.

Comparison of Nimodipine Delivery Routes in Cerebral Vasospasm
After Subarachnoid Hemorrhage: An Experimental Study in Rabbits 23
Onal, M.B., Civelek, E., Kircelli, A., Solmaz, I., Ugurel, S.,
Narin, F., Isikay, I., Bilginer, B., and Yakupoglu, H.

Effect of Recombinant Osteopontin on Cerebral Vasospasm After
Subarachnoid Hemorrhage in Rats 29
Suzuki, H., Hasegawa, Y., Kanamaru, K., and Zhang, J.H.

The Effect of Intracisternal Zn (II) Protoporphyrin IX on Vasospasm
Process in the Experimental Subarachnoid Hemorrhage Model 33
Isikay, I., Bilginer, B., Narin, F., Soylemezoglu, F., and Akalan, N.

Temporal Profile of the Effects of Intracisternal Injection of Magnesium
Sulfate Solution on Vasodilation of Spastic Cerebral Arteries in the Canine
SAH Model 39
Mori, K., Miyazaki, M., Hara, Y., Aiko, Y., Yamamoto, T.,
Nakao, Y., and Esaki, T.

Comparison of Intrathecal Cilostazol and Nimodipine Treatments in Subarachnoid Hemorrhage: An Experimental Study in Rabbits 43
Onal, M.B., Bilginer, B., Narin, F., Ziyal, M.I.,
Soylemezoglu, F., and Ozgen, T.

Blocking Cerebral Lymphatic Drainage Deteriorates Cerebral Oxidative Injury in Rats with Subarachnoid Hemorrhage 49
Sun, B.-l., Xie, F.-m., Yang, M.-f., Cao, M.-z., Yuan, H.,
Wang, H.-t., Wang, J.-r., and Jia, L.

Comparison of Intrathecal Dotarizine and Nimodipine Treatments in Cerebral Vasospasm After Subarachnoid Hemorrhage: An Experimental Study in Rabbits 55
Onal, M.B., Solmaz, I., Civelek, E., Kircelli, A., Tehli, O.,
Izci, Y., Erdogan, E., and Gonul, E.

Changes of Blood–Brain Barrier Permeability Following Intracerebral Hemorrhage and the Therapeutic Effect of Minocycline in Rats 61
Shi, W., Wang, Z., Pu, J., Wang, R., Guo, Z., Liu, C.,
Sun, J., Gao, L., and Zhou, R.

Comparison of Intrathecal Flunarizine and Nimodipine Treatments in Cerebral Vasospasm After Experimental Subarachnoid Hemorrhage in Rabbits 69
Civelek, E., Solmaz, I., Onal, M.B., Kircelli, A.,
Temiz, C., Secer, H.I., Izci, Y., and Gonul, E.

Treatment with Ginsenoside Rb1, A Component of *Panax Ginseng*, Provides Neuroprotection in Rats Subjected to Subarachnoid Hemorrhage-Induced Brain Injury 75
Li, Y., Tang, J., Khatibi, N.H., Zhu, M., Chen, D.,
Tu, L., Chen, L., and Wang, S.

The Effects of Intrathecal Nicergoline and Nimodipine in Cerebral Vasospasm: An Experimental Study in Rabbits 81
Solmaz, I., Onal, M.B., Civelek, E., Kircelli, A.,
Ongoru, O., Ugurel, S., Erdogan, E., and Gonul, E.

Metabolic Reflow as a Therapy for Ischemic Brain Injury 87
Manabe, H., Wang, Y., Yoshimura, R., Cai, Y.,
Fitzgerald, M., Clarke, R., and Lee, K.S.

Section VIII: Surgical & Endovascular Treatment for Cerebral Vasospasm

The Influence of Cisternal and Ventricular Lavage on Cerebral Vasospasm in Patients Suffering from Subarachnoid Hemorrhage: Analysis of Effectiveness 95
Hänggi, D. and Steiger, H.-J.

Dural Arteriovenous Fistulae at the Craniocervical Junction: The Relation Between Clinical Symptom and Pattern of Venous Drainage 99
Chen, G., Wang, Q., Tian, Y., Gu, Y., Xu, B.,
Leng, B., and Song, D.

Surgical Procedure and Results of Cisternal Washing Therapy for the Prevention of Cerebral Vasospasm Following SAH 105
Nakagomi, T., Furuya, K., Nagashima, H., Tanaka, J.-i., Ishii, T., Takanashi, S., Shinohara, T., Watanabe, F., Ogawa, A., Fujii, N., and Tamura, A.

Objective Evaluation of the Treatment Methods of Intracranial Aneurysm Surgery 111
Xu, R., Zhu, J., Sun, X.-c., He, Z.-h., and Zhang, X.-d.

Recurrent Vasospasm After Endovascular Treatment in Subarachnoid Hemorrhage 117
Frontera, J.A., Gowda, A., Grilo, C., Gordon, E., Johnson, D., Winn, H.R., Bederson, J.B., and Patel, A.

Endovascular Embolization for Intracranial Aneurysms: Report of 162 Cases 123
Tang, W., Feng, H., Chen, Z., Miu, H., Pan, J., Lin, J., and Zhu, G.

Treatment of Post-hemorrhagic Cerebral Vasospasm: Role of Endovascular Therapy 127
Grande, A., Nichols, C., Khan, U., Pyne-Geithman, G., Abruzzo, T., Ringer, A., and Zuccarello, M.

Delayed Intracranial Hemorrhage Associated with Antiplatelet Therapy in Stent-Assisted Coil Embolized Cerebral Aneurysms 133
Zhang, X.-d., Wu, H.-t., Zhu, J., He, Z.-h., Chai, W.-n., and Sun, X.-c.

Microsurgical Treatment of Ruptured Intracranial Aneurysm: A 120-Case Analysis 141
Tang, W., Feng, H., Chen, Z., Miu, H., Pan, J., Lin, J., and Zhu, G.

Section IX: Clinical Management of Subarachnoid Hemorrhage

Clazosentan: Prevention of Cerebral Vasospasm and the Potential to Overcome Infarction 147
Beck, J. and Raabe, A.

Current Management of Subarachnoid Hemorrhage in Advanced Age 151
Shimamura, N., Munakata, A., and Ohkuma, H.

A Numerical Approach to Patient-Specific Cerebral Vasospasm Research 157
Ho, H., Zhang, C., Xie, X., and Hunter, P.

Evidenced Based Guidelines for the Management of Good Grade Subarachnoid Haemorrhage Patients in Leeds, UK 161
Quinn, A.C., Hall, G., Marsh, S., Clark, M., and Ross, S.

Clinical Trial of Nicardipine Prolonged-Release Implants for Preventing Cerebral Vasospasm: Multicenter Cooperative Study in Tokyo 165
Kasuya, H.

Intravenous Magnesium Sulfate After Aneurysmal Subarachnoid Hemorrhage: Current Status 169
Chu Wong, G.K., Vai Chan, M.T., Gin, T., and Poon, W.S.

**Predictors Analysis of Symptomatic Cerebral Vasospasm
After Subarachnoid Hemorrhage** 175
Yin, L., Ma, C.Y., Li, Z.K., Wang, D.D., and Bai, C.M.

**Intra-arterial Administration of Fasudil Hydrochloride for
Vasospasm Following Subarachnoid Haemorrhage: Experience of 90 Cases** 179
Iwabuchi, S., Yokouchi, T., Hayashi, M., Sato, K., Saito, N., Hirata, Y.,
Harashina, J., Nakayama, H., Akahata, M., Ito, K., Kimura, H., and Aoki, K.

Role of Controlled Lumbar CSF Drainage for ICP Control in Aneurysmal SAH 183
Murad, A., Ghostine, S., and Colohan, A.R.T.

Chronic Hydrocephalus After Aneurysmal Subarachnoid Space Hemorrhage 189
Huo, G., Tang, M.-y., Feng, Q.-l., Zheng, L.-p., and Yang, G.

**Statins in the Management of Aneurysmal Subarachnoid Hemorrhage:
An Overview of Animal Research, Observational Studies, Randomized
Controlled Trials and Meta-analyses** 193
Kramer, A.H.

New Modalities to Assess Efficacy of Triple-H Therapy: Early Experience 203
Bhargava, D., Al-Tamimi, Y., Quinn, A., and Ross, S.

Nicardipine Pellets for the Prevention of Cerebral Vasospasm 209
Thomé, C., Seiz, M., Schubert, G.A., Barth, M., Vajkoczy, P.,
Kasuya, H., and Schmiedek, P.

Part IV: Imaging Studies

Section X: Neural Imaging for Subarachnoid Hemorrhage

**Neuromonitoring in Intensive Care: A New Brain Tissue Probe for
Combined Monitoring of Intracranial Pressure (ICP) Cerebral
Blood Flow (CBF) and Oxygenation** 217
Keller, E., Froehlich, J., Muroi, C., Sikorski, C., and Muser, M.

Vasospasm After Subarachnoid Hemorrhage: A 3D Rotational Angiography Study ... 221
Yao, G.-E., Li, Q., Jiang, X.-J., Liu, J., Li, J.-L.,
Zhang, L.-L., Li, L.-L., Zhang, J., and Xie, P.

Value of Noninvasive Imaging in Follow-Up of Intracranial Aneurysm 227
Jiang, L., He, Z.-h., Zhang, X.-d., Lin, B., Yin, X.-h., and Sun, X.-c.

Neuroimaging Research on Cerebrovascular Spasm and Its Current Progress 233
Chen, F., Wang, X., and Wu, B.

**Detection and Characterization of Intracranial Aneurysms
with Dual-Energy Subtraction CTA: Comparison with DSA** 239
Lv, F., Li, Q., Liao, J., Luo, T., Shen, Y., Li, J., Zhang, J., and Xie, P.

Author Index 247

Subject Index 251

Table of Contents (Vols. 1 and 2) 257

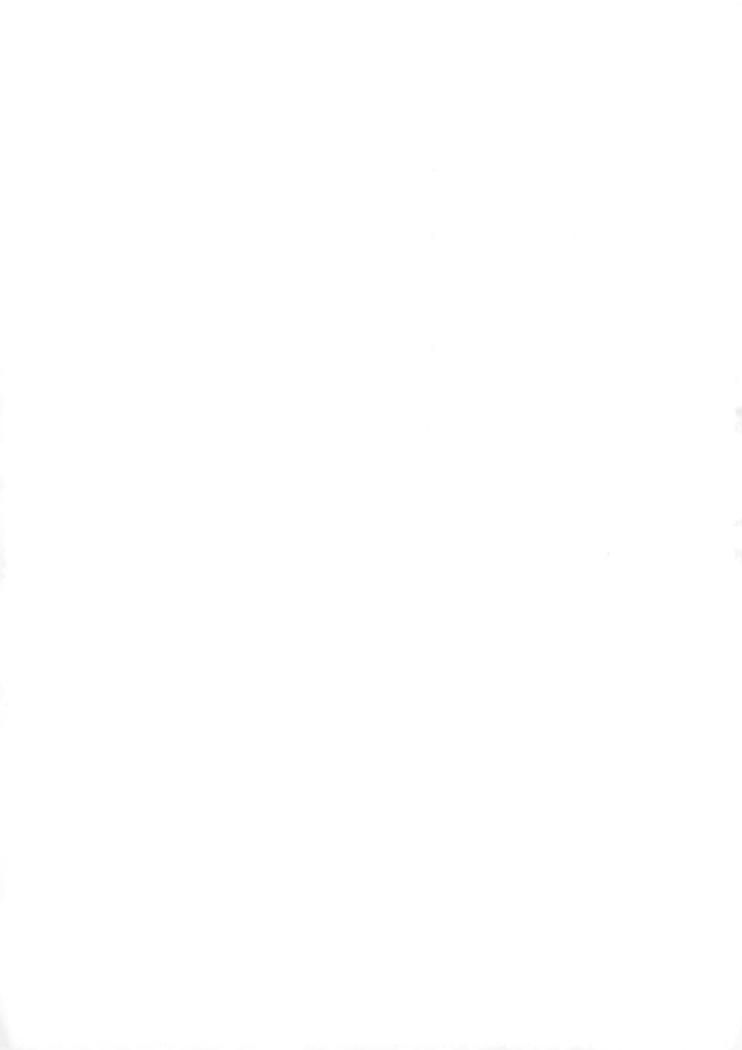

Printing: Ten Brink, Meppel, The Netherlands
Binding: Stürtz, Würzburg, Germany